Case Studies in Critical Care

Case Studies in Pediatric Critical Care

Edited by

Peter J. Murphy
Stephen C. Marriage
Peter J. Davis

CAMBRIDGE
UNIVERSITY PRESS

CAMBRIDGE UNIVERSITY PRESS
Cambridge, New York, Melbourne, Madrid, Cape Town,
Singapore, São Paulo, Delhi

Cambridge University Press
The Edinburgh Building, Cambridge CB2 8RU, UK

Published in the United States of America by
Cambridge University Press, New York

www.cambridge.org
Information on this title: www.cambridge.org/
9780521878340

First published 2009

Printed in the United Kingdom at the University Press,
Cambridge

A catalog record for this publication is available from the
British Library

ISBN 978-0-521-87834-0 paperback

Contents

Contributors

Sanjay M. Bhananker
Assistant Professor in Anesthesiology
University of Washington School of Medicine
Harborview Medical Center
Seattle, WA
USA

Farhan Bhanji
Staff Specialist, Critical Care Medicine
The Montreal Children's Hospital
Montreal, Quebec
Canada

Emma J. Bould
Paediatric and Neonatal Intensive Care Units
Great Ormond Street Hospital for Children
London, UK

Michael Burch
Consultant Paediatric Cardiologist
Department of Cardiothoracic Transplant
Great Ormond Street Hospital NHS Trust
London, UK

Anthony C. Chang
Associate Professor & Chief, Critical Care
Cardiology
The Lillie Frank Abercrombie Section of
Cardiology
Department of Pediatrics
Baylor College of Medicine Director
Pediatric Cardiac Intensive Care Unit
Texas Children's Hospital
Houston Texas USA

Laura J. Coates
Fellow in Paediatric Intensive Care
Bristol Royal Hospital for Children
Bristol, UK

Gordon Cohen
Children's Hospital & Regional Medical Center
Seattle, USA

Mehrengise Cooper
Consultant in Paediatric Intensive Care
PICU
St. Mary's Hospital
London, UK

Peter J. Davis
Consultant in Paediatric Intensive Care
Paediatric Intensive Care Unit
Bristol Royal Hospital for Children
Bristol, UK

Heather A. Dickerson
Assistant Professor, Critical Care
Cardiology
Department of Pediatrics, Baylor College of
Medicine
The Lillie Frank Abercrombie Section of
Cardiology
Texas Children's Hospital
Houston, TX
USA

Heather Duncan
Consultant in Paediatric Intensive Care
Diana, Princess of Wales Children's
Hospital
Paediatric Intensive Care Unit
Birmingham, UK

Lisa Dyke
Division of Emergency Medicine
British Columbia's Children's Hospital
Vancouver, BC
Canada

Matthew Fenton
Department of Cardiothoracic Transplant
Great Ormond Street Hospital NHS Trust
Great Ormond Street
London, UK

Peter J. Fleming
FSID Research Unit
Institute of Child Life and Health
St Michaels Hospital
Bristol, UK

Adrian Y. Goh
Associate Professor in Pediatric Intensive
Care
Pediatric Intensive Care
University of Malaya Medical Centre
Kuala Lumpur
Malaysia

David J. Grant
Consultant in Paediatric Intensive Care
Bristol Royal Hospital for Children
Bristol, UK

Mark Hatherill
Consultant Paediatric Intensivist
Red Cross Children's Hospital and School
of Child & Adolescent Health,
Klipfontein Road, Rondebosch
University of Cape Town
Cape Town
South Africa

Ian A. Jenkins
Consultant in Paediatric Anaesthesia and
Intensive Care
Bristol Royal Hospital for Children
Bristol, UK

Roger Langford
Fellow in Paediatric Cardiac Anaesthesia
and Intensive Care
Bristol Royal Hospital for Children
Bristol, UK

Stephen C. Marriage
Associate Specialist in Paediatric
Intensive Care
Paediatric Intensive Care Unit
Bristol Royal Hospital for Children
Bristol, UK

Lynn D. Martin
Professor of Anesthesiology & Pediatrics
(adjunct)
Department of Anesthesiology & Pain
Medicine
Children's Hospital & Regional Medical
Center
Seattle, WA

Robert Mazor
Department of Pediatrics
Pediatric Critical Care Medicine
Children's Hospital & Regional Medical
Center
Seattle, WA
USA

Duncan McAuley
Consultant Emergency Medicine,
Addenbrooke's Hospital,
Cambridge, UK

Andrew A. M. Morris
Consultant in Metabolic Medicine
Royal Manchester Children's Hospital
Hospital Road, Pendlebury
Manchester, UK

Peter J. Murphy
Consultant in Paediatric Anaesthesia and
Intensive Care
Bristol Royal Hospital for Children
Bristol, UK

Simon Nadel
Consultant in Paediatric Intensive Care
PICU
St. Mary's Hospital
London, UK

Gabrielle A. Nuthall
Consultant
Paediatric Intensive Care Unit
Starship Children's Hospital
Auckland
New Zealand

Roddy O'Donnell
Consultant Paediatrician
Paediatric Intensive Care Unit
Addenbrooke's Hospital
Cambridge, UK

Matt Oram
Consultant Anaesthetist
Cheltenham General Hospital
Sandford Road, Cheltenham,
Gloucestershire, UK

Mark J. Peters
Consultant in Paediatric Intensive Care
Paediatric and Neonatal Intensive Care
Units
Great Ormond Street Hospital for
Children
London, UK

Stephen D. Playfor
Consultant Paediatric Intensivist
Paediatric Intensive Care Unit
Royal Manchester Children's Hospital
Hospital Road, Pendlebury
Manchester, UK

Trevor Richens
Consultant Cardiologist
Royal Hospital for Sick Children
Yorkhill NHS Trust
Glasgow, UK

Michael Roe
Consultant Paediatrician
Paediatric Intensive Care Unit
Addenbrooke's Hospital
Cambridge, UK

Robert Ross Russell
Consultant Paediatric Intensive Care Unit,
Addenbrooke's Hospital,
Hill's Road
Cambridge, UK

Margrid Schindler
Consultant in Paediatric Intensive Care
Bristol Royal Hospital for Children
Bristol, UK

Sam R. Sharar
Professor of Anesthesiology
University of Washington School of
Medicine
Harborview Medical Center
Department of Anesthisology
Seattle, WA, USA

Lara Shekerdemian
Director
Paediatric Intensive Care Unit
Royal Children's Hospital,
Melbourne, Australia.

Sam D. Shemie
Staff Specialist, Critical Care Medicine
The Montreal Children's Hospital
Montreal, Quebec
Canada

Peter Skippen
Staff Specialist
Division of Critical Care
British Columbia's Children's Hospital
Vancouver, BC
Canada

Mike South
Specialist in Intensive Care
Director, Department of General
Medicine,
Royal Childrens Hospital
Deputy Head of Paediatrics, University of
Melbourne
Royal Children's Hospital,
Parkville, Victoria
Australia

Christian Stocker
Staff Specialist
Queensland Paediatric Intensive Care Service,
Royal Childrens Hospital,
Herston Road,
Herston,
Australia

Ulf Theilen
Consultant in Paediatric Intensive
Care
Paediatric Intensive Care Unit
Royal Hospital for Sick Children,
Edinburgh, UK

Joshua C. Uffman
Acting Assistant Professor
Department of Anesthesiology
University of Washington School of
Medicine
Attending Anesthesiologist, Children's
Hospital & Regional Medical Center and
Harborview Medical Center
Seattle, WA
USA

Monica S. Vavilala
Associate Professor
Departments of Anesthesiology, Pediatrics,
and Neurological Surgery (Adj)
University of Washington School of
Medicine
Attending Anesthesiologist, Harborview
Medical Center
Attending Emergency Physician, Children's
Hospital & Regional Medical Center
Seattle, WA
USA

Patricia M. Weir
Consultant in Paediatric Anaesthesia and
Intensive Care
Bristol Royal Hospital for Children
Bristol, UK

Andrew R. Wolf
Professor of Paediatric Anaesthesia and
Intensive Care
Bristol Royal Hospital for Children
Bristol, UK

Foreword

In pediatric intensive care, as in most areas of clinical practice, we learn best by experience. No textbook can hope to replace the learning process that occurs from long hours of clinical practice, the experience of decision-making (whether right or wrong), and the deeply ingrained learning that comes from the process of clinical apprenticeship.

This book, with its very practically oriented chapters dealing with both common and less common clinical problems, and illustrated with structured case studies, goes a long way in helping the novice (or experienced) intensivist to focus, get to grips with, and learn from the experience and knowledge of recognized experts in the field.

The editors and chapter contributors have carefully avoided the usual uninspiring "politically correct" forms used in many publications to present systematic reviews and meta-analyses, but have not sacrificed any of the clinical or epidemiological rigor inherent in those standard forms of presentation.

This book, with its refreshing and helpful emphasis on the human and humane as well as on the scientific aspects of pediatric intensive care will, I believe, have an important role in the training of future intensivists. For those clinicians involved in the care of children, but who are not usually directly involved in the field of pediatric intensive care, this book will also provide the reader with useful insights into the processes of caring for critically ill children.

Professor Peter J Fleming
FSID Research Unit
Bristol UK

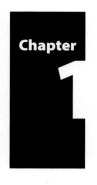

Chapter 1

Respiratory syncytial virus bronchiolitis

Roddy O'Donnell and Michael Roe

Introduction

Respiratory Syncytial Virus (RSV) bronchiolitis is the leading cause of admission to hospital in children under the age of 1 year in developed countries.[1] RSV is identified as the cause in the overwhelming majority (75%) of cases of bronchiolitis. However, other viruses such as parainfluenza, influenza, adenovirus, and human metapneumovirus may also cause a clinically indistinguishable illness. In the USA it has been estimated that RSV causes 51 000–82 000 admissions annually with 200 to 500 associated deaths.[2,3]

RSV appears to infect almost all children by the time they are about 2 to 3 years old. Having older siblings or attending day care is associated with earlier primary infection.[3] Primary RSV infections are rarely believed to be asymptomatic but very few children require hospitalization. In the developed world, however, admission rates appear to be rising. Over the last 20 years, admission rates have more than doubled to about 3%, although length of admission may have fallen from above 5 days to about 3 days.[4] Up to 15% of infants hospitalized with bronchiolitis require intensive care and about half of these will require mechanical ventilation. As well as causing misery for children and their families, RSV bronchiolitis accounts for a great deal of healthcare expenditure.[5] In children who are otherwise well, recovery from severe RSV bronchiolitis is frequently associated with chronic and recurrent wheezing in response to subsequent respiratory virus infection. Pulmonary function abnormalities have been shown to persist for decades following severe bronchiolitis.[6]

Although most children admitted with RSV have previously been well, children with congenital heart disease, chronic lung disease, or immunosuppression are at increased risk of severe disease.[7]

The management of bronchiolitis is primarily supportive and, although there are a number of therapeutic options that may be explored, clear evidence of the beneficial effects of many therapies has been difficult to obtain.

Case history

A 10-month-old female infant presented in January to her local hospital with a 7-day history of cough, mild pyrexia, and wheeze. She has a history of multiple episodes of cough and wheeze, some of which required admission to hospital, that were treated with inhaled bronchodilators – both β2 agonists and ipratropium bromide – and steroids.

She was born prematurely by cesarean section at 28 weeks' gestation because of maternal placenta praevia. She had a birth weight of 1050 grams. In the neonatal period, she was managed with nasal Continuous Positive Airway Pressure (CPAP) and supplemental oxygen and did not require intubation and ventilation. At 8 weeks of age (36 weeks' post-conceptual age), she was discharged home and required no supplemental oxygen. She had received all

Case Studies in Pediatric Critical Care, ed. Peter. J. Murphy, Stephen C. Marriage, and Peter J. Davis. Published by Cambridge University Press. © Cambridge University Press 2009.

her routine immunizations to date, had no known allergies, and had reached appropriate developmental milestones.

On admission to local hospital:

Examination

Temperature	37.8 °C
Respiratory rate	48 breaths.min^{-1}
Saturations	88%–92% in air, rising to 96% in 2 litres of oxygen
Chest	Moderate subcostal/intercostal recession widespread expiratory wheeze and fine crackles

Investigations

Chest X-ray	Hyperexpanded with areas of atelectasis in both lung fields
Nasopharyngeal aspirate	Negative for respiratory viruses

On this admission she was treated with oxygen and given a trial of salbutamol and ipratropium bromide inhalers as metered dose inhalers using a spacer device. Both salbutamol and ipratropium bromide were felt to have some therapeutic benefit. She was allowed to continue with normal feeding and appeared to tolerate feeds well.

Over the next 24 hours, there were episodes of increased respiratory distress and rising oxygen requirements. Oral clarithromycin was commenced and feeds were given by nasogastric tube.

By the second day of admission, respiratory distress had worsened and there was an increasing requirement for oxygen. Enteral feeds were discontinued and intravenous fluids (80 ml kg^{-1} per day of 0.45% saline with 5% dextrose) were started. A capillary blood gas was undertaken which showed: pH = 7.39, pCO_2 = 6.28 kPa, BE = −3.1. Nasal Continuous Positive Airway Pressure (nCPAP) using nasal prongs was started.

A few hours later, she further deteriorated with a respiratory rate above 60 breaths min^{-1}. There was head-bobbing and severe recession. She had become pale, sweaty and was noted to have become lethargic. A repeat capillary gas now showed respiratory acidosis: pH = 7.17, pCO_2 = 9.07 kPa, BE = −3.4. It was decided that she was no longer able to cope and invasive ventilatory support should be instituted.

She was referred to the regional Pediatric Intensive Care Unit (PICU). Prior to transfer she was anesthetized with sevoflurane, fentanyl, and rocuronium and was intubated uneventfully. Sedation, analgesia and muscle relaxation were maintained with morphine, midazolam, and vecuronium. Intermittent positive pressure ventilation was started with settings of 27 cmH$_2$O PIP and 6 cmH$_2$O PEEP, to generate a tidal volume of 6–7 ml kg^{-1}. Central venous and arterial access was established. Nebulized salbutamol was administered. There was evidence of partially compensated shock with a tachycardia of 135 b min^{-1} and peripheral vasoconstriction. A 20 ml kg^{-1} 0.9% NaCl bolus was given and dopamine started at 8 mcg kg^{-1} per min to maintain a normal blood pressure. Intravenous cefotaxime was added to her antibiotic regime. The retrieval team transferred her uneventfully to the regional PICU.

Progress on pediatric intensive care unit (Table 1.1)

Respiratory

On admission, she had a strikingly prolonged expiratory phase with wheeze and inspiratory crackles. Since salbutamol had appeared to be associated with improvement at her referring hospital, a salbutamol infusion was commenced beginning at 1 mcg kg^{-1} per min. Over the following 12 hours, oxygen requirements remained high. After further discussion, a trial of High Frequency Oscillatory Ventilation (HFOV) was commenced. After initiating HFOV there was marked hemodynamic instability, necessitating increased inotropic and vaso-pressor support and it was necessary to return to BIPAP.

A second trial of HFOV on the following day was also abandoned because of hemodynamic instability. On the third day of intensive care, she continued to deteriorate and PEEP had to be increased to 8 cm H_2O. The inspired oxygen fraction to maintain saturations greater than 88% was 0.8–0.9. At this time, the oxygenation index was 19.0 and the Alveolar Arterial Difference in Oxygen (AaDO$_2$) 520 mmHg. She was placed in a prone position.

The therapeutic options were reconsidered and nitric oxide, steroids, surfactant, and ECMO discussed.

Nitric oxide

It was decided to initiate a therapeutic trial of Nitric Oxide (NO) starting at 5 ppm. There was a concomitant fall in inspired oxygen from 0.95 to 0.65 with a resultant fall in the oxygenation index to 11.8. The NO was increased to 10 ppm with no further associated improvement. Nitric oxide was continued until day 12 at settings between 5 and 12 ppm. Weaning of NO was in accordance with improving ventilation. Ventilatory pressures remained high until the tenth day, when weaning to pressures of 18/6 was possible.

Table 1.1. *Findings on admission to PICU*

Airway	4.5 uncuffed oral endotracheal tube fixed 11.5 cm at lips
Breathing	BIPAP, Pressures 28/6, rate 24,
	Inspiratory time = 0.8 seconds
	FiO$_2$ = 70%
Gas	pH = 7.32, pCO_2 = 6.65 kPa, pO_2 = 12.22 kPa, BE = −1.3.
Circulation	Pulse = 136 b min^{-1}, BP = 88/44 mmHg (MAP = 56)
	Warm and well perfused; peripheral capillary refill time <2 s
	Dopamine @ 8 mcg kg^{-1} per min Glucose = 2.7 mmol l^{-1}, therefore 5 ml kg^{-1} 10% dextrose given
	Urine output = 2 ml kg^{-1} per h
Neurology	Pupils small but equal and react briskly to light
Investigations	Hb = 9.4 g dl^{-1}, WCC = 11.4 × 10^9 l^{-1}, Plts = 294 × 10^9 l^{-1}
	Na = 140 mmol l^{-1}, K = 4.1 mmol l^{-1}, U = 1.3 mmol l^{-1}, Cr = 17 μmol l^{-1}, CRP = 45 mg l^{-1}

Extra-corporeal membrane oxygenation (ECMO)

After deciding to initiate a trial of NO, the supra-regional ECMO center was contacted in accordance with our normal local practice. Daily contact was maintained, but she remained adequately oxygenated and did not meet the criteria for ECMO (oxygenation index >25).

Corticosteroids

Despite NO, her clinical condition still gave cause for concern. She remained very unstable, requiring high ventilatory pressures after 5 days of intensive care. It was decided to initiate a therapeutic trial of corticosteroids. Intravenous methylprednisolone ($2 \, mg \, kg^{-1}$ per day) was commenced and continued at high dose for 7 days and then weaned over the following week.

Surfactant

On the ninth day of intensive care, 4 days after starting corticosteroids and 6 days after starting NO, she had a prolonged period of respiratory acidosis and required increasing inspired inflation pressures. After further discussion, it was decided to give a single trial dose of surfactant (Curosurf (Poractant Alfa, Chiesi)). The dose was instilled into the trachea in a weight-appropriate dose in accordance with the manufacturer's instructions. Over the following 6 to 8 hours, no significant improvement in ventilation was felt to have occurred and no further doses were administered.

Cardiovascular and fluids

Dopamine was continued at a rate of $5–10 \, mcg \, kg^{-1}$ per min for 5 days to maintain adequate blood pressure. No other inotropes were required. The patient was generally hemodynamically stable except for a brief period when high frequency oscillation ventilation was tried.

Fluid and electrolyte balance

Intravenous fluids were initially restricted to $70 \, ml \, kg^{-1}$ per day. Enteral feeds were commenced on Day 4 and fluid allowance was increased the following day to $100 \, ml \, kg^{-1}$ per day. Regular furosemide ($0.5 \, mg \, kg^{-1}$ q6) was started on Day 3 to keep the overall fluid balance negative and urine output greater than $1 \, ml \, kg^{-1}$ per h. This was changed to a continuous furosemide infusion on Day 9, which was continued for 3 days before converting back to intermittent dosing. Serum sodium levels were $140–145 \, mmol \, L^{-1}$ during the period of difficult ventilation and urea and creatinine levels remained in the normal range.

Microbiology

Initial viral and bacterial investigations were negative, although RSV was isolated on Day 4 of hospitalization. Microbiological culture of a tracheal aspirate grew *Haemophilus influenzae* spp. on one occasion, but all other bacterial and fungal cultures, from sputum and blood, were negative. A 7-day course of cefotaxime was given. Clarithromycin was given for 3 days. The CRP rose to a maximum of 115 on day two of PICU.

Other

She was paralyzed with a continuous infusion of vecuronium for the first 12 days on PICU. She was sedated according to a local protocol with morphine and midazolam, and fentanyl was substituted for morphine from the ninth day of intensive care. Clonidine and chloral hydrate were used from the 12th PICU day onwards to allow weaning of intravenous sedation and manage withdrawal symptoms.

Weaning and discharge

She gradually improved after the 10th day of intensive care and was weaned sufficiently to allow elective extubation on the 16th day after admission. For the next day, she required a small amount of supplemental oxygen, which was steadily reduced and then stopped. She was discharged from the intensive care unit after 17 days and was transferred back to her referring hospital on the following day to complete her recovery.

Discussion

In temperate and continental climates such as most of Europe and North America RSV bronchiolitis occurs in annual epidemics at the coldest point of the year. To date, it is believed that man is the only natural host and that no animal reservoir exists. Nonetheless, it is unclear why there are very few cases at other times of the year or where the virus goes. Recently, some evidence has emerged from animal models that RSV may be able to persist in the lung after primary infection raising the possibility of reactivation.[8]

Most children admitted will be between 3 and 6 months of age during primary RSV infection and the case was slightly older than most. Preterm infants are generally admitted at a younger post presented conceptual age and it has been noted that the peak age of admission corresponds in time with waning passive maternal antibody levels. During the winter months the number of children presenting to pediatric intensive care can be so great that bed availability is stretched and this impacts on the availability of beds for elective or routine procedures. Most transmission is by direct inoculation of the mucous membranes of the eye and nose; both have respiratory epithelium, the mouth does not. Aerosol spread is probably uncommon.[9] Nosocomial spread is well recognized and RSV has been shown to be able to remain infectious for hours on surfaces and other fomites.[10] For vulnerable infants in hospital, this can represent a real threat.

Presentation of RSV bronchiolitis

Respiratory syncytial virus infection may present in several ways. The first isolates from a child were in a case of croup. However, RSV more commonly presents with symptoms or signs of a coryzal illness or upper respiratory tract infection (URTI), together with evidence of Lower Respiratory Tract Infection (LRTI). In some infants obstruction to airflow is pronounced and wheeze is common. In very young infants apnoea may be a striking feature.

Central, prolonged apnea can be the first sign of RSV infection in young infants in the absence of other respiratory symptoms, the mechanism of which is unclear. It has not been possible to detect viral genome in CSF to confirm direct infection.[11] Those under 2 months of age are most likely to present with RSV associated apnea. Apnea at admission increases the risk of recurrent apnea and the need for supportive ventilation significantly increases in children who suffer from recurrent apnea.[12]

Understanding immunity to RSV

RSV is poorly cytopathic *in vitro* and probably causes relatively little direct cell damage during infection. Infection is mainly confined to the respiratory epithelial cells lining the eye, nose, middle ear and lower respiratory tract.

In the 1960s a number of vaccine trials were undertaken in children using a formalin-inactivated preparation of the virus. This vaccine was created using the same techniques that had proven so successful in vaccinating against polio. In these studies children showed good serum antibody responses and cell-mediated lymphocyte responses after vaccination. During subsequent natural RSV infection, however, illness appeared to be enhanced.[13–16] There were increased admissions and some children died with evidence at postmortem of a vigorous inflammatory response in the lung.

In the 1980s and 1990s, with greater understanding of the role of lymphocytes and with animal models, it was possible to show that, during RSV infection, both CD4 helper and CD8 cytotoxic T cells were important in controlling RSV infection. Removing either subset was associated with prolonged shedding of virus but interestingly with reduced illness.[17,18] Further studies have confirmed that T-cells are essential in controlling primary RSV infection, but are also associated with an inflammatory response that produces the illness we refer to as bronchiolitis. Removing specific cytokines that can be produced by T cells in particular TNF-α has also been shown to ameliorate illness in animal models.[19]

Specific T-cell subsets may be primed by different proteins of RSV. In particular the attachment surface "G" protein has been associated with T-helper 2 responses.[20] This may have great importance in designing any future vaccine. The RSV genome appears to be somewhat distinct from the other paramyxoviruses and intriguingly the nucleoprotein and polymerase show closer sequence homology to filoviruses like Ebola and Marburg suggesting a possible common ancestor.[21]

Fluid and electrolyte balance

In infants admitted to hospital with bronchiolitis, water overload and hyponatremia may complicate fluid and electrolyte management. RSV bronchiolitis is associated with both increased ADH secretion and hyper-reninemia with secondary hyperaldosteronism.[22] These may lead to water retention. In some series hyponatremia has been associated with seizures.[23] Close control of fluid balance and usually fluid restriction are employed by many PICUs.[24]

Corticosteroids

Corticosteroids have been used in clinical practice for the treatment of many inflammatory diseases for many decades. The predominant mechanism of action is via corticosteroid receptors that are expressed very widely throughout the body.[25] Corticosteroids affect multiple steps in immune activation: they inhibit antigen presentation, cytokine production, and lymphocyte proliferation. Lymphocyte, monocyte, and basophil counts decrease in response to corticosteroids, while neutrophil counts increase.[26] The striking similarities in some of the clinical features that acute bronchiolitis has with acute asthma has led to the hypothesis that corticosteroids may have a therapeutic role. It is known that acute RSV bronchiolitis is associated with a measurable acute stress response that has similarities to, and differences from, other severe infections such as bacterial sepsis. Cortisol levels are elevated in acute bronchiolitis, but there is no evidence that these levels are higher in children who go on to need intensive care.[27]

For at least 40 years researchers have been attempting to show whether corticosteroids may be of benefit in acute bronchiolitis.[28] Even today there have been advocates for and against. A recent editorial in the *Journal of Pediatrics* [29] strongly advocated the early use corticosteroids following the publication of a randomized control trial of oral prednisolone in the same journal.[30] Conversely, in a recent Cochrane review and meta-analysis,[31] the authors found no benefits in either length of stay or clinical score in infants and young children treated with systemic glucocorticoids as compared with placebo. They also found no significant differences in any of the subanalyses or in return to hospital or readmission rates. Therefore, at present it would seem there is inadequate data to recommend the routine use of steroids in bronchiolitis. The long period of research without demonstrating a clear benefit suggests that, if there is a benefit of corticosteroids, it is unlikely to be clinically very significant.

Surfactant

There are several strands of evidence of the importance of surfactant in bronchiolitis. Knockout animal models have suggested that surfactant protein A may have a role in clearance of RSV.[32] Surfactant protein concentrations may be lower in those with severe bronchiolitis.[33] An association may exist between certain surfactant protein A polymorphisms[34] and severe bronchiolitis. RSV infects and causes the apoptosis *in vitro* of type 2 pneumocytes that produce pulmonary surfactant.[35]

These pieces of data taken together have suggested to some clinicians that there may be a role for the administration of exogenous surfactant in severely ill infants with bronchiolitis. Although reported as individual cases, very few studies have been undertaken using what is still a relatively expensive therapy. Recently, Tibby *et al.* have described a small series of patients in whom some improvement of oxygenation was found after exogenous surfactant in bronchiolitis.[36] At present, there is inadequate data to recommend the routine use of surfactant, and cost and potential adverse effects suggest that larger studies will be needed.

Bronchodilators: salbutamol, ipratropium bromide, and adrenaline

For over 30 years clinicians have tried to determine the effectiveness of bronchodilators in bronchiolitis. The consistent finding of airflow obstruction and some similarities in presentation to older children with wheezing has suggested that perhaps bronchospasm may play a role.

A review by Schindler[37] commented that, in the 1990, there were 12 randomized control trials, involving many hundreds of infants, examining beta-agonists in bronchiolitis. Nine showed that bronchodilators had no effect and three showed a small transient improvement in the acute clinical score. She also noted that ipratropium bromide had no significant effect.

Two large meta-analyses in 1996[38] and 2000[39] have concluded that bronchodilator recipients did not show improvement in oxygenation, the rate of hospitalization, or duration of hospitalization. The authors conclude that, at best, bronchodilators produce modest short-term improvement in clinical scores.

Epinephrine has been shown to improve respiratory system resistance but not oxygenation or ventilation. Compared with beta-agonists, adrenaline (epinephrine) was not associated with lower admission rates or/and improved oxygen saturation, although it has been suggested that, soon after treatment, respiratory rate may be lower than after treatment with other bronchodilators. A large recent meta-analysis has concluded that "there is insufficient evidence to support the use of epinephrine for the treatment of bronchiolitis."[40]

Ribavirin

Ribavirin is a synthetic guanosine analog that inhibits RSV replication during the active replication phase. Introduced into clinical practice in the 1980s after great promise *in vitro*, aerosolized Ribavirin was purported to be associated with improved oxygenation, improved clinical scores, and diminished levels of secretory mediators of inflammation associated with severe wheezing and disease.[41] However, its use was limited initially because of expense and, over the last 20 years, a number of investigators have been unable to convincingly show a beneficial effect on clinical outcome. More studies have been undertaken to determine whether those who had received Ribavirin had better or worse long-term outcomes. No significant differences in outcome following Ribavirin therapy have been demonstrated using outcome measures such as response to methacholine challenge; reported wheezing; severity of recurrent lower respiratory tract illness; oxygen saturation; peak expiratory flow or spirometry,[42,43] although, in one follow-up study, weighted severity scores suggested a possible long-term beneficial effect.[44] More recent understandings of the role of the immune response in causing the clinical manifestations of bronchiolitis may indicate why interference with viral replication might have, at most, a limited therapeutic role.

RSV-specific immunoglobulin

It has been noted that the peak incidence of hospitalization with RSV bronchiolitis appears to coincide with the nadir of humoral immunity, as passively acquired maternal antibody wanes. This observation led to studies showing that infants born with higher levels of passive maternal antibody to RSV had a degree of protection against severe RSV bronchiolitis. In the 1990s a preparation of pooled RSV-specific immunoglobulin from donors was developed. Studies suggested that given prophylactically to high-risk infants, the duration and severity of hospitalizations due to RSV may be reduced.

Subsequently, a humanized monoclonal antibody preparation has been produced for use in high risk groups (Palivizumab™, Abbott Laboratories). Data from large randomized controlled studies show some evidence for protection with passive immunization. Some centers have begun to offer Palivizumab to very high-risk infants. However, as Buck *et al.* have suggested,[45] relatively few children admitted to PICU with RSV bronchiolitis are likely to fall into the groups considered eligible for immunization. The costs of offering this therapy compared with the likely benefits need to be carefully considered.

Despite the potential drawbacks of immunoglobulin from pooled human donations, there may be one group who may still benefit from its use. Progression to pneumonia in pre-engraftment recipients of bone marrow transplants due to RSV is associated with an overall mortality of 60%–80%. There is some evidence that the combination of intravenous immunoglobulin and Ribavirin may significantly reduce mortality in this group.[10,46]

Nitric oxide

Inhaled nitric oxide (NO) has been used for over a decade in acute lung injury or acute respiratory distress. However, there is little evidence from clinical trials to support its use. It is recognized that, as therapy with NO begins, oxygenation is frequently improved and this is principally due to better matching of ventilation and perfusion. In the context of a child in whom oxygenation cannot be maintained despite maximal ventilation, it is easy to understand why clinicians see a role for its use despite a lack of detailed evidence. Children who are as sick as the child described in this chapter are relatively rare and studies of adequate power hard to achieve. In a recent Cochrane review, inhaled NO had no impact on survival and only transient effects on oxygenation.[47]

Co-infection and the use of antibiotics

Many studies in the developed world have noted that bacterial co-infection during RSV bronchiolitis is unusual. Despite this, in children who require pediatric intensive care, antibiotic use is almost universal.[48] It is frequently suggested that antibiotics may be being overused and that measures should be taken to reduce this.[49] However, diagnosis of co-infection can be delayed, is more common in children requiring intensive care and is associated with a more severe course.[50] In addition, a recent report has suggested that tracheal colonization with *Haemophilus influenzae* may be associated with a worse PIC course in RSV bronchiolitis.[51] Co-infection with *Bordatella pertussis*[52] or *Streptococcus pneumoniae*[53] are unusual, but not rare, and should be considered. Co-infection with viruses such as human metapneumovirus and human bocavirus have recently been emerging as another potential cause of more severe illness during the bronchiolitis season[54] and can be diagnosed by PCR.

Summary

The child described happily appears to have completely recovered from a life-threatening episode of bronchiolitis due to RSV infection. Recent epidemiological data regarding bronchiolitis mortality in the United States makes concerning reading. Although childhood deaths associated with any respiratory disease decreased steadily between 1979 and 1997, the number of deaths associated with bronchiolitis among children showed no similar reduction. It was also found that most children dying with bronchiolitis were not concurrently diagnosed with underlying prematurity or pulmonary or cardiac conditions.[3]

There is evidence of considerable variation in the use of different therapies between institutions but resulting in very little difference in the lengths of stay.[55] Treatment will therefore remain essentially supportive as we have a great deal still to learn about this illness.

Learning points

- RSV is the dominant respiratory pathogen in infants children needing pediatric intensive care.

- The presentation of RSV bronchiolitis is varied but falls into clinically recognizable patterns.

- The immune response to infection is complex and, although essential in controlling infection, it may be the cause of the clinical illness.

- There may be specific problems related to fluid and sodium balance.

- High-risk groups who may suffer severe illness can be identified and some preventative strategies considered including passive immunization.

- Infection control is important to protect vulnerable infants.

- Proven therapeutic interventions are few and treatment remains essentially supportive.

- Co-infection with viral or bacterial pathogens is associated with more severe illness.

- Long-term pulmonary sequelae occur in the majority of infants following RSV bronchiolitis.

References

1. Leader S, Kohlhase K. Respiratory syncytial virus-coded pediatric hospitalizations, 1997 to 1999. *Pediatr Infect Dis J* 2002; **21**: 629–32.
2. Shay DK, Holman RC, Newman RD, Liu LL, Stout JW, Anderson LJ Bronchiolitis-associated hospitalizations among US children, 1980–1996. *J Am Med Assoc* 1999; **282**: 1440–6.
3. Shay DK, Holman RC, Roosevelt, GE, Clarke MJ, Anderson LJ. Bronchiolitis-associated

mortality and estimates of respiratory syncytial virus-associated deaths among US children, 1979–1997. *J Infect Dis* 2001.; **183** (1): 16–22.

4. Langley JM, LeBlanc JC, Smith B, Wang EE Increasing incidence of hospitalization for bronchiolitis among Canadian children, 1980–2000. *J Infect Dis* 2003; **188**: 1764–7.

5. Langley JM, Wang EE, Law BJ *et al.* Economic evaluation of respiratory syncytial virus infection in Canadian children: a Pediatric Investigators Collaborative Network on Infections in Canada (PICNIC) study. *J Pediatr* 1997; **131**: 113–17.

6. Piippo-Savolainen E, Remes S, Kannisto S, Korhonen K, Korppi M. Asthma and lung function 20 years after wheezing in infancy: results from a prospective follow-up study. *Arch Pediatr Adolesc Med* 2004; **158**: 1070–6.

7. Hall CB Respiratory syncytial virus and parainfluenza virus. *N Engl J Med* 2001; **344**: 1917–28.

8. Schwarze J, O'Donnell DR, Rohwedder A, Openshaw PJ. Latency and persistence of respiratory syncytial virus despite T cell immunity. *Am J Respir Crit Care Med* 2004; **169**: 801–5.

9. Hall CB, Douglas RGJ, Schnabel KC, Geiman JM. Infectivity of respiratory syncytial virus by various routes of inoculation. *Infect Immun* 1981; **33**: 779–83.

10. Hall CB, Douglas RG, Jr, Geiman JM. Possible transmission by fomites of respiratory syncytial virus. *J Infect Dis* 1980; **141**: 98–102.

11. O'Donnell DR, McGarvey MJ, Tully JM, Balfour-Lynn IM, Openshaw PJ. Respiratory syncytial virus RNA in cells from the peripheral blood during acute infection. *J Pediatr* 1998; **133**: 272–4.

12. Kneyber MC, Brandenburg AH, de Groot R *et al.* Risk factors for respiratory syncytial virus associated apnoea. *Eur J Pediatr* 1998; **157**: 331–5.

13. Chin J, Magoffin RL, Shearer LA, Schieble JH, Lennette EH. Field evaluation of a respiratory syncytial virus vaccine and a trivalent parainfluenza virus vaccine in a pediatric population. *Am J Epidemiol* 1969; **89**: 449–63.

14. Fulginiti VA, Eller JJ, Sieber OF, Joyner JW, Minamitani M, Meiklejohn G. Respiratory virus immunization. I. A field trial of two inactivated respiratory virus vaccines; an aqueous trivalent parainfluenza virus vaccine and an alum-precipitated respiratory syncytial virus vaccine. *Am J Epidemiol* 1969; **89**: 435–48.

15. Kapikian AZ, Mitchell RH, Chanock RM, Shvedoff RA, Stewart CE. An epidemiologic study of altered clinical reactivity to respiratory syncytial (RS) virus infection in children previously vaccinated with an inactivated RS virus vaccine. *Am J Epidemiol* 1969; **89**: 405–21.

16. Kim HW, Canchola JG, Brandt CD *et al.* Respiratory syncytial virus disease in infants despite prior administration of antigenic inactivated vaccine. *Am J Epidemiol* 1969; **89**: 422–34.

17. Graham BS, Bunton LA, Wright PF, Karzon DT Role of T lymphocyte subsets in the pathogenesis of primary infection and rechallenge with respiratory syncytial virus in mice. *J Clin Invest* 1991; **88**: 1026–33.

18. Openshaw PJ. Immunopathological mechanisms in respiratory syncytial virus disease. *Springer Semin Immunopathol* 1995; **17**: 187–201.

19. Hussell T, Pennycook A, Openshaw PJ Inhibition of tumor necrosis factor reduces the severity of virus-specific lung immunopathology. *Eur J Immunol* 2001; **31**: 2566–73.

20. Openshaw PJ, Culley FJ, Olszewska W. Immunopathogenesis of vaccine-enhanced RSV disease. *Vaccine* 2001; **20** Suppl 1: S27–31.

21. Barr J, Chambers P, Pringle CR, Easton AJ. Sequence of the major nucleocapsid protein gene of pneumonia virus of mice: sequence comparisons suggest structural homology between nucleocapsid proteins of pneumoviruses, paramyxoviruses, rhabdoviruses and filoviruses. *J Gen Virol* 1991; **72**: 677–85.

22. Gozal D, Colin AA, Jaffe M, Hochberg Z. Water, electrolyte, and endocrine homeostasis in infants with bronchiolitis. *Pediatr Res* 1990; **27**: 204–9.

23. Hanna S, Tibby SM, Durward A, Murdoch IA. Incidence of hyponatraemia and hyponatraemic seizures in severe respiratory syncytial virus bronchiolitis. *Acta Paediatr* 2003; **92**: 430–4.

24. Poddar U, Singhi S, Ganguli NK, Sialy R. Water electrolyte homeostasis in acute bronchiolitis. *Indian Pediatr* 1995; **32**: 59–65.

25. O'Malley BW. Mechanisms of action of steroid hormones. *N Engl J Med* 1971; **284**: 370–7.
26. Fauci AS. Mechanisms of corticosteroid action on lymphocyte subpopulations. II. Differential effects of in vivo hydrocortisone, prednisone and dexamethasone on in vitro expression of lymphocyte function. *Clin Exp Immunol* 1976; **24**: 54–62.
27. Tasker RC, Roe MF, Bloxham DM, White DK, Ross-Russell RI, O'Donnell DR. The neuroendocrine stress response and severity of acute respiratory syncytial virus bronchiolitis in infancy. *Intens Care Med* 2004; **30**: 2257–62.
28. Danus O. [Bronchiolitis. Analysis of 30 cases treated with Meticorten]. *Pediatria. (Santiago.)* 1965; **8**: 113–20.
29. Weinberger M. Corticosteroids for first-time young wheezers: current status of the controversy. *J Pediatr* 2003; **143**: 700–2.
30. Csonka P, Kaila M, Laippala P, Iso-Mustajarvi M, Vesikari T, Ashorn P. Oral prednisolone in the acute management of children age 6 to 35 months with viral respiratory infection-induced lower airway disease: a randomized, placebo-controlled trial. *J Pediatr* 2003; **143**: 725–30.
31. Patel H, Platt R, Lozano JM, Wang EE. Glucocorticoids for acute viral bronchiolitis in infants and young children. *Cochrane Database Syst Rev* 2004; CD004878.
32. LeVine AM, Gwozdz J, Stark J, Bruno M, Whitsett J, Korfhagen T. Surfactant protein-A enhances respiratory syncytial virus clearance in vivo. *J Clin Invest* 1999; **103**: 1015–21.
33. Dargaville PA, South M, McDougall PN. Surfactant abnormalities in infants with severe viral bronchiolitis. *Arch Dis Child* 1996; **75**: 133–6.
34. Lofgren J, Ramet M, Renko M, Marttila R, Hallman M. Association between surfactant protein A gene locus and severe respiratory syncytial virus infection in infants. *J Infect Dis* 2002; **185**: 283–9.
35. O'Donnell DR, Milligan L, Stark JM Induction of CD95 (Fas) and apoptosis in respiratory epithelial cell cultures following respiratory syncytial virus infection. *Virology* 1999; **257**: 198–207.
36. Tibby SM, Hatherill M, Wright SM, Wilson P, Postle AD, Murdoch IA. Exogenous surfactant supplementation in infants with respiratory syncytial virus bronchiolitis. *Am J Respir Crit Care Med* 2000; **162**: 1251–6.
37. Schindler M Do bronchodilators have an effect on bronchiolitis? *Crit Care* 2002; **6**: 111–12.
38. Kellner JD, Ohlsson A, Gadomski AM, Wang EE. Efficacy of bronchodilator therapy in bronchiolitis. A meta-analysis. *Arch Pediatr Adolesc Med* 1996; **150**: 1166–72.
39. Kellner JD, Ohlsson A, Gadomski AM, Wang EE. Bronchodilators for bronchiolitis. *Cochrane Database Syst Rev* 2000; CD001266.
40. Hartling L, Wiebe N, Russell K, Patel H, Klassen TP. Epinephrine for bronchiolitis. *Cochrane Database Syst Rev* 2004; CD003123.
41. Collins PL, McIntosh K, Channock RM. Respiratory syncytial virus. In: Fields BN, Knipe DM, Howley RM *et al.*, eds. *Fields Virology*. Philadelphia, Lippincott-Raven, 1996; 1313–51.
42. Krilov LR, Mandel FS, Barone SR, Fagin JC. Follow-up of children with respiratory syncytial virus bronchiolitis in 1986 and 1987: potential effect of ribavirin on long term pulmonary function. The Bronchiolitis Study Group. *Pediatr Infect Dis J* 1997; **16**: 273–6.
43. Long CE, Voter KZ, Barker WH, Hall CB. Long term follow-up of children hospitalized with respiratory syncytial virus lower respiratory tract infection and randomly treated with ribavirin or placebo. *Pediatr Infect Dis J* 1997; **16**: 1023–8.
44. Rodriguez WJ, Arrobio J, Fink R, Kim HW, Milburn C. Prospective follow-up and pulmonary functions from a placebo-controlled randomized trial of ribavirin therapy in respiratory syncytial virus bronchiolitis. Ribavirin Study Group. *Arch Pediatr Adolesc Med* 1999; **153**: 469–74.
45. Buck JJ, Debenham P, Tasker RC. Prophylaxis for respiratory syncytial virus infection: missing the target. *Arch Dis Child* 2001; **84**(4): 375.
46. Ghosh S, Champlin RE, Englund J. *et al.* Respiratory syncytial virus upper respiratory tract illnesses in adult blood and marrow transplant recipients:

combination therapy with aerosolized ribavirin and intravenous immunoglobulin. *Bone Marrow Transpl* 2000; **25**(7): 751–5.

47. Sokol J, Jacobs SE, Bohn D. Inhaled nitric oxide for acute hypoxemic respiratory failure in children and adults. *Cochrane Database Syst Rev* 2000; CD002787.

48. Kneyber MC, Oud-Alblas HB, van Vliet M, Uiterwaal CS, Kimpen JL, van Vught AJ. Concurrent bacterial infection and prolonged mechanical ventilation in infants with respiratory syncytial virus lower respiratory tract disease. *Intens Care Med* 2005; **31**: 680–5.

49. Purcell K Fergie J. Concurrent serious bacterial infections in 2396 infants and children hospitalized with respiratory syncytial virus lower respiratory tract infections. *Arch Pediatr Adolesc Med* 2002; **156**: 322–4.

50. Duttweiler L, Nadal D, Frey B. Pulmonary and systemic bacterial co-infections in severe RSV bronchiolitis. *Arch Dis Child* 2004; **89**: 1155–7.

51. Flamant C, Hallalel F, Nolent P, Chevalier JY, Renolleau S. Severe respiratory syncytial virus bronchiolitis in children: from short mechanical ventilation to extracorporeal membrane oxygenation. *Eur J Pediatr* 2005; **164**: 93–8.

52. Crowcroft NS, Booy R, Harrison T *et al*. Severe and unrecognised: pertussis in UK infants. *Arch Dis Child* 2003; **88**: 802–6.

53. Korppi M, Leinonen M, Koskela M, Makela PH, Launiala K. Bacterial coinfection in children hospitalized with respiratory syncytial virus infections. *Pediatr Infect Dis J* 1989; **8**: 687–92.

54. Konig B, Konig W, Arnold R, Werchau H, Ihorst G, Forster J. Prospective study of human metapneumovirus infection in children less than 3 years of age. *J Clin Microbiol* 2004; **42**: 4632–5.

55. Wang EE, Law BJ, Boucher FD *et al*. Pediatric Investigators Collaborative Network on Infections in Canada (PICNIC) study of admission and management variation in patients hospitalized with respiratory syncytial viral lower respiratory tract infection. *J Pediatr* 1996; **129**: 390–5.

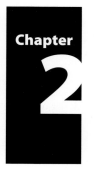

Chapter 2

The infant with meningococcal septicemia

Mehrengise Cooper and Simon Nadel

Introduction

Meningococcal septicemia is associated with a high morbidity and mortality. Following the introduction of the meningococcal C vaccine, there has been a reduction in the incidence of disease, with the majority of the disease now being caused by *Neisseria meningitidis* group B. In 2003–2004, 969 cases of meningococcal disease in children under 15 years were notified to the Health Protection Agency in England and Wales.[1] Prompt recognition and early aggressive management of children has been shown to reduce both morbidity and mortality, with the majority surviving without long-term sequelae.

Case history

A previously well 10-month-old boy was admitted to his local hospital having been non-specifically unwell for 2 days with a fever. Initial blood results were unremarkable and he was admitted to the ward for observation. Two hours later, two petechial spots were noted on his neck. At this time, his heart rate (HR) was 160 b min^{-1}; he was normotensive and had a capillary refill time (CRT) <2 seconds. He continued to be closely observed. Four hours later, the rash was noted to be more florid, and both maculo-papular and petechial in nature; his skin was mottled, and CRT had increased to 4–5 seconds. His vital signs were: HR 180–200 b min^{-1}, Blood Pressure (BP) 80/42 mmHg, Respiratory rate (RR) 60 breaths min^{-1}, maintaining SpO$_2$ at 100% in 10 l min^{-1} O$_2$ via facemask. His temperature was recorded at 39.5 °C via tympanic thermometer. He was responsive only to painful stimuli. A capillary blood gas showed a pH of 7.1, with a base excess of –10 mmol l^{-1} and pCO$_2$ of 3.5 kPa. Intravenous ceftriaxone 80 mg kg^{-1} was administered. Over the preceding 30 minutes, he received intravascular fluid administration in three aliquots – one bolus of 10 ml kg^{-1} 4.5% Human Albumin Solution (HAS), and two boluses of 20 ml kg^{-1} 4.5% HAS. He had not passed urine for 8 hours.

Repeat blood tests were taken for Full Blood Count (FBC), C-Reactive Protein (CRP), urea, electrolytes and Liver Function Tests (LFTs), and Arterial Blood Gas analysis (ABG); blood cultures were sent to the laboratory.

At this time the regional pediatric intensive care unit (PICU) was contacted for advice, with a view to retrieval for a patient with presumed meningococcal septicemia in septic shock. In addition to the resuscitation, which had already been given, the PICU team advised the following actions be taken:

1. Elective tracheal intubation – rapid sequence, with volume support.

2. Commence inotropes – with mean blood pressure guidance.

3. Correction of electrolyte abnormalities – K$^+$, ionized Ca^{2+}, Mg^{2+}, HCO$_3^-$.

4. Order Fresh Frozen Plasma (FFP) for the likely present coagulopathy.

5. Placement of nasogastric tube and urinary catheter.

Case Studies in Pediatric Critical Care, ed. Peter. J. Murphy, Stephen C. Marriage, and Peter J. Davis. Published by Cambridge University Press. © Cambridge University Press 2009.

Table 2.1. *Blood results*

Na (mmol l^{-1})	137
K (mmol l^{-1})	3.3
Cl (mmol l^{-1})	109
Urea (mmol l^{-1})	3.9
Creatinine (μmol l^{-1})	38
Calcium (mmol l^{-1})	2.24
Bilirubin (μmol l^{-1})	16
Albumin (g dl^{-1})	39
CRP (mg l^{-1})	7.5
AST (U l^{-1})	43
ALP (U l^{-1})	279
Hb (g dl^{-1})	11.6
WBC ($\times 10^9$ l^{-1})	3
Neutrophils ($\times 10^9$ l^{-1})	1.6
Platelets ($\times 10^9$ l^{-1})	319
pH	7.29
pCO$_2$ (kPa)	3.12
pO$_2$ (kPa)	26.5
HCO$_3$ (mmol l^{-1})	11.7
BE	-12

The local consultant anesthetist intubated his trachea via a rapid sequence induction of anesthesia, using IV atropine, thiopentone and suxamethonium. The airway was straightforward to manage at this time with a Grade 1 direct laryngoscopy; an oral endotracheal tube of 4.0 mm internal diameter was placed and secured; this was shown to be in a good position by chest radiograph. The initial ventilator settings he was placed on were: intermittent mandatory ventilation, with pressure control:

PIP 20 cmH$_2$O

PEEP 5 cmH$_2$O

Rate 30 bpm

Inspiratory time 1.0 second

FiO$_2$ 0.6

A dobutamine infusion was commenced via peripheral venous line at 5 mcg kg^{-1} min^{-1} and subsequently increased to 10 mcg kg^{-1} min^{-1}, and his mean BP was maintained at ≥60 mmHg. He received intravenous bicarbonate replacement (1 mmol kg^{-1}), and further colloid resuscitation.

The Retrieval team arrived shortly after the above measures had taken place. In order to facilitate as safe a transfer as possible, he was reassessed. He had a safe and stable artificial

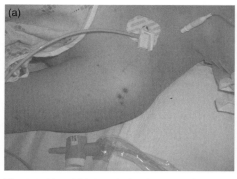
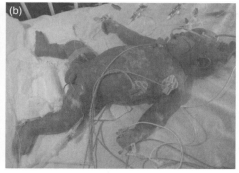

Fig. 2.1. (a) and (b): Petechial rash, purpura fulminans. (see color plate section).

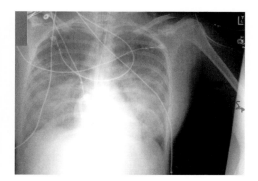

Fig. 2.2. CXR – pulmonary edema.

airway, with ETT in a good position. His SpO$_2$ deteriorated to <90% and a chest radiograph was consistent with pulmonary edema; his ventilator settings were optimized to PIP 28 cm H$_2$O, PEEP 8 cmH$_2$O and an increased FiO$_2$, with good effect. A left femoral arterial line was sited and arterial blood gas analysis at this time was: pH 7.34, pCO$_2$ 4.8 kPa, pO$_2$ 27 kPa, HCO$_3^-$ 19 mmol l^{-1}, BE −6.5 mmol.l^{-1}. Central venous access was gained through the left femoral vein and the inotropes were administered via this route. An adrenaline infusion was commenced in order to maintain his mean BP ≥60 mm Hg and improve his presumed poor cardiac output; this infusion was commenced at 0.1 mcg kg^{-1} per min and increased to 0.5 mcg kg^{-1} per min due to refractory hypotension. His extremities remained poorly perfused. He was commenced on intravenous morphine and midazolam infusions.

Repeat FBC at this stage revealed: Platelets 11 × 10^9 l^{-1}, Hb 8 g dl^{-1}, WBC 4.2 × 10^9 l^{-1}, and clotting analysis showed INR 1.8 and APTR 2.0. He received a platelet transfusion of 15 ml kg^{-1}, FFP 20 ml kg^{-1}, and packed red blood cells of 15 ml kg^{-1}. A further 10 ml kg^{-1} of 4.5% HAS was administered.

His urine output had improved, and by now he was passing 1 ml kg^{-1} per h. He received further IV electrolyte replacements to correct plasma calcium, magnesium, and potassium levels (Figs. 2.1(a), (b), 2.2).

At this point he was felt to be safe for transfer and was transferred by the retrieval team to the PICU. The journey took 90 minutes and he was stable throughout. Maximal infusions of

Table 2.2. *Investigations and results on admission to PICU*

Na (mmol l^{-1})	144
K (mmol l^{-1})	3.9
Urea (mmol l^{-1})	10.9
Creatinine (μmol l^{-1})	87
Calcium (mmol l^{-1})	2.01
Bilirubin (μmol l^{-1})	22
Albumin (g dl^{-1})	26
CRP (mg l^{-1})	58
Hb (g dl^{-1})	9.7
WBC ($\times 10^9$ l^{-1})	4.8
Neutrophils ($\times 10^9$ l^{-1})	1.7
Platelets ($\times 10^9$ l^{-1})	63
INR	1.4
TT (s)	1.5
Lactate (mmol l^{-1})	3.5
Glucose (mmol l^{-1})	2.9
Rapid antigen screen	Positive for meningococcus
Blood cultures	Group B meningococcus

dobutamine and adrenaline were 10 mcg kg^{-1} per min and 2 mcg kg^{-1} per min, respectively during transfer, in order to maintain a mean arterial BP ≥55 mmHg. This was felt to be an age-appropriate level of blood pressure in order to try to maintain end-organ perfusion. Two further 4.5% HAS boluses were administered *en route*.

Progress and management on PICU

On arrival on PICU he was reviewed. On examination, he was edematous, and had areas of confluent purpura over his trunk and neck; his peripheral perfusion was very poor, with a CRT >5 seconds and white/blue appearance to his digits. His hands and feet were severely mottled and ischemic looking, with palpable peripheral pulses. His vital signs were the following: temperature 38.9 °C, HR 200 b min^{-1}, mean BP >65 mmHg, SpO$_2$ 100%, RR 30 breaths min^{-1}. He had normal heart sounds with no murmur, good bilateral air entry, and a distended abdomen, with a 3 cm liver edge palpable. He was well sedated and pupils were pinpoint.

Medications on admission: dobutamine 5 mcg kg^{-1} per min, adrenaline (epinephrine) 1.5 mcg kg^{-1} per min, morphine 40 mcg kg^{-1} per h, midazolam 2 mcg kg^{-1} per min, Ceftriaxone 80 mg kg^{-1} daily. He was also receiving intravenous fluids as 0.45% saline/5% dextrose at 80% of maintenance. He had received 250 ml kg^{-1} of fluid resuscitation as boluses over the preceding 12-hour period.

Admission investigations taken on PICU included: FBC, U&E, LFTs, CRP, coagulation profile, blood cultures, rapid antigen screen, meningococcal PCR; throat swab for bacteriology.

Table 2.3. *Blood results at 24 hours*

Na (mmol l^{-1})	140
K (mmol l^{-1})	3.4
Urea (mmol l^{-1})	6.9
Creatinine (μmol l^{-1})	75
Calcium (mmol l^{-1})	2.23
Bilirubin (μmol l^{-1})	19
Albumin (g dl^{-1})	28
CRP (mg l^{-1})	259
Hb (g dl^{-1})	20.3
WBC ($\times10^9$ l^{-1})	22.4
Neutrophils ($\times10^9$ l^{-1})	20.3
Platelets ($\times10^9$ l^{-1})	159
INR	1.4
TT (s)	22.9

Following his arrival on the PICU, in the next 2 hours he became progressively more difficult to oxygenate and ventilate despite FiO_2 of 1.0, high peak inspiratory pressures, and increasing peak end expiratory pressure. ABG analysis showed: pH 7.18, pCO_2 8.0 kPa, pO_2 10 kPa, HCO_3 21 mmol l^{-1}, BE –5 mmol l^{-1}. He was then commenced on High Frequency Oscillatory Ventilation (HFOV) with an initial frequency of 8 Hz, mean airway pressure (MAP) 26 cmH_2O, amplitude (ΔP) 55, and FiO_2 0.8. Following this, oxygenation and ventilation improved.

Over the next 2 hours he became progressively more hypotensive, with decreasing diastolic BP and his inotropic management was changed – dobutamine discontinued, and noradrenaline (norepinephrine) commenced at 0.5 mcg kg^{-1} per min. Hydrocortisone was commenced (1 mg kg^{-1} every 6 hours). He required further colloid boluses in the form of 4.5% HAS, FFP and platelets.

Over this same 2-hour period he became progressively oliguric and then anuric, despite an adequate mean BP. His renal function had deteriorated over the same period of time in keeping with an Acute Tubular Necrosis (ATN). A vascular access catheter was placed in the right femoral vein, and Continuous Veno-Venous Haemofiltration (CVVH) was commenced in order to optimize fluid management. Enteral feeds were commenced via nasojejunal tube.

His overall condition improved over the next 24 hours, with improving ventilation parameters, weaning off noradrenaline with a reduction in blood product and colloid requirements. However, his hands and feet had showed marked ischemic damage. Vital signs at 24 hours following admission were: HR 160 b min^{-1}, mean BP 80, temperature 36.5 °C, SpO2 96%. Ventilation: HFOV – MAP 29 cmH_2O, Frequency 8 Hz, ΔP 62, FiO_2 0.55, with ABG – pH 7.37, pCO_2 6.65 kPa, PO$_2$ 15.6 kPa, HCO_3 27 mmol l^{-1}, BE +3 mmol l^{-1}, lactate 2.2 mmol l^{-1} (Table 2.3).

He was converted back to conventional ventilation after 5 days and adrenaline was discontinued on day 11. He was able to be extubated on day 12. His urine output improved after 4 days, and CVVH was discontinued after 6 days, with furosemide support. He received a 7-day course of ceftriaxone.

His extremities showed changes consistent with dry gangrene, and he was reviewed by the orthopedic, vascular and plastic surgery teams. It was important to allow the ischemic areas to demarcate in order to assess the areas of viable skin present.

He was discharged to the pediatric ward after 2 weeks of intensive care. He initially remained in hospital with ongoing occupational therapy, physiotherapy, and dietary input and later underwent surgical debridement of necrotic tissue, all toes, and finger tips of all fingers. In recovery, support was arranged through being supported by orthotic and rehabilitation teams.

Discussion

In severe cases of meningococcal septicemia, there is a rapid deterioration in clinical status leading to multi-organ failure. With aggressive early management, the mortality has decreased from 30% to 5% over the last 10 years.[2,3] Although the majority survive intact, some children develop sequelae with long-term consequences, including neurological dysfunction, limb, digit or skin loss, and frequent psychological disturbance.

Severe sepsis occurs following the coordinated activation of the innate immune response triggered by endotoxin released from proliferating meningococci in the bloodstream. This process then leads to the activation and mobilization of leucocytes and platelets, secretion of pro- and anti-inflammatory cytokines, activation of endothelial cells, coagulation and inhibition of fibrinolysis, and increased cellular apoptosis.[4,5] The thrombin generated by the inflammatory process causes fibrin to be deposited in the microvasculature, and also promotes further inflammation. Unfortunately, although a coordinated, controlled response may be appropriate in an attempt to protect the host from severe infection, an uncontrolled host inflammatory response occurring in the bloodstream is deleterious. Endothelial cell dysfunction leads to capillary injury with profound capillary leak into extravascular spaces, reduction in Systemic Vascular Resistance (SVR), together with microvascular and macrovascular thromboses. In addition, cardiac dysfunction occurs which is multifactorial in origin. These processes lead to the clinical features of sepsis, multi-organ failure, skin and peripheral necrosis, and eventually death.

While these pathophysiological processes occur in all forms of sepsis, meningococcal septicemia is characterized by the rapidity of disease progression. This may be due to the relatively high levels of endotoxin found in the bloodstream of patients with meningococcal septicemia and the extent of activation of the inflammatory and coagulation cascades.[4]

Initial assessment and management on PICU

The typical presentation of a child with meningococcal septicemia includes non-specific signs and symptoms of fever, vomiting, abdominal pain, headache, and myalgia.[6] These may be present for a few hours or longer. Once the typical hemorrhagic rash is present, the diagnosis is more obvious and is usually associated with a rapid deterioration into shock. The rash seen in meningococcemia is petechial, purpuric, and non-blanching in 80%. In 20% there may be a more atypical rash which may be maculo-papular in nature, or rarely there may be no rash seen.[6] Meningitis alone is present in around 50% of patients with meningococcal disease, whilst septicemia alone is present in 10%; 40% have a mixed picture.[7]

Initial investigations that are recommended for a full assessment of severity include: full blood count and differential, urea and electrolytes, glucose, C-reactive protein, liver function tests, coagulation screen, and arterial or venous blood gases. In addition, microbiological assessment may include serum rapid antigen screen, EDTA blood for meningococcal PCR, blood cultures, and throat swab for *Neisseria meningitidis*.

Features associated with a poor prognosis are: age <6 months, the absence of clinical or laboratory features of meningitis, coma, hypotension, peripheral WBC <10 000/cm^3, CRP <50 mg l^{-1}, ESR <10 mm h^{-1} the presence of thrombocytopenia and DIC, and metabolic acidosis.[8,9]

Where meningococcal infection is suspected, antibiotics must be given as soon as possible. In the absence of venous access, IM benzylpenicillin or ceftriaxone can be given.

The initial assessment includes an evaluation of ABC. Children with meningococcal shock need immediate resuscitation and restoration of circulating volume.[10] First, the airway must be assessed for patency and security. Supplemental oxygen at high concentration, via face mask or endotracheal tube, should be given even if there is reasonable transcutaneous oxygen saturation. Secure and efficient vascular access must be obtained. Even if major signs of shock are not present, all children with meningococcal septicemia will have a degree of hypovolemia. This should be promptly treated by infusing fluid; 40–60 ml kg^{-1} of 0.9% saline or 4.5% HAS may be given in the first hour without an increased risk of pulmonary or cerebral edema.[11] The degree of hypovolemia is usually underestimated, and it is not uncommon for children with meningococcal shock to require several times their circulating volume of fluid resuscitation in the first 24 hours. Such volumes can only be given safely with invasive monitoring of central venous and arterial pressure, continuous measurement of urine output and continuous clinical and laboratory assessment. This is best undertaken by a PICU team familiar with the interpretation of hemodynamic monitoring.

The treatment of shock includes replacement of circulating volume. Initially, 0.9% saline may be used as a bolus of 10–20 ml kg^{-1}, given over 5–10 minutes; in septic shock, colloid solutions may be more effective than crystalloid solutions as they may remain intravascular longer, and be more effective at restoring circulating volume. The colloid of choice in childhood sepsis is 4.5% human albumin solution.[10] Fluid boluses may improve the clinical parameters of shock, but these effects may only be temporary and continual assessment of the airway, breathing and circulation is paramount. A recent study comparing the use of 5% HAS against 0.9% saline as the resuscitation fluid of choice in critically ill adult patients found no difference in overall outcome at 28 days. However, subgroup analysis in patients with severe sepsis showed that those patients who were randomized to receive HAS appeared to have a better outcome than those in the saline group.[12]

Capillary leak often leads to pulmonary edema. Elective early tracheal intubation and mechanical ventilation should be considered when 40–60 ml kg^{-1} of resuscitation fluid has been given, particularly if there is evidence of ongoing fluid requirement. The optimal mode of ventilation depends upon the degree of pulmonary capillary leak and pulmonary edema. Relatively high Positive End-Expiratory Pressure (PEEP) should be used to optimize oxygenation. Where high PEEP and inflation pressures are increasing with little improvement in oxygenation, High Frequency Oscillatory Ventilation (HFOV) may be required to improve oxygenation.

The inflammatory process also leads to myocardial dysfunction, together with an increased myocardial oxygen demand due to shock. Poorly characterized myocardial depressant factors are found in the serum of patients with sepsis. A recent report has identified Interleukin 6 (IL-6) as a major myocardial depressant factor in patients with meningococcal septicemia.[13]

In patients with shock who require large volumes of fluid with signs of ongoing circulatory insufficiency, vasoactive agents for circulatory support are necessary. The optimal agent for use in children with septic shock is not known. Dobutamine, adrenaline and noradrenaline were all used on the patient described. Each has its advantages and disadvantages, and the choice is dependent on the clinical scenario. Dobutamine and adrenaline have both inotropic and vaso-dilator properties, depending on the dosages used, and usually increase cardiac output. However, they may also increase myocardial oxygen requirements and cause myocardial failure. Adrenaline and noradrenaline may act as vasopressors and increase systemic vascular resistance. While maintenance of blood pressure is important, vasopressors may worsen myocardial function in the face of a low cardiac output state seen in pre-terminal sepsis, and reduce perfusion to ischemic areas of skin and distal extremities, and to the splanchnic circulation. Newer agents being evaluated in the maintenance of the circulation include vasopressin by infusion in inotrope unresponsive vasodilatation due to sepsis, and milrinone in low cardiac output conditions.[14–16]

A study of the use of Early Goal-Directed Therapy (EGDT) in septic adult patients showed a significant reduction in mortality, when compared with standard therapy.[16] The EGDT included: fluids administered to achieve a CVP between 8 and 12 mmHg; where the mean blood pressure was low, vasopressors were used; if the mean arterial pressure was high, vasodilators were administered, and patients were transfused up to a hematocrit of 30%. The patients in the EGDT group showed improved central venous oxygen saturation, reduction in lactate levels, lower base deficit, higher pH, and a higher urine output when compared with standard therapy. The patients in the study group, randomized to receive EGDT, had a significantly lower mortality than those treated with standard therapy.

Cellular oxygen extraction is increased in patients with septic shock. The mixed venous oxygenation saturation provides a surrogate marker for cardiac index as an objective marker of the effectiveness of cardiac output in the delivery of oxygen to the tissues. Mixed venous oxygen saturation is best measured in the pulmonary artery using a pulmonary artery catheter. However, this technique is difficult and often impractical in children. Central venous oxygenation saturation ($ScvO_2$) is more easily measured, and is related to mixed venous oxygen saturation. $ScvO_2$ is therefore used clinically, and a value of <70% (with arterial oxygen saturation >90%) indicates an increase in tissue oxygen consumption. In order to improve the $ScvO_2$, dobutamine is commonly used to try to improve oxygen delivery to the tissues.

Where hypotension becomes refractory, despite increasing vasopressor support, cortico-steroids may be used. The hypothalamic–pituitary–adrenal axis is activated in children with severe sepsis and this leads to high levels of cortisol and its precursor, Adrenocorticotrophic Hormone (ACTH). However, low serum cortisol concentrations, combined with high ACTH concentrations have been found in some children with meningococcal septicemia who had an increased risk of death.[18,19]

In adults with septic shock, low-dose corticosteroids are now recommended in patients where vasopressors are required for the maintenance of an adequate blood pressure, despite adequate fluid replacement.[20] The reasoning for this is based upon several factors including relative adrenal insufficiency, peripheral steroid resistance, the effects of steroids on vascular tone, and steroid effects on immune response. There is no evidence of benefit from high-dose corticosteroids in patients with septic shock; in fact, there may be some evidence of harm.

Fluid management

Acute Tubular Necrosis (ATN) develops where there is a reduction in renal perfusion pressure and this occurs commonly in patients with septic shock. Oliguria or anuria may develop with an increase in serum urea and creatinine. The large volumes of resuscitation fluid required in sepsis may lead to widespread edema; this may affect pulmonary compli-ance, and peripheral perfusion with the development of compartment syndrome.

Diuretic therapy may optimize urine output in more stable patients; however, renal replacement therapy with CVVH allows fluid management to be more accurately controlled. CVVH allows easier administration of ongoing fluid and electrolyte replacement, optimizing nutritional requirements, and potentially removal of circulating proinflammatory cytokines, and tissue metabolites such as lactate and urea. There is some evidence that high volume hemofiltration may be beneficial in patients with septic shock and acute renal failure, with a putative mechanism of the removal of inflammatory mediators.[21] There is no consensus on the use of plasma- or hemofiltration in removal of cytokines from the circulation in patients with septic shock. Further studies remain to be carried out.[22]

Hyperglycemia possibly due to insulin resistance and the effects of catecholamines often occurs in critically ill children. Hyperglycemia occurring in critically ill adults has been shown to be associated with an increase in morbidity – such as increase in nosocomial infection, multi-organ failure – and in mortality. It has been shown that tight control of plasma glucose in critically ill adult surgical patients is associated with a reduction in morbidity and mortality.[23] In this study, plasma glucose levels were maintained between 4.4 and 6.1 mmol l^{-1}. Therefore, when hyperglycemia occurs in children with septic shock, insulin infusion may be required to achieve normoglycemia.

Where there is meningitis at presentation, appropriate neuroprotection must be included in management. It is important to achieve a blood pressure which will achieve a Cerebral Perfusion Pressure (CPP) of >40 mmHg, where there is the probability of the presence of raised Intracranial Pressure (ICP), (CPP = MAP–ICP). Lumbar puncture is contraindicated where there is clinical suspicion of raised ICP, and in patients with hemodynamic instability and coagulopathy. A CT scan may show cerebral edema, but is an insensitive guide to the presence of raised ICP. Where there is an acute neurological deterioration with signs of impending brainstem herniation, management includes the administration of mannitol or other hyperosmolar therapy and short-term hyperventilation.[24,25]

The management of children with a mixed picture of both raised ICP and septicemia presents a major challenge. The priorities are to maintain CPP by preservation of MAP, at the same time as attempting to reduce development of cerebral edema by limiting fluid administration. In this situation, maintenance of the circulation is the priority as, without an adequate blood pressure, cerebral perfusion is impaired.

Public health

One of the priorities following the admission of a child with meningococcal disease is informing the local public health department. *Neisseria meningitidis* is carried in the nasopharynx of healthy people. The organism is spread by droplets via close contact. Any individual who has been in close (kissing) contact with a child who has developed meningococcal disease must be contacted urgently and be given appropriate prophylactic antibiotics. Consultants in Communicable Disease Control assist in contact tracing and should be informed of any child admitted with suspected or proven meningococcal disease.

Ongoing management on PICU

Cardiorespiratory support

As the clinical circumstances allow, mechanical ventilation is tailored to achieve normal gas exchange and weaned as this is achieved. In the acute setting, patients have pulmonary capillary leak and pulmonary edema. This often requires increasing support where there is ongoing capillary leak and, as the fluid moves back into the intravascular space, ventilation may be weaned.

Inotropic support is continued in order to maintain adequate end-organ perfusion, and may require optimization in different clinical circumstances. Commonly used methods of assessment of the circulation, such as continuous Central Venous Pressure (CVP) monitoring, Transesophageal Doppler measurement of cardiac output,[26] and indwelling arterial monitors using the Fick principle (PICCO™, Philips) are useful in the measurement of cardiac indices (Cardiac Index, Systemic Vascular Resistance) in septic patients and may provide a useful guide to management of inotropes and fluids.[27] Nevertheless, one of the more valuable guides to cardiac output remains urine output.[11] Where an inotrope is required, dobutamine and adrenaline are titrated to effect; where vasoconstriction is required, for example, in a vasodilated (low SVR) state with a wide pulse pressure, noradrenaline is the agent of choice. Once again, these agents are weaned as the shock improves.

Fluid management

Maintenance fluids are administered at 80% of total maintenance fluid requirements; our fluid of choice is 0.45% saline with 5% dextrose. Enteral feeding should be instituted early. This may be carried out by either the nasogastric or nasojejunal route. We commence trophic feeds early and then grade up to full enteral feeds when tolerated.

Skin and limb care

Meningococcal septicemia is characterized by a hemorrhagic rash, which may progress to areas of confluent purpura. Areas of the skin and limbs – in particular extremities – may become necrotic. A compartment syndrome may develop in the acute situation where there is severe capillary leak threatening the perfusion of underlying muscle. It is important to involve vascular, orthopedic, and plastic surgical teams early. Fasciotomy should only be performed if deemed absolutely necessary, where compartment pressures have been demonstrated to be high and arterial pulses are absent. Most of the skin and limb necrosis that occurs is usually due to microvascular thrombosis, and fasciotomy rarely, if ever, has any benefit.[28] In order to have optimal functional recovery of limbs and extremities, the decision to perform amputation and debridement is best made in the convalescent phase of the illness and must involve a multidisciplinary team approach.

Newer therapies

Much work has focused on the use of therapeutic agents that act as adjuncts to the current supportive therapies used in the management of meningococcal septicemia. The adjunctive agents that have been used to modulate the inflammatory response include anti-endotoxin agents, such as recombinant bactericidal-permeability increasing protein (rBPI$_{21}$)[29] and anticoagulants such as Antithrombin III[30] and Activated Protein C (APC). Activated Protein C is an endogenous regulator of coagulation and inflammation. Once Protein C is activated by the thrombin–thrombomodulin complex, it is able to exert both antithrombotic and profibrinolytic effects. Patients with severe sepsis have been demonstrated to have a reduction or absence of protein C, which is associated with an increased risk of morbidity and mortality.[31,32] Drotrecogin alfa (activated) is a recombinant form of human APC and in the recently published PROWESS trial,[33] was administered to adults with severe sepsis. This multi-centre double-blind, randomized, placebo-controlled trial compared APC to placebo. The trial drug was administered for a total of 96 hours. There was a statistically significant reduction in 28-day all-cause mortality, with a relative risk reduction of 19.4% in those adults who received APC when compared with the placebo group. This was the first study of an adjunctive therapy in severe sepsis to show a survival advantage in the overall patient population. APC is now licensed for use in adults with severe sepsis.

Following a safety, pharmacokinetic and pharmacodynamic study in children, APC has been shown to have a safety profile similar to that seen in adults.[34,35] A multicentre, double-blind, randomized, placebo-controlled trial study, comparing APC with placebo in children with severe sepsis, stopped enrolling patients in 2005.[36] An external, independent Data Monitoring Committee recommended that the trial be stopped due to futility, following an interim analysis which revealed that the use of APC was unlikely to show an improvement over placebo in the primary endpoint of "Composite Time to Complete Organ Failure Resolution" over 14 days. In addition, there appeared to be an increase in the rate of Central Nervous System (CNS) bleeding in the APC group. There appeared to be no difference in mortality or the rate of other serious complications between the two groups.

Learning points

- With aggressive early management, the mortality from meningococcal septicemia has significantly reduced over the last 10 years.
- Early recognition and prompt management reduces the number of sequelae that occur.
- Initial management requires careful assessment of airway, breathing, and circulation.
- For the management of shock, fluid resuscitation is necessary for the replacement of circulating volume – colloid (4.5% HAS) is the fluid of choice.
- Once 40–60 ml kg^{-1} of fluid has been administered, and ongoing fluid resuscitation is felt necessary, elective tracheal intubation is advised.
- Early administration of vasoactive agents is beneficial for vascular and myocardial dysfunction; by monitoring CVP, BP, lactate, urine output, and $ScvO_2$, therapy may be optimized.
- Where shock is refractory to vasopressor support, low-dose corticosteroids may be of benefit.
- If the child becomes oligo-anuric with a poor response to diuretic therapy, CVVH should be commenced.
- Insulin infusion is likely to be of benefit where there is hyperglycemia.
- The consultant in communicable disease control should be contacted for contact tracing on admission.
- Ongoing intensive care management is largely supportive. Orthopedic, vascular, and plastic surgical teams should be involved as necessary for extensive purpuric lesions, where limbs may be affected by a compartment syndrome and where digits or facial areas are affected.
- Newer adjunctive therapies which modulate the inflammatory response in children with septic shock are currently under investigation, and the results of these studies are keenly awaited.

Early Management of Meningococcal Disease in Children*

6th Edition

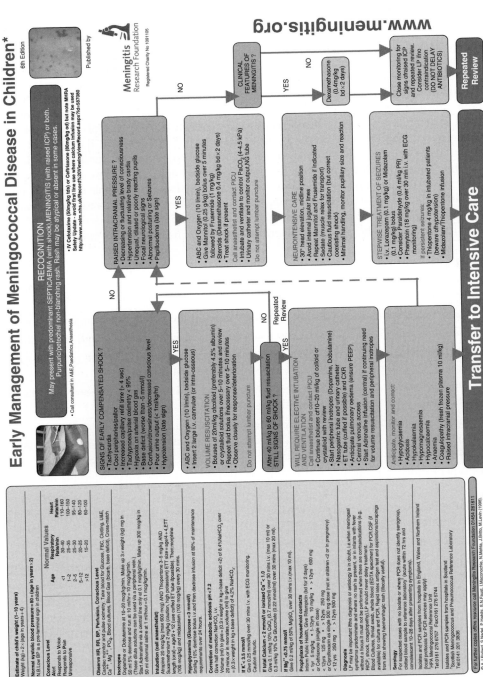

Published by

Meningitis Research Foundation

Registered Charity No 1091105

www.meningitis.org

RECOGNITION

May present with predominant SEPTICAEMIA (with shock),MENINGITIS (with raised ICP) or both.
Purpuric/petechial non-blanching rash. Rash may be atypical or absent in some cases.

* Call consultant in A&E, Paediatrics, Anaesthesia

• IV Cefotaxime (50mg/kg tds) or Ceftriaxone (80mg/kg od) but note MHRA
Safety Update - avoid first line use where calcium infusion may be used
http://www.nelm.nhs.uk/Record%20viewing/viewRecord.aspx?id=587060

SIGNS OF EARLY COMPENSATED SHOCK ?
• Tachycardia
• Cool peripheries/pallor
• Increased capillary refill time (> 4 sec)
• Tachypnoea/pulse oximetry < 95%
• Hypoxia on arterial blood gas
• Base deficit (worse than –5 mmol/l)
• Confusion/drowsiness/decreased conscious level
• Poor urine output (< 1ml/kg/hr)
• Hypotension (late sign)

NO → **RAISED INTRACRANIAL PRESSURE ?**
• Decreasing or fluctuating level of consciousness
• Hypertension and relative bradycardia
• Unequal, dilated or poorly reacting pupils
• Focal neurological signs
• Abnormal posturing or Seizures
• Papilloedema (late sign)

YES

• ABC and Oxygen (10 l/min), bedside glucose
• Insert 2 large i.v. cannulae (or intra-osseous)

VOLUME RESUSCITATION
• Boluses of 20ml/kg olcolloid (preferably 4.5% albumin)
or crystalloid solutions over 5–10 minutes and review
• Repeat fluid bolus if necessary over 5–10 minutes
• Observe closely for response/deterioration

Do not attempt lumbar puncture

After 40 ml/kg to 60 ml/kg fluid resuscitation
STILL SIGNS OF SHOCK ?

NO → Repeated Review

YES

**WILL REQUIRE ELECTIVE INTUBATION
AND VENTILATION**
Call anaesthetist and contact PICU
• Continue boluses of 10–20 ml/kg of colloid or
crystalloid with review
• Start peripheral inotropes (Dopamine, Dobutamine)
• Nasogastric tube and urinary catheter
• ET tube (cuffed if possible) and CXR
• Anticipate pulmonary oedema (ensure PEEP)
• Central venous access
• Start Adrenaline infusion (central) if continuing need
for volume resuscitation and peripheral inotropes

Anticipate, monitor and correct:
• Hypoglycaemia
• Acidosis
• Hypokalaemia
• Hypomagnesaemia
• Hypocalcaemia
• Anaemia
• Coagulopathy (fresh frozen plasma 10 ml/kg)
• Raised intracranial pressure

YES

• ABC and Oxygen (10 l/min), bedside glucose
• Give Mannitol (0.25 g/kg) bolus over 5 minutes
followed by Frusemide (1 mg/kg)
• Steroids (Dexamethasone 0.4 mg/kg bd x 2 days)
• Treat shock if present
Call anaesthetist and contact PICU
• Intubate and ventilate to control PaCO₂ (4.4–5 kPa)
• Urinary catheter and monitor output,NG tube
Do not attempt lumbar puncture

NEUROINTENSIVE CARE
• 30° head elevation, midline position
• Avoid internal jugular lines
• Repeat Mannitol and Frusemide if indicated
• Sedate (muscle relax for transport)
• Cautious fluid resuscitation (but correct
coexisting shock)
• Minimal handling, monitor pupillary size and reaction

STEPWISE TREATMENT OF SEIZURES
• i.v. Lorazepam (0.1 mg/kg) or Midazolam
(0.1 mg/kg) bolus
• Consider Paraldehyde (0.4 ml/kg PR)
• Phenytoin (18 mg/kg over 30 min i.v. with ECG
monitoring)
If persistent seizures:
• Thiopentone 4 mg/kg in intubated patients
(beware of hypotension)
• Midazolam/Thiopentone infusion

**CLINICAL
FEATURES OF
MENINGITIS ?**

NO

YES → **Dexamethasone
(0.4 mg/kg
bd x 2 days)**

Close monitoring for
signs ofraised ICP
and repeated review.
Consider LP (no
contraindications)
(DO NOT DELAY
ANTIBIOTICS)

→ **Repeated
Review**

Transfer to Intensive Care

Estimate of child's weight (1–10 years)
Weight (kg) = 2 × (age in years + 4)
N.B.Low BP is a pre-terminal sign in children

Normal systolic blood pressure = 80 + (age in years × 2)

Conscious Level		Normal Values		
	Age	Respiratory Rate/min	Heart Rate/min	
Alert	<1	30–40	110–160	
Responds to Voice	1–2	25–35	100–150	
Responds to Pain	2–5	25–30	95–140	
Unresponsive	5–12	20–25	80–120	
	>12	15–20	60–100	

Observe HR, RR, BP, Perfusion, Conscious Level
Cardiac monitor and pulse oximetry. Take blood for Glucose, FBC, Clotting, U&E,
Ca²⁺, Mg²⁺, PO₄, Blood cultures. Blood Gas (bicarb, base deficit), Cross-match

Inotropes
Dopamine or Dobutamine at 10–20 mcg/kg/min. Make up 3 × weight (kg) mg in
50 ml 5% dextrose and run at 10 ml/hr = 10 mcg/kg/min.
(These dilute solutions can be used via a peripheral vein.)
Start Adrenaline via a central line only at 0.1 mcg/kg/min. Make up 300 mcg/kg in
50 ml ofnormal saline at 1 ml/hour = 0.1 mcg/kg/min.

Intubation (call anaesthetist)
Atropine 20 mcg/kg (max 600 mcg) AND Thiopentone 3–5 mg/kg AND
Suxamethonium 2 mg/kg (caution: high potassium) ETT size = age/4 + 4,ETT
length (oral) age/2 + 12 (use cuffed ET tube ifpossible). Then morphine
(100 mcg/kg) and midazolam (100 mcg/kg) every 30 mins.

Hypoglycaemia (Glucose < 3 mmol/l)
5ml/kg 10% dextrose bolus i.v. and then dextrose infusion at 80% of maintenance
requirements over 24 hours.

Correction of metabolic acidosis pH <7.2
Give 8.4% NaHCO₃ i.v.
Volume (ml) to give = (0.3 × weight in kg – base deficit ÷2 of 8.4%NaHCO₃ over
20 mins or in neonates,volume (ml) to give
= (0.3 × weight in kg × base deficit) of 4.2% NaHCO₃.

If K⁺ <3.5 mmol/l
Give 0.25 mmol/kg over 30 mins i.v. with ECG monitoring.
Caution Potassium.

If total Calcium < 2 mmol/l or ionized Ca²⁺ < 1.0
Give 0.1 ml/kg 10% CaCl₂ (0.7 mmol/ml) over 30 mins i.v. (max 10 ml) or
0.3 ml/kg 10% Ca Gluconate (0.22 mmol/ml) over 30 min (max 10 ml).

If Mg²⁺ <0.75 mmol/l
Give 0.2 ml/kg of 50% MgSO₄ over 30 mins i.v.(max 10 ml).

Prophylaxis of household contacts
Inform Public Health. Give Rifampicin (bd for 2 days)
< 1yr 5 mg/kg   • 1–12yrs 10 mg/kg   • > 12yrs 600 mg
or Ceftriaxone (single im dose)
< 12yrs 125 mg   •   > 12yrs 250 mg
or Ciprofloxacin as single oral dose (not in children <2 or in pregnancy)
< 12 yrs 250 mg   •   > 12yrs 500 mg

Diagnosis
LP may be important if the diagnosis or aetiology is in doubt, i.e when meningeal
symptoms predominate and where no rash is present, or in infants with fever
without a focus.It must not be performed when there are contraindications (e.g.
RICP, shock, coagulopathy).LP should never delay treatment.
Blood Cultures, throat swab, whole blood (EDTA specimen) for PCR,CSF (if
available) for culture and PCR. Rapid latex antigen test and aspirations/scrapings
from skin showing haemorrhagic rash (iflocally useful).

Serology
For suspected cases with no isolate or where PCR does not identify serogroup,
clotted blood for serology is useful(acute within 72 hrs and
convalescent 10–28 days after presenting symptoms).
Isolates and PCR samples from hospitals in England, Wales and Northern Ireland
(local protocols for PCR services may apply)
HPA Meningococcal Reference Unit
Tel 0161 276 6757   Fax 0161 276 6744
Isolates and PCR samples from hospitals in Scotland
†Scottish Meningococcus and Pneumococcus Reference Laboratory
Tel 0141 201 3836

For further copies of this resource call Meningitis Research Foundation 01454 281811
© A.J.Pollard, S.Nadel, P Habibi, S.N Faust, I.Maconochie, N.Mehta, J.Britto, M.Levin (1998).
Department of Paediatrics, Imperial College School of Medicine, St Mary's Hospital, London W2
(*Arch Dis Child Apr 2007;92:283-6)

References

1. Health Protection Agency Homepage. Meningococcal Reference Unit Laboratory Confirmed Neisseria Meningitidis: England and Wales, by Age Group, 1989/1990 to 2003/2004.
2. Booy R, Habibi P, Nadel S et al. Reduction in the case fatality rate from meningococcal disease associated with improved healthcare delivery. Arch Dis Child 2001; 85: 386–90.
3. Thorburn K, Baines P, Thomson A, Hart CA. Mortality in severe meningococcal disease. Arch Dis Child 2001; 85: 382–5.
4. Nadel S, Levin M, Habibi P. Treatment of meningococcal disease in child hood. In Cartwright K, ed. Meningococcal Disease. Chichester, Wiley, 1995; 207–43.
5. Pathan N, Faust S, Levin M. Pathophysiology of meningococcal meningitis and septicaemia. Arch Dis Child 2003; 88: 601–7.
6. Steven N, Wood M. The clinical spectrum of meningococcal disease. In Cartwright K, ed. Meningococcal Disease. Chichester, Wiley, 1995; 177–205.
7. Kirsch EA, Barton RP, Kitchen L, Giroir BP. Pathophysiology, treatment and outcome of meningococcemia: a review and recent experience. Pediatr Infect Dis J 1996; 15: 967–78.
8. Steihm ER, Damrosch DS. Factors in the prognosis of meningococcal infection infection. Review of 63 cases with emphasis on recognition and management of the severely ill patient. J Pediatr 1966; 68: 457–67.
9. Sinclair JF, Skeoch CH, Hallworth D. Prognosis of meningococcal septicaemia Lancet 1987; 2(8549): 38.
10. Pollard AJ, Britto J, Nadel S et al. Emergency management of meningococcal disease. Arch Dis Child 2001; 85: 386–90.
11. Carcillo JA, Fields AI, Task Force Committee Members. Clinical practice parameters for hemodynamic support of pediatric and neonatal patients in septic shock. Crit Care Med 2002; 30: 1365–78.
12. Finfer S, Bellomo R, Boyce N et al. A comparison of albumin and saline for fluid resuscitation in the intensive care unit. N Engl J Med 2004; 350(22): 2247–56.
13. Pathan N, Hemingway CA, Alizadeh AA et al. Role of interleukin 6 in myocardial dysfunction of meningococcal septic shock. Lancet 2004; 363: 203–9.
14. Beale RJ, Hollenberg SM, Vincent J-L, Parillo JE. Vasopressor and inotropic support in septic shock: An evidence-based review. Crit Care Med 2004; 32(Suppl.): S455–65.
15. Heinz G, Geppert A, Delle Karth G et al. IV milrinone for cardiac output increase and maintenance:comparison in nonhyperdynamic SIRS/sepsis and congestive heart failure. Intens Care Med 1999; 25: 620–4.
16. Rich N, West N, McMaster P, Alexander J. Milrinone in meningococcal sepsis. Pediatr Crit Care Med 2003; 4: 394–5.
17. Rivers E, Nguyen B, Havstad S et al. Early goal-directed therapy in the treatment of severe sepsis and septic shock. N Engl J Med 2001; 345: 1368–77.
18. De Kleijn ED, Joosten KFM Van Rijn B et al. Low serum cortisol in combination with high adrenocorticotrophic hormone concentrations are associated with poor outcome in children with severe meningococcal disease. Pediatr Infect Dis J 2002; 21: 330–6.
19. Riordan FAI, Thomson APJ, Ratcliffe JM, Sills JA, Diver MJ, Hart AC. Admission cortisol and adrenocorticotrophic hormone levels in children with meningococcal disease: evidence of adrenal insufficiency? Crit Care Med 1999; 27: 2257–61.
20. Keh D, Sprung CL. Use of corticosteroid therapy in patients with sepsis and septic shock: an evidence-based review. Crit Care Med 2004; 32(Suppl.): S527–53.
21. Ronco C, Bellomo R, Homel P et al. Effects of different doses in continuous veno-venous haemofiltration on outcomes of acute renal failure: a prospective randomised trial. Lancet 2000; 356: 26–30.
22. McMaster P, Shann F. The use of extracorporeal techniques to remove humoral factors in sepsis. Pediatr Crit Care Med 2003; 4: 2–7.
23. Van den Berghe G, Wouters P, Weekers F et al. Intensive Insulin Therapy in Critically Ill patients. N Engl J Med 2001; 345: 1359–67.
24. Use of hyperosmolar therapy in the management of severe pediatric traumatic brain injury. From Guidelines for the acute

medical management of severe traumatic brain injury in infants, children and adolescents. *Pediatr Crit Care Med* 2003; **4**: S40-4.

25. Use of hyperventilation in the acute management of severe pediatric traumatic brain injury. From Guidelines for the acute medical management of severe traumatic brain injury in infants, children and adolescents. *Pediatr Crit Care Med* 2003; **4**: S45–8.

26. Tibby SM, Hatherill M, Durward A, Murdoch IA. Are transoesophageal Doppler parameters a reliable guide to paediatric haemodynamic status and fluid management? *Intens Care Med* 2001; **27**: 201–5.

27. Mohan UR, Britto J, Habibi P, De Munter C, Nadel S. Noninvasive measurement of cardiac output in critically ill children. *Pediatr Cardiol* 2002; **23**: 58–61.

28. Davies MS, Nadel S, Habibi P *et al.* The orthopaedic management of peripheral ischaemia in meningococcal septicaemia in children. *J Bone Joint Surg* 2000; **82**: 383–6.

29. Levin M, Quint PA, Goldstein B *et al.* Recombinant bactericidal permeability-increasing protein (rBPI21) as adjunctive treatment for children with meningococcal sepsis: a randomised trial. *RBPI21 Meningococcal Sepsis Study Group.* Lancet 2000; **356**: 961–7.

30. Opal S. Therapeutic rationale for antithrombin III in sepsis. *Crit Care Med* 2000; **28**(Suppl.): S34–7.

31. Fourrier F, Chopin C, Goudemand J *et al.* Septic shock, multiple organ failure, and disseminated intravascular coagulation. Compared patterns of antithrombin III, protein C, and protein S deficiencies. *Chest* 1992; **101**: 816–23.

32. Leclerc F, Hazelzet J, Jude B *et al.* Protein C and S deficiency in severe infectious purpura of children: a collaborative study of 40 cases. *Intens Care Med* 1992; **18**: 202–5.

33. Bernard GR, Vincent JL, Laterre PF *et al.* Efficacy and safety of recombinant human activated protein C for severe sepsis. *N Engl J Med* 2001; **344**: 699–709.

34. Barton P, Kalil AC, Nadel S *et al.* Safety, pharmacokinetics, and pharmacodynamics of drotrecogin alfa (activated) in children with severe sepsis. *Pediatrics* 2004; **113**: 7–17.

35. Weiss KD. Safety, Pharmacokinetics, and pharmacodynamics of drotrecogin alfa (activated) in children with severe sepsis – commentary. *Pediatrics* 2004; **113**: 134.

36. 2005 Safety Alert: Xigris [drotrecogin alfa (activated)]. US Food and Drug Administration. http://www.fda.gov/medwatch/safety/2005/Xigris_dearhcp_4-21-05.pdf.

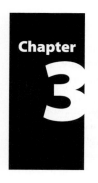

Chapter 3

A 2-year-old child with acute bacterial meningitis

Stephen C. Marriage and Laura J. Coates

Introduction

Infectious illnesses are consistently one of the most frequent causes of unplanned admission to pediatric intensive care. Acute bacterial meningitis – despite developments in antimicrobial therapy and intensive care – persists in having both a high mortality and a high incidence of resultant neurological sequelae. The development of highly efficacious conjugate vaccines has had a significant impact on the incidence of meningitis caused by *Haemophilus influenzae* type B, serogroup C *Meningococcus* and *Pneumococcus* in those countries with sufficient resources to have a universal vaccination schedule;[1-3] however, their high cost precludes their use in many developing countries. Intensive care units will continue to see children with acute bacterial meningitis: in young infants; in children born in countries without universal vaccination; in children of families who opt not to choose vaccination and in children with immunosuppression. Optimizing their acute management and care will help minimize mortality and morbidity.

Case history

A 2-year-old girl developed a vomiting illness whilst on holiday. The vomiting became marked and associated with a fever. Away from home, the family sought medical attention only after 36 hours had passed. She was normally a well child and had no relevant past medical history. The girl was seen by a primary care physician, who noted that the child was hot, not very responsive, and not able to recognize her parents. No parenteral antibiotics were administered at this initial consultation. She was referred to the emergency department of the local hospital.

On arrival at the emergency department the child was triaged and immediately referred to the on-call pediatric team. Initial observations revealed a child with tachypnea of 40 breaths min^{-1}, a tachycardia of 145 beats min^{-1}, and a central capillary refill time of 5 seconds. There was no rash and the blood pressure was not measured. The child responded neither to voice nor painful stimuli, although she did spontaneously open her eyes. Her pupillary responses to light were sluggish, but equal. She seemed unaware of her surroundings. A capillary blood gas analysis revealed a base deficit of −8.5 with a degree of respiratory compensation.

A presumptive diagnosis of meningoencephalitis was made. She was given high-flow oxygen and the anesthetic team called to secure her airway. An intra-osseous (IO) needle was inserted because of difficulty in establishing venous access and 100 mg kg^{-1} cefotaxime administered via the IO route, followed by 250 ml of 0.9% saline. The anesthetic team performed a rapid sequence induction using atropine, thiopentone and suxamethonium. A 4.5 mm endotracheal (ET) tube was placed and she was bagged in 100% oxygen using a T-piece, as no suitable ventilator was available in the department. A chest X-ray confirmed

Case Studies in Pediatric Critical Care, ed. Peter. J. Murphy, Stephen C. Marriage, and Peter J. Davis. Published by Cambridge University Press. © Cambridge University Press 2009.

the ET tube to be in a good position and no other diagnostic features were revealed. Unsuccessful attempts were then made to establish arterial access. Eventually, a single lumen 20 g cannula was inserted in the left femoral vein; this was used to undertake further laboratory studies, including a blood glucose, which was low at 2.4 mmol l^{-1}. A bolus of 5 ml kg^{-1} dextrose 10% was administered and maintenance fluids commenced. The child began to breathe against the ventilator and an infusion of morphine was instituted at 20 mcg kg^{-1} per h, together with intermittent boluses of atracurium 500 mcg kg^{-1} per dose.

Contact was made with the regional pediatric intensive care unit and arrangements made to retrieve the child. Whilst the transfer team were travelling out, it was suggested that aciclovir be added to the antimicrobial therapy and that an urgent computerized tomographic (CT) scan be arranged to exclude the possibility of abscess, subdural effusion or other space-occupying lesion. It was emphasized that, even should the scan prove normal, no lumbar puncture should be taken at this stage.[4] Cranial CT imaging was undertaken and revealed generalized cerebral edema and small frontal effusions bilaterally, but no focal features. The child returned to the emergency department, where she continued to be ventilated by hand.

On arrival of the PICU team, an assessment of the child's overall condition was made. She was placed on a transport ventilator and capnographic monitoring established, with an aim of maintaining normocapnia (4.5–5.0 kPa). Arterial access was established, and invasive blood pressure monitoring immediately revealed a blood pressure of 115/88 mmHg. Despite the morphine infusion, her pupils were dilated to 4–5 mm and responded sluggishly to light. Fundoscopy proved difficult in the brightly lit emergency department. Her fluids were restricted to two-thirds maintenance and a bolus of 0.25 g kg^{-1} mannitol administered. A urinary catheter was placed and a small residual urine volume noted. As steroids had neither been given before, nor with, the first dose of antibiotics, it was decided not to add them to the therapeutic regime.

The child was transferred back to the regional center via road ambulance. Infusions of morphine (30 mcg kg per h), midazolam (100 mcg kg per h) and vecuronium (120 mcg kg per h) were given to maintain stability during transfer. During the journey, an episode of hypertension (arterial BP 120/91 mmHg) with an associated bradycardia of 98 b min^{-1} was noted and a second dose of mannitol administered. The episode resolved and the transfer completed uneventfully. The child was transferred to an intensive care bed; the head of the bed was elevated to an angle of 30 °, and the child's head kept in the midline position. Normocapnic ventilation was maintained. Antimicrobial therapy was continued with ceftriaxone 80 mg kg^{-1} daily as a single antibacterial agent[5] and aciclovir 500 mg m^{-2} 8 hourly. Laboratory analyses were undertaken and the low plasma sodium concentration noted. The possibility of inappropriate ADH secretion was considered and a fluid restriction of two-thirds maintenance prescribed. Because of ongoing pyrexia, the child was cooled to normothermia. Muscle relaxation was discontinued to enable neurological evaluation and to prevent the masking of seizures, but the infusions of morphine and midazolam were maintained. Because of the clinical signs of raised intracranial pressure, lumbar puncture was deferred.

Later that night, tonic–clonic seizure activity was noted. The seizure was terminated with lorazepam 100 mcg kg^{-1} and she was subsequently loaded with phenytoin 18 mg kg^{-1}. Continuous EEG monitoring was commenced using a 12-channel monitor. Phenytoin 5 mg kg^{-1} twice daily was then continued throughout her ITU stay.

Following treatment for seizures, it was noted that her blood pressure had settled significantly to 80/50 mmHg (mean 62 mmHg). It was assumed that her intracranial pressure would be raised and that cerebral perfusion pressure would therefore be inadequate.[6]

Intracranial pressure was not measured directly, but an infusion of noradrenaline was commenced at 0.04 mcg kg^{-1} per min and titrated to achieve a mean arterial pressure of 75 mmHg.[7] Assuming the intracranial pressure to be 25 mmHg, this would give a resultant cerebral perfusion pressure of 50 mmHg.

Over the next 48 hours her clinical condition settled. Seizures became less frequent and the infusion of noradrenaline was able to be discontinued. Blood cultures were positive for a fully sensitive *Pneumococcus* sp. and her antibiotics were rationalized to high-dose benzyl penicillin 60 mg kg^{-1} four times daily.[8] She was weaned from the ventilator on the fifth day of admission and discharged from intensive care the following day. Plans were made to continue antibiotics for 14 days and to formally evaluate hearing 6 weeks' post-discharge.

Discussion

Epidemiology

Acute Bacterial Meningitis (ABM) is a disease that has predominated in children until the advent of the highly immunogenic conjugate vaccines in the past 20 years. In 1986, 79% of all episodes of bacterial meningitis in the United States occurred in children under the age of 18: by 1995, with the introduction of immunization against *Haemophilus influenzae* type B, this had fallen below 50%.[9] This proportion can be expected to fall further as other conjugate vaccines are introduced.[1] In such a rapidly moving period of medical advance, estimates of the incidence of ABM are hard to establish: for example, by 1995 the incidence of Hib meningitis in the United States and Canada had fallen by over 95% compared with pre-vaccination data.[10] A similar decrease in the incidence of invasive pneumococcal disease – including meningitis – has occurred in those areas where heptavalent pneumococcal vaccination has been introduced.[11]

Recently published data from the UK, following a programme of enhanced surveillance for pneumococcal disease before the introduction of pneumococcal conjugate vaccine, estimated the incidence of pneumococcal meningitis to be 0.7 per 100 000 of the population per year.[12] The figure was as high as 5.7 per 100 000 for children under the age of 5 years. In other populations the incidence is much higher: in Burkina Faso, the annual incidence has been calculated as 41 per 100 000 in children under the age of 5 years[13] and in Western Australia the incidence of pneumococcal meningitis has been reported as being over 77 per 100 000 in indigenous children under the age of 2.[14]

Antimicrobial therapy

In a rapidly progressive case of meningitis with associated features of systemic illness, presumptive antibiotic therapy will often have to be initiated without knowledge of the causative organism. In such cases the initial choice of antibiotics will to some extent be driven by associated features – such as the classical rash of meningococcaemia – but more frequently by knowledge of local epidemiology and antibiotic sensitivities. The age of the patient is crucial in dictating choice of treatment, as this will determine the likely causative organisms.[15] Outside the neonatal period, the two most likely organisms to cause ABM are *Pneumococcus* and *N. meningitidis*. Third-generation cephalosporins such as ceftriaxone or cefotaxime cross the blood–brain barrier readily and are effective against all meningococcal serogroups. In the UK, pneumococcal resistance to cephalosporins is rare and therefore they may confidently be used as an effective single agent in empiric therapy. In other countries, most notably Spain, South Africa, and in some parts of the Americas, cephalosporin resistance has become an increasing problem and vancomycin has to be included as part of empiric therapy until sensitivities become known.

Aciclovir was used as an additional antiviral agent in this case as the diagnosis of bacterial meningitis had not been confirmed. If the differential diagnosis includes the possibility of herpes encephalitis, aciclovir should always be used from the outset. It can be stopped if an alternative infectious agent has been proven, or in the absence of serological, electrophysiological or polymerase chain reaction evidence of infection.

Lumbar puncture

The performance – or non-performance – of a lumbar puncture often divides opinion between intensivists and infectious disease specialists. There are specific contraindications to lumbar puncture that should be strictly adhered to (Table 3.1). It is unusual for a child, sick enough to require the services of the intensive care unit, not to fulfill several of these criteria and for the investigation to need to be postponed.

The reasons for postponing the investigation have been classically demonstrated in a series looking at episodes of tentorial herniation, and relating them temporally to the performance of a lumbar puncture.[16] In the majority of cases the only safe option is to delay obtaining CSF, to start empiric therapy, and to use other techniques such as PCR, blood cultures, and throat swabs to confirm the diagnosis.[17] In the majority of cases, the clinical condition of the child will improve sufficiently to allow the investigation merely to be deferred until clinically stable. Much useful information may still be derived from the investigation up to 48 hours after presentation.

Steroids

There is no clear answer as to whether steroids should be used routinely as part of adjunctive therapy in acute bacterial meningitis. Early use of dexamethasone has been demonstrated to result in a decreased incidence of hearing loss in children with Hib meningitis,[18] which may also be true, though less clearly so, for pneumococcal meningitis.[19] Dexamethasone therapy has also resulted in improved outcomes for adults with pneumococcal meningitis.[20] The most recent Cochrane Review of the available evidence recommends the use of adjunctive steroids in adults and in children from high-income countries. There were insufficient data to make a similar recommendation for children from low-income countries.[21]

If steroids are to be used, it seems clear that they should be given before, or with, the first dose of antibiotics. The timing is critical, as their theoretical mechanism of action is to blunt the actions of cytokines and chemokines released at the time of initial bacterial killing, thereby preventing secondary neuronal damage due to the resultant inflammatory cascade. The majority of damage in ABM arises from inflammation that is triggered by products released by bacterial cell-wall breakdown. A complex cytokine/chemokine cascade is initiated, which leads to the influx of inflammatory cells and the breakdown of the blood–brain barrier, with local vasculitis, loss of cerebrovascular autoregulation, and cerebral edema.[22] In this instance, antibiotics had been given at the referring centre without adjunctive corticosteroids. By the time the transfer team had arrived, it was felt that it was already too late to derive benefit from their administration.

Cerebral perfusion

It is now well established that the monitoring of Intracranial Pressure (ICP) and Cerebral Perfusion Pressure (CPP) are good predictors of death in pediatric patients with *traumatic* brain injury, although absolute criteria for what constitutes an adequate CPP have not been determined. This whole area of study has been thoroughly reviewed with the recommendation that higher levels of CPP should be actively maintained, using strategies both to increase mean arterial pressure – with pressors – and to reduce intracranial pressure, with osmotherapy, positioning and attempts to minimize cerebral metabolism through the use of cooling and sedation.[23]

The data in patients with non-traumatic coma, including ABM, are less clear. In a group of children with non-traumatic coma – some of whom had meningitis – a CPP of less than 38 mmHg was a predictor of a poorer outcome, although the specificity of the observation was not high – some children had poor outcomes in whom the CPP was never shown to be low.[24] These findings were supported by a study of 27 children with acute meningitis and encephalitis, in whom the ICP and CPP were significantly different when stratified into survivors and non-survivors.[6] What remains unclear is whether or not a CPP-modifying strategy confers any benefit in ABM (or any other cause of coma).[25]

SIADH

Studies have shown that a very high proportion of patients with ABM may develop inappropriate secretion of antidiuretic hormone (SIADH) as a complication.[26] Treatment consists of fluid restriction in the first instance; in this case a restriction of two-thirds maintenance was adopted. Care should be taken, however, when restricting fluids in children with ABM. They are often dehydrated (in which case the secretion of ADH would be entirely appropriate) and cerebral perfusion, as discussed above, may be compromised by a too-vigorous regime of fluid restriction. Fluid restriction in ABM as a first-line management strategy has been shown to confer no benefit.[26]

Seizures

The potential causes of seizures in ABM are manifold and include the inflammatory process itself, electrolyte imbalance, fever, and cerebral edema. Generalized seizures should prompt immediate management with short-acting benzodiazepines followed by a longer-acting anticonvulsant such as phenytoin or a barbiturate. Both drugs have the advantage that they can be introduced quickly and are amenable to monitoring of therapeutic levels. Cranial imaging and electrophysiological studies are warranted to exclude directly treatable etiologies such as subdural effusions or intracranial abscesses. Focal seizures are of greater prognostic significance and may be caused by focal infarction or ischemia. Again, they warrant immediate cranial imaging.

Summary

Acute bacterial meningitis, and specifically pneumococcal meningitis, is a devastating disease with a high mortality and incidence of neurological sequelae. Apart from appropriate empiric antibiotic therapy, necessary because of the frequent postponement of a definitive lumbar puncture, therapeutic options include the early administration of steroids, management of raised intracranial pressure and the control of seizures. In high-income countries the introduction of powerful, conjugate vaccines against all of the commonest forms of bacterial meningitis offer a new hope of the elimination of the majority of cases.

Table 3.1. *Contraindications to lumbar puncture*

Presence of shock
Glasgow Coma Score <13
Signs of raised intracranial pressure
Abnormal pupillary signs
Abnormal tone or posturing
Respiratory abnormalities
Papilledema
Hypertension /relative bradycardia
Seizures
Coagulopathy
Local skin infection over LP site

Learning points

- Acute bacterial meningitis – despite developments in antimicrobial therapy and intensive care – persists in having both a high mortality and a high incidence of resultant neurological sequelae.

- Outside the neonatal period, the two most likely organisms to cause ABM are *Pneumococcus* and *N. meningitidis*.

- If the differential diagnosis includes the possibility of herpes encephalitis, aciclovir should always be used from the outset.

- There are specific contraindications to lumbar puncture that should be strictly adhered to (Table 3.1).

- There is no clear answer as to whether or not steroids should be used routinely as part of adjunctive therapy in acute bacterial meningitis.

- It remains unclear whether or not a CPP-modifying strategy confers any benefit in ABM.

- A high proportion of patients with ABM may develop inappropriate secretion of anti-diuretic hormone (SIADH) as a complication.

- In ABM generalized seizures should prompt immediate management with short-acting benzodiazepines followed by a longer-acting anticonvulsant such as phenytoin or a barbiturate.

- In high-income countries the introduction of powerful, conjugate vaccines against all of the commonest forms of bacterial meningitis offer a new hope of the elimination of the majority of cases.

References

1. Davison KL, Ramsay ME. The epidemiology of acute meningitis in children in England and Wales. *Arch Dis Child* 2003; **88**(8): 662–4.

2. Balmer P, Borrow R., Miller, E. Impact of meningococcal C conjugate vaccine in the UK. *J Med Microbiol* 2002; **51**(9): 717–22.

3. Dubos F, Marechal I, Husson MO, Courouble C, Aurel M, Martinot A. Decline in pneumococcal meningitis after the introduction of the heptavalent-pneumococcal conjugate vaccine in northern France. *Arch Dis Child* 2007; **92**(11): 1009–12.

4. Shetty AK, Desselle BC, Craver RD, Steele RW. Fatal cerebral herniation after lumbar puncture in a patient with a normal computed tomography scan. *Pediatrics* 1999; **103**(6 Pt 1): 1284–7.

5. Saez-Llorens X, McCracken Jr. GH, Bacterial meningitis in children. *Lancet* 2003; **361** (9375): 2139–48.

6. Rebaud P, Berthier JC, Hartemann E, Floret D. Intracranial pressure in childhood central nervous system infections. *Intens Care Med* 1988; **14**(5): 522–5.

7. Moller K, Larsen FS, Quist J *et al.* Dependency of cerebral blood flow on mean arterial pressure in patients with acute bacterial meningitis. *Crit Care Med* 2000; **28** (4): 1027–32.

8. Pneumococcal infections. *Red Book* 2006; **2006**(1): 525–537.

9. Schuchat A, Robinson K, Wenger JD *et al.* Bacterial meningitis in the United States in 1995. Active Surveillance Team. *N Engl J Med* 1997; **337**(14): 970–6.

10. Wenger JD. Epidemiology of *Haemophilus influenzae* type b disease and impact of *Haemophilus influenzae* type b conjugate vaccines in the United States and Canada. *Pediatr Infect Dis J* 1998; **17**(9 Suppl): S132–6.

11. Black S, France EK, Isaacman D *et al.* Surveillance for invasive pneumococcal disease during 2000–2005 in a population of children who received 7-valent pneumococcal conjugate vaccine. *Pediatr Infect Dis J* 2007; **26**(9): 771–7.

12. Foster D, Knox K, Walker AS *et al.* Invasive pneumococcal disease: epidemiology in children and adults prior to implementation of the conjugate vaccine in the Oxfordshire region, England. *J Med Microbiol* 2008; **57** (4): 480–7.

13. Parent du Chatelet I, Traore Y, Gessner BD *et al.* Bacterial meningitis in Burkina Faso: surveillance using field-based polymerase chain reaction testing. *Clin Infect Dis* 2005; **40**(1): 17–25.

14. King BA, Richmond P. Pneumococcal meningitis in Western Australian children: Epidemiology, microbiology and outcome. *J Paediatr Child Hlth* 2004; **40**(11): 611–15.

15. McCracken GH Jr, Nelson JD, Kaplan SL, Overtwf GD, Rodriguez WJ, Steele RW. Consensus report: antimicrobial therapy for bacterial meningitis in infants and children. *Pediatr Infect Dis J* 1987; **6**(6): 501–5.

16. Rennick G, Shann F, de Campo J. Cerebral herniation during bacterial meningitis in children. *Br Med J*, 1993; **306**(6883): 953–5.

17. Riordan FAI, Cant AJ. When to do a lumbar puncture. *Arch Dis Child* 2002; **87** (3): 235–7.

18. Lebel MH, Freij BJ, Syrogiannopoulos GA *et al.* Dexamethasone therapy for bacterial meningitis. Results of two double-blind, placebo-controlled trials. *N Engl J Med* 1988; **319**(15): 964–71.

19. Kanra GY, Ozen H, Secmeer G, Ceyhan M, Ecevit Z, Belgin E. Beneficial effects of dexamethasone in children with pneumococcal meningitis. *Pediatr Infect Dis J* 1995; **14**(6): 490–4.

20. de Gans J, van de Beek D. Dexamethasone in adults with bacterial meningitis. *N Engl J Med* 2002; **347**(20): 1549–56.

21. van de Beek D, de Gans J, McIntyre P, Prasad K. Corticosteroids for acute bacterial meningitis. *Cochrane Database Syst Rev*, 2007(1): CD004405.

22. Meli DN, Christen S, Leib SL, Tauber MG. Current concepts in the pathogenesis of meningitis caused by Streptococcus pneumoniae. *Curr Opin Infect Dis* 2002; **15** (3): 253–7.

23. Chambers IR, Kirkham FJ. What is the optimal cerebral perfusion pressure in children suffering from traumatic coma? *Neurosurg Focus* 2003; **15**(6): E3.

24. Tasker RC, Matthew DJ, Helms P, Dinwiddie R, Boyd S. Monitoring in non-traumatic coma. Part I: Invasive intracranial measurements. *Arch Dis Child* 1988; **63**(8): 888–94.

25. Czosnyka M, Pickard JD. Monitoring and interpretation of intracranial pressure. *J Neurol Neurosurg Psychiatry* 2004; **75**(6): 813–21.

26. Feigin RD, Dodge PR, Bacterial meningitis: newer concepts of pathophysiology and neurologic sequelae. *Pediatr Clin North Am* 1976; **23**(3): 541–56.

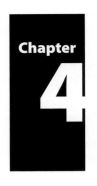

Chapter 4

Management of a neonate with hypoplastic left heart syndrome

Ulf Theilen and Lara Shekerdemian

Introduction

Until little over two decades ago, Hypoplastic Left Heart Syndrome (HLHS) was considered an inoperable and fatal condition, with most deaths occurring in early infancy, and almost all infants dying before their first birthday. However, the advent of surgical palliation and advances in peri-operative intensive care, have dramatically changed the prognosis of this condition.

Whilst many of these babies are antenatally diagnosed, others present with clinical signs of systemic hypoperfusion, acidosis and hypotension, most commonly during the first days of life. The primary goal of early intensive care of the infant with a known or suspected diagnosis of HLHS is to act pre-emptively, with management aimed at optimizing systemic oxygen delivery and organ perfusion. There is little doubt that early intensive care plays a key role in the ultimate survival of this challenging group of infants.

This case follows the early clinical course of an infant with a prenatal diagnosis of HLHS, transferred during the first few hours of life to a cardiac center for intensive care management, surgery, and subsequent post-operative care.

Case history

A 30-year-old lady presented for a routine fetal anomaly scan during an uncomplicated pregnancy. The four-chamber view of the fetal heart suggested that the left heart was underdeveloped, and she was therefore referred for a fetal echocardiogram. No other abnormalities were seen. The fetal echo confirmed a diagnosis of HLHS. After discussions with the pediatric cardiologist, the decision was made to continue with the pregnancy with a view to postnatal surgical palliation. The mother had regular ultrasound examinations to follow the fetal development, and adequacy of the interatrial communication. At 39 weeks' gestation, the mother was transferred to an obstetric unit with a level 4 neonatal intensive care unit. The obstetrician contacted the consultant pediatric cardiologist to inform him of the imminent delivery. Labour was induced, and a 2.7 kg boy was delivered by spontaneous vaginal delivery. A neonatologist was in attendance at the delivery.

Examination and initial management in neonatal ICU

The infant was born in good condition. No oxygen or bag–mask–valve ventilation was administered in the delivery room. Pulsoximeter and ECG monitor leads were attached. Initial observations were: oxygen saturation 84%, PR 145, non-invasive blood pressure 62/29. An umbilical venous catheter was inserted by the neonatalogist while still in the delivery room, and a prostaglandin E_1 infusion was commenced at 10 ng kg^{-1} per min. The infant was transferred to the neonatal intensive care unit.

Case Studies in Pediatric Critical Care, ed. Peter. J. Murphy, Stephen C. Marriage, and Peter J. Davis. Published by Cambridge University Press. © Cambridge University Press 2009.

Shortly after admission to the NICU, the infant became apnoeic and desaturated. Bag–mask ventilation was delivered using air, with immediate improvement in saturations and heart rate, and the infant was given 3 mcg kg^{-1} fentanyl and 0.1 mg kg^{-1} pancuronium for intubation. Oral intubation with a 3.5 endotracheal tube was uncomplicated and it was secured at 9.5 cm at the lips. Further peripheral intravenous access was obtained, and a 24 G cannula inserted in the right radial artery. A nasogastric tube and urinary catheter were also inserted. An infusion with morphine at 20 mcg kg^{-1} per hr was commenced, and maintenance fluids (10% dextrose, at 60 ml kg^{-1} per day) were started. Prostaglandin infusion was continued at 10 ng kg^{-1} per min.

Ventilation was set at pressures of 18/4, with a respiratory rate of 22, inspiratory time of 0.7 s in 21% oxygen. The initial arterial blood gas was: pH 7.23, pCO$_2$ 41 mmHg, pO$_2$ 42 mm Hg, bicarbonate 16 mmol l^{-1}, BE –9. Oxygen saturation at the time was 82%. Further results of interest were Hb 15.7 g dl^{-1}, sodium 141 mmol l^{-1}, potassium 4.4 mmol l^{-1}, calcium 2.13 mmol l^{-1}, magnesium 0.97 mmol l^{-1} and glucose 4.7 mmol l^{-1}. Blood lactate was 4.6 mmol l^{-1}. The infant was given a bolus of 10 ml kg^{-1} of normal saline. A chest X-ray confirmed well-positioned endotracheal and nasogastric tubes. Lung fields were radiologically clear.

The neonatal retrieval service was contacted to transport the infant to the pediatric intensive care unit at the nearby pediatric cardiac surgical center. The receiving pediatric cardiologist and intensive care physician were also contacted and further details were given about the infant's condition.

The retrieval team arrived 2 hours later, and gave the infant a further dose of pancuronium (0.1 mg kg^{-1}) and transferred him to the incubator and transport ventilator, using the same ventilatory settings as those above. The transport ventilator was operated with E-sized cylinders of medical air (FiO$_2$ 0.21). Peripheral oxygen saturation remained around 75% throughout, with no significant changes in blood pressure. The infant was transferred by road ambulance to the PICU at the nearby cardiac center.

Progress in pediatric intensive care unit

On arrival at PICU, the cardiologist performed an echo which confirmed the diagnosis of HLHS with aortic atresia, and showed a widely patent arterial duct, and a non-restrictive atrial septal defect. The right ventricular function was normal, and there was mild tricuspid regurgitation.

Over the following 2 hours there was a worsening of the metabolic acidosis, with an arterial gas at 8 hours of age showing pH 7.19, pCO$_2$ 38 mmHg, pO$_2$ 52 mmHg, bicarbonate 15 mmol l^{-1}, BE –12. Lactate was 5.7 mmol l^{-1}. Further observations at the time were: oxygen saturation 92%, pulse rate 152 per minute, blood pressure 44/29 mmHg, mean 35. There was no urine output. A repeat echocardiogram at this time demonstrated moderate impairment of right ventricular function. The PICU physician was concerned that this instability was due to systemic hypoperfusion resulting from excessive pulmonary blood flow and ventricular dysfunction. A dobutamine infusion was therefore commenced at 5 mcg kg^{-1} per min, and nitrogen was added to the inspired gas to reduce FiO$_2$ to 0.19. Oxygen saturations subsequently fell to 80%, and 2 hours later the mean blood pressure was 40 mmHg, and the arterial gas had improved, with a lactate of 3.5. The infant remained stable, and at 12 hours of age, the lactic acidosis had completely resolved.

The following day, the infant had ultrasound examinations of his head and abdomen, which were normal, and was commenced on parenteral nutrition which was delivered via the umbilical line.

Stage I palliation was performed on day 4. Anesthesia was induced using the existing lines, deliberately avoiding the need for an internal jugular line. A modification of the Norwood procedure was performed, using a 5 mm conduit placed between the right ventricle and the pulmonary artery. No major complications occurred intra-operatively; however, the infant's chest was not closed at the end of surgery, according to the institutional protocol. The umbilical venous catheter was exchanged for a double-lumen direct atrial line, which was placed by the cardiac surgeon. A 4F optical catheter was also inserted into the right atrium, with its tip lying in the low SVC, for continuous measurement of mixed venous oxygen saturation. A Tenckhoff catheter was inserted to enable peritoneal dialysis to be started if required. The infant returned to the PICU on an infusion of dobutamine 10 mcg kg^{-1} per min, and sodium nitroprusside 0.5 mcg kg^{-1} per min.

The following observations were made on arrival in intensive care after surgery: central temperature 37.3 °C, heart rate 153, blood pressure 56/28 mmHg, mean 39, CVP 9 mmHg, systemic oxygen saturation 79%, mixed venous oxygen saturation 54%. The following ventilatory settings were used: pressures 23/5, rate 20 breaths per minute, inspiratory time 0.90 s, FiO$_2$ 0.35. An initial arterial blood gas showed pH 7.35, pCO$_2$ 41 mmHg, pO$_2$ 37 mmHg, BE −3.1 mmol l^{-1}, lactate 3.2 mmol l^{-1}, hemoglobin 14.1 g dl^{-1}, coagulation normal, sodium 139 mmol l^{-1}, potassium 5.5 mmol l^{-1}, ionized calcium 1.25 mmol l^{-1}, magnesium 1.12 mmol l^{-1}. Analgesia and anesthesia were continued after surgery using intravenous infusions of morphine (40 mcg kg^{-1} per h) and midazolam (1 mcg kg^{-1} per min); pancuronium (0.1 mg kg^{-1}) was given as required.

In view of the early hyperkalemia, in the context of a long operation with aortic cross-clamp, peritoneal dialysis was commenced 1 hour after arrival in PICU. Chest X-ray, 12-lead ECG and atrial electrogram showed no significant abnormalities. The patient was started on 50 ml kg^{-1} per day of total fluids. Chest drain losses were 2–3 ml kg^{-1} per h over the first 3 hours, then decreased. Heparin was started at 10 U kg^{-1} per h.

There was little change over the next 4 hours; however, after midnight, arterial gases showed a worsening lactic acidosis: pH 7.35, pCO$_2$ 41 mmHg, pO$_2$ 38 mmHg, BE −1.2, lactate 5.9 mmol l^{-1}, hemoglobin 11.8 g dl^{-1}. Systemic oxygen saturation was 75%, mixed venous oxygen saturation was 48%, and mean blood pressure was 44 mmHg. An echocardiogram was requested, which revealed mild right ventricular dysfunction with moderate tricuspid regurgitation. Two maneuvers were performed with the aim of improving systemic oxygen delivery. First, a blood transfusion was given (15 ml kg^{-1} packed cells over 2 hours), and a bolus of phenoxybenzamine (0.5 mg kg^{-1} over 1 hour). An arterial blood gas 4 hours later was somewhat better: pH 7.38, pCO$_2$ 40 mmHg, pO$_2$ 43 mmHg, BE −2.7, lactate 1.7 mmol l^{-1}. Hemoglobin had increased to 14.5 g dl^{-1}, and mixed venous saturation increased to 58%. Phenoxybenzamine was continued regularly thereafter.

On the first post-operative day, muscle relaxants were stopped, and sedation was reduced. The total fluid allowance was increased to 70 ml kg^{-1} per day, and TPN was re-commenced. 24 hours after surgery, urine output had started to improve. Diuresis was encouraged with intravenous frusemide (1 mg kg^{-1} 6-hourly), and this allowed cessation of peritoneal dialysis. On the second post-operative day, the infant's chest was closed. Inspiratory pressures were increased in anticipation of this procedure. Following chest closure, the intensivists were able to begin weaning ventilation. On the fourth post-operative day, enteral feeds were commenced, and captopril was introduced (0.1 mg kg^{-1} three times per day, with increasing doses thereafter). On day 6, the infant was extubated successfully. Dobutamine was weaned off over the next 24 hours, and the infant was transferred to the cardiology ward the following day.

Discussion

The primary goal of the peri-operative care of the neonate undergoing stage I palliation (Norwood operation or its modifications) is to optimize systemic oxygen delivery and organ perfusion. This is achieved using expert anticipatory care commencing before delivery, continuing postnatally in the neonatal unit, and subsequently after transfer to the cardiac center.

This case illustrates an infant in whom prenatal diagnosis allowed for a well-planned delivery, with appropriate communication between medical teams, prompt medical intervention, and early transfer to the cardiac unit. The infant did, however, encounter an episode of low systemic cardiac output before surgery, which was associated with pulmonary over-circulation and mild ventricular dysfunction. The post-operative course was complicated by an early episode of reduced systemic perfusion, due to a combination of factors: a relative anemia, myocardial dysfunction, and tricuspid regurgitation. This occurred at a time-point after surgery where a "nadir" of cardiac output is typically seen. These episodes of compromised systemic perfusion were promptly addressed, and appropriate investigations and interventions were performed. More significant sequelae were therefore avoided. The subsequent post-operative recovery was relatively slow but not unusual for this group of infants.

Diagnosis and immediate management

Prenatal diagnosis allows for more careful planning of delivery and immediate postnatal care of infants with HLHS. Prenatal diagnosis rates vary greatly between institutions, from around 35% to 70%.[1,2] Although the reported impact of prenatal diagnosis on overall survival is variable, prenatal diagnosis is associated with improved neurological outcome[1] and with a lower incidence of pre-operative acidosis and ventricular dysfunction requiring inotropic support.[3] These results reinforce the important contribution of early, focused management in these challenging infants.

In the absence of a prenatal diagnosis, babies with HLHS usually present with circulatory shock during the first days of life with severe acidosis, hypotension, and poor perfusion. There may be evidence of end-organ impairment, with acute tubular acidosis, necrotizing enterocolitis, liver failure, and cerebral ischemia.[4] These infants may also be hypoglycemic and coagulopathic. The presentation can be clinically indistinguishable from other causes of neonatal collapse including sepsis, inborn errors of metabolism, arrhythmias, and other causes of obstructed systemic circulation, e.g. critical aortic stenosis, severe aortic coarctation. A study that assessed the usefulness of clinical findings to distinguish between sepsis and an obstructed systemic circulation suggested that all clinical findings (including a murmur and weak pulses) either alone or in combination with other clinical findings, were not sensitive enough to allow a reliable differential diagnosis.[5] Given the insensitivity of clinical examination, echocardiography will be instrumental in guiding the differential diagnosis.

Ventricular dysfunction secondary to coronary ischemia and acidosis is common in these patients with HLHS without a prenatal diagnosis, and an inotrope such as dobutamine is often required. The subsequent prognosis will also depend on the degree to which end-organ failure caused by systemic hypoperfusion is recoverable.

The arterial duct is the main source of systemic blood flow, and provides retrograde filling to the aortic arch, diminutive ascending aorta, and coronary arteries. Prostaglandin E should be commenced in the delivery room, or in the absence of a prenatal diagnosis, as soon as the diagnosis is suspected.

Early survival in infants with HLHS also depends on a non-restrictive Atrial Septal Defect (ASD). An important minority of newborn infants with HLHS may have a restrictive ASD. This may have already been diagnosed on prenatal ultrasound examinations, in which case delivery should take place at a cardiac centre capable to urgently institute cardiopulmonary bypass. A restrictive ASD should also be suspected in the infant with HLHS, who rapidly develops profound hypoxemia and acidosis, unresponsive to usual measures such as mechanical ventilation, high inspired oxygen fractions, or nitric oxide. A chest X-ray typically shows severe pulmonary venous congestion.

These infants will die without urgent intervention,[6,7] and must be transferred without delay to the pediatric cardiac center, in order for urgent atrial decompression to be performed. Following relief of inter-atrial restriction by open surgical septectomy, or by the transcatheter route, a few days should be allowed before undergoing stage 1 palliation. This allows resolution of organ damage secondary to severe hypoxia, and for improvement in lung function.[8]

Optimizing systemic perfusion

The systemic, pulmonary, and coronary circulations of infants with HLHS run in parallel, and are all supplied by the right ventricle. The balance between pulmonary and systemic flow is critically important: an excess of one will compromise the other.[9] Systemic hypoperfusion in the pre-operative setting most commonly results from a circulatory imbalance in favour of the pulmonary circulation, with relative systemic vasoconstriction. This may also be associated with right ventricular dysfunction. The pulmonary blood flow of neonates is exquisitely sensitive to alveolar oxygen, carbon dioxide, and pH. The key to the management of systemic hypoperfusion is early recognition of disturbances of oxygen saturations and acid–base balance using blood gas analysis; and monitoring of ventricular function and competence of the tricuspid valve using echocardiography.

The pre-operative optimization of systemic perfusion in infants with HLHS can, to a great extent, be achieved by routinely avoiding factors that increase pulmonary flow such as excessive oxygen administration and respiratory alkalosis. In addition, there may be roles for early intervention using ventilatory strategies aimed at controlling pulmonary vascular resistance; for the careful use of systemic vasodilators; and, where appropriate, for the administration of inotropic agents.

Pre-operative mechanical ventilation is not mandatory in stable infants with HLHS. Indications for intubation are given below (Table 4.1): apnoeas or severe respiratory distress, worsening metabolic acidosis, pulmonary overcirculation *with* signs of systemic hypoperfusion, and significant myocardial dysfunction. Intubation can be associated with important morbidity in infants with HLHS, and should, where possible, be performed by senior clinicians, using appropriate anesthetic agents.[10] Acute distress, pain or agitation should be avoided as these can produce rapid elevations in systemic vascular resistance in infants with HLHS, resulting in important morbidity and mortality.[11]

A common, early sign of pulmonary overcirculation may be an increase in arterial oxygen saturation. Seemingly minor increases in oxygen saturation can reflect major elevations of pulmonary flow, at the expense of systemic perfusion.[12] If left untreated, the later manifestations of systemic hypoperfusion – diastolic hypotension, myocardial and other end-organ dysfunction – may result. Mesenteric ischemia leading to severe necrotizing enterocolitis,[13] and hypoxic-ischemic or hemorrhagic cerebral damage can ultimately preclude surgical intervention.

Table 4.1. *Indications for intubation of pre-operative infants with HLHS*

Apneas or severe respiratory distress
Worsening metabolic acidosis
Pulmonary overcirculation *with* signs of systemic hypoperfusion
Significant myocardial dysfunction

Table 4.2. *Guide to immediate respiratory management of infants prior to surgery for HLHS; if ventilated, use initially FiO₂ 0.21, PEEP 4–5 cm H₂O*

Target blood gases	
• $PaCO_2$	35–45 mmHg
• pH	7.35–7.40
• PaO_2	33–45 mmHg
• SaO_2 (systemic)	70–80%

Table 4.2 gives a guide to target blood gases in infants with HLHS. However, it must be remembered that elevated oxygen saturations in an otherwise stable, non-acidotic infant, are not necessarily an indication for escalation of medical therapy.

Pulmonary overcirculation with signs of systemic hypoperfusion in the pre-operative setting can be managed using ventilatory manipulations aimed at controlling the pulmonary vascular resistance. If necessary, hypoxic gas mixtures can be delivered by adding nitrogen to ventilator or ambient gases, resulting in inspired oxygen of less than 21%.[14] Arterial pCO_2 can be deliberately increased with the administration of additional carbon dioxide to ventilator gases.[15] In the only published clinical comparison of hypoxia (17%) and hypercarbia (FiCO₂ 2.7%), in infants with unoperated HLHS, both maneuvers similarly decreased the pulmonary blood flow and arterial oxygen saturation.[16] Interestingly, however, hypercarbia, but not hypoxia, increased the mixed venous and cerebral oxygen saturation, suggesting improved systemic oxygen delivery.

In infants after surgery, while it is still important to avoid pulmonary overcirculation, changing management strategies have lessened the need for active manipulation of the pulmonary vascular resistance. These strategies are first modifications of the stage I operation: the use of limiting Blalock–Taussig shunts in the classical Norwood circulation; the recent advent of the right ventricle-to-pulmonary artery conduit; and second, in the post-operative patient the more routine use of systemic vasodilators. Thus, intervention with additional ventilator gases (nitrogen or carbon dioxide) is very rarely, if ever, required post-operatively.

Inotropes and vasodilators can help optimize systemic oxygen delivery in infants with HLHS. Inotropes can be beneficial in some infants prior to surgery: in particular, those with a metabolic acidosis, and those with coronary ischemia secondary to pulmonary overcirculation are at particular risk of developing early right ventricular dysfunction. In this situation, a low-dose infusion of an inotrope such as dobutamine (5–10 mcg kg^{-1} per min) may be useful. The majority of patients after stage I palliation will require inotropes to maintain cardiac contractility in the early post-operative period. Dobutamine and dopamine are both appropriate for this role, though the additional vasodilatation afforded by dobutamine would make this the drug of choice for many clinicians.

Intravenous vasodilators produce systemic vasodilatation and therefore can directly improve systemic perfusion in infants with HLHS. Also, through their beneficial effects on ventricular afterload, vasodilators can be especially useful in management of infants with ventricular dysfunction, and tricuspid regurgitation.

Two main classes of intravenous vasodilators are commonly used in infants with HLHS. Sodium nitroprusside, a nitrovasodilator, has a rapid onset of action, with the advantage of a relatively titratable dose-dependent effect, and a short half-life.[4] Phenoxybenzamine, an α-adrenergic receptor blocker, reduces Qp:Qs and improves systemic oxygen delivery, and has even been associated with increased survival in infants with HLHS.[17–20] Interestingly, higher levels of arterial oxygen are much better tolerated in the presence of aggressive afterload reduction.[21,22] Systemic vasodilators should always be used carefully in order to avoid excessive hypotension, which can, to an extent, be avoided if the intravascular volume status is adequate. Once enteral feeds have been established, an oral vasodilator such as captopril can be introduced.

The important contribution of hemoglobin to systemic oxygen delivery should always be remembered. In the infant with HLHS, where systemic saturation is relatively low, hemoglobin should be maintained around $14–16\,g\,dl^{-1}$ to maximize tissue oxygen delivery.

The adequacy of systemic oxygen delivery, which is so critical, and so variable, is paradoxically difficult to assess. An increasing or persistent metabolic acidosis, or an elevated serum lactate may confirm that perfusion is under threat or already compromised. These parameters are not continuously monitored, and therefore give only periodic information. Mixed venous oxygen saturation provides a useful, continuous surrogate measure of adequacy of systemic oxygen delivery in the functionally univentricular circulation,[23] and can be used to guide therapy with systemic vasodilators.[17,18]

In some centers, mixed venous saturation is continuously monitored after stage I palliation using a co-oximeter placed at the time of surgery.[19] Although the absolute numbers obtained by this method are not always accurate, the trend in data generated by a well-positioned co-oximeter can be useful, with subtle changes potentially preceding changes in other parameters. A fall in saturation would suggest increased tissue oxygen extraction, and impaired oxygen delivery[24] and should stimulate us to search for a cause.[18]

Surgical options and considerations for HLHS

Staged surgical palliation for HLHS remains the mainstay of treatment and begins with the Norwood operation, or one of its modifications. Stage I palliation is ideally performed at around day 4 of life, or a few days later in the infant presenting with a restrictive ASD. The aim of stage I palliation is to enlarge the aorta and to establish its continuity with the right ventricle; to provide free mixing of the pulmonary and systemic venous blood through an atrial septectomy; and to provide the lungs with forward flow.

Until recently, the only way to achieve forward flow to the lungs was via a modified Blalock–Taussig (BT) shunt. More recently, the so-called "Sano" modification has been introduced and is increasingly used in cardiac surgical units around the world. This approach involves the placement of a small (4–6 mm) conduit between the right ventricle and pulmonary artery, in place of a BT shunt.[25,26] The conduit offers the potential advantage of maintenance of diastolic coronary perfusion, avoiding the unwanted diastolic "run-off" associated with a BT shunt, leading to preservation of myocardial function in patients with a conduit. This hypothesis is supported by a number of observational studies which have reported a higher diastolic pressure in patients with a conduit;[26-29] echocardiographic data demonstrating that infants with conduit palliation have no diastolic flow reversal in the aortic arch; and tissue Doppler data and catheterization data suggest improved ventricular performance after the conduit operation.[29,30]

Early clinical data on the newer surgical approach are also encouraging. Retrospective series from a number of centers report improved early post-operative physiology with a smoother clinical course[31,32] and even improved survival[27] in infants with a conduit rather than a BT shunt. Active manipulation of pulmonary blood flow (beyond standard measures) is also rarely necessary with this modification.[25]

In some centers, the option of heart transplantation in early infancy is offered as an alternative to stage I palliation. Centers routinely performing transplantation have previously reported impressive early survival figures which would favor this option over stage I palliation.[33] For the single reason of limited donor organ supply, primary transplantation is not a realistic option in most institutions outside North America. If available, transplantation is not an easy option either. Most infants awaiting transplantation require long-term therapy with prostaglandin and may need repeated septal decompressions, and potentially other extracardiac procedures. Also, transplantation introduces a new set of considerations: the need for lifelong immune suppression, the accelerated onset of coronary artery disease, and the unknown question of the long-term viability of a neonatal donor heart. Moreover, with improving survival rates for staged palliation, the relative benefits of heart transplantation have narrowed over the past decade. Thus, a study from the US, of 2264 infants diagnosed with HLHS, demonstrated a reduction in the proportion being transplanted during the last decade.[34]

Extra-Corporeal Life Support (ECLS) has been used to support many children with refractory cardiopulmonary dysfunction after surgery for congenital heart disease, with a hospital survival of around 40%. Historically, the survival for the subgroup requiring ECLS after stage 1 palliation for HLHS has been much lower, at less than 30%. In fact many centers, until very recently, considered HLHS to be a relative contraindication for ECLS. However, it is becoming increasingly recognized that the period of myocardial "rest," and optimal systemic perfusion afforded by ECLS may have advantages over high-dose inotrope therapy in borderline patients. In some centers this approach is becoming much more routine, with very encouraging outcomes.[35] Therefore, although carrying a significant risk, ECLS can, if initiated promptly, improve the outcome in infants with impaired cardiopulmonary function after stage 1 palliation.[36]

Infants with HLHS require central venous access during the peri-operative period. Ideally, umbilical venous access will be secured early after delivery; and this reliable form of access can be used for drug infusions and parenteral nutrition before surgery. Line-related venous thrombosis is a well-recognized complication of central venous catheters, and this can have important consequences in infants with HLHS. In particular, thrombosis of the superior caval vein can result in the development of chylothorax; and may also preclude further staged palliation. For this reason, many cardiac units have now moved away from placing internal jugular central venous catheters at the time of surgery, in favor of direct atrial lines, with subsequent removal of umbilical venous catheters. Although there is little evidence base in the current literature, it would be worth considering the routine use of low-dose intravenous heparin in infants with HLHS who have central venous lines.

In summary, survival of patients with hypoplastic left heart syndrome has improved dramatically over the last 20 years, with many centers now quoting a survival after stage I palliation of over 75%.[1,5,22,37] However, mortality for these infants remains higher than for other congenital heart defects requiring surgical intervention in the neonatal period. Three main reasons for this have been identified: pre-operative instability, mainly caused by inadequate systemic oxygen delivery, mortality following stage I palliation and out-of-hospital mortality whilst waiting for stage II palliation.[38] Pre-emptive management aimed at optimizing systemic perfusion in the pre- and post-operative phase and refinement of surgical techniques should help to further narrow the gap in prognosis between babies with HLHS and other infants with congenital heart disease.

Learning points

- Secure venous access should be obtained immediately after delivery.
- The circulation of infants with HLHS is critically dependent on a patent arterial duct. Prostaglandin E should be started as soon as possible after delivery.
- A restrictive ASD should be suspected in infants with suspected HLHS who do not respond to early resuscitation with prostaglandin, ventilation, and inspired oxygen.
- HLHS patients with restrictive ASD require urgent intervention (surgical septectomy or transcatheter approach). If diagnosed antenatally, delivery should take place in or near a center capable to perform these interventions.
- The main goal of peri-operative intensive care of infants with HLHS is to optimize systemic perfusion, while avoiding pulmonary overcirculation.
- Routine pre-operative management should be aimed at avoiding factors which increase pulmonary flow.
- Pulmonary blood flow can be limited with the use of hypoxic gas mixtures or additional carbon dioxide in the pre-operative phase.
- Systemic flow in the pre- and post-operative periods can be optimized with the careful use of intravenous vasodilators.
- A lower arterial pressure in the infant who is systemically vasodilated is preferable to systemic hypertension with systemic vasoconstriction.
- Careful monitoring of blood gases, acid–base balance, lactate, and surrogate markers of systemic blood flow and echocardiography should be used to guide medical interventions.
- Early data suggests that the RV–PA conduit may offer the advantage of a less complicated post-operative course, and possibly improved early survival.
- ECLS, if initiated promptly, can improve outcome in HLHS patients with significantly impaired cardiopulmonary function after stage I palliation.
- Pre-emptive management, early investigation, and early intervention, are crucial aspects of the intensive care of these infants.

References

1. Mahle WT, Clancy RR, McGaurn SP, Goin JE, Clark BJ. Impact of prenatal diagnosis on survival and early neurologic morbidity in neonates with the hypoplastic left heart syndrome. *Pediatrics* 2001; **107**: 1277–82.

2. Bull C. Current and potential impact of fetal diagnosis on prevalence and spectrum of

serious congenital heart disease at term in the UK. *Lancet* 1999; **354**: 1242–7.

3. Tworetzky W, McElhinney DB, Reddy VM, Brook MM, Hanley FL, Silverman NH. Improved surgical outcome after fetal diagnosis of hypoplastic left heart syndrome. *Circulation* 2001; **103**: 1269–73.

4. Norwood WI, Jr. Hypoplastic left heart syndrome. *Ann Thorac Surg* 1991; **52**: 688–95.

5. Pickert CB, Moss MM, Fiser DH. Differentiation of systemic infection and congenital obstructive left heart disease in the very young infant. *Emerg Care* 1998; **14**: 263–7.

6. Bove EL, Lloyd TR. Staged reconstruction for hypoplastic left heart syndrome. Contemporary results. *Ann Surg* 1996; **224**: 387–95.

7. Canter CE, Moorehead S, Huddleston CB, Spray TL. Restrictive atrial septal communication as a determinant of outcome of cardiac transplantation for hypoplastic left heart syndrome. *Circulation* 1993; **88**(5 Pt 2): II456–60.

8. Atz AM, Feinstein JA, Jonas RA, Perry SB, Wessel DL. Preoperative management of pulmonary venous hypertension in hypoplastic left heart syndrome with restrictive atrial septal defect. *Am J Cardiol* 1999; **83**: 1224–8.

9. Lawrenson J, Eyskens B, Vlasselaers D, Gewillig M. Manipulating parallel circuits: the perioperative management of patients with complex congenital cardiac disease. *Cardiol Young* 2003; **13**: 316–22.

10. Nicolson SC, Jobes DR. Hypoplastic left heart syndrome. In: Lake CL ed. *Pediatric Cardiac Anesthesia*. Norwalk, Connecticut, Appleton & Lange, 1993.

11. Wright GE, Crowley DC, Charpie JR, Ohye RG, Bove EL, Kulik TJ. High vascular resistance and sudden cardiovascular collapse in Norwood patients. *Ann Thorac Surg* 2004; **77**: 48–52.

12. Barnea O, Santamore WP, Rossi A, Salloum E, Chien S, Austin EH. Estimation of oxygen delivery in newborns with a univentricular circulation. *Circulation* 1998; **98**: 1407–13.

13. McElhinney DB, Hedrick HL, Bush DM *et al.* Necrotizing enterocolitis in neonates with congenital heart disease: risk factors and outcomes. *Pediatrics* 2000; **106**: 1080–7.

14. Shime N, Hashimoto S, Hiramatsu N, Oka T, Kageyama K, Tanaka Y. Hypoxic gas therapy using nitrogen in the preoperative management of neonates with hypoplastic left heart syndrome. *Pediatr Crit Care Med* 2000; **1**: 38–41.

15. Jobes DR, Nicolson SC, Steven JM, Miller M, Jacobs ML, Norwood WI, Jr. Carbon dioxide prevents pulmonary overcirculation in hypoplastic left heart syndrome. *Ann Thorac Surg* 1992; **54**: 150–1.

16. Tabbutt S, Ramamoorthy C, Montenegro LM *et al.* Impact of inspired gas mixtures on preoperative infants with hypoplastic left heart syndrome during controlled ventilation. *Circulation* 2001; **104**(12 Suppl 1): I159–64.

17. Tweddell JS, Hoffman GM, Fedderly RT *et al.* Phenoxybenzamine improves systemic oxygen delivery after the Norwood procedure. *Ann Thorac Surg* 1999: **67**: 161–7.

18. Tweddell JS, Hoffman GM, Mussatto KA *et al.* Improved survival of patients undergoing palliation of hypoplastic left heart syndrome: lessons learned from 115 consecutive patients. *Circulation* 2002; **106** (12 Suppl 1): I82–9.

19. Tweddell JS, Hoffman GM, Fedderly RT, *et al.* Patients at risk for low systemic oxygen delivery after the Norwood procedure. *Ann Thorac Surg* 2000; **69**: 1893–9.

20. Poirier NC, Drummond-Webb JJ, Hisamochi K, Imamura M, Harrison AM, Mee RB. Modified Norwood procedure with a high-flow cardiopulmonary bypass strategy results in low mortality without late arch obstruction. *J Thorac Cardiovasc Surg* 2000; **120**: 875–84.

21. Hoffman GM, Tweddell JS, Ghanayem NS *et al.* Alteration of the critical arteriovenous oxygen saturation relationship by sustained afterload reduction after the Norwood procedure. *J Thorac Cardiovasc Surg* 2004; **127**: 738–45.

22. Bradley SM, Atz AM, Simsic JM. Redefining the impact of oxygen and hyperventilation after the Norwood procedure. *J Thorac Cardiovasc Surg* 2004; **127**: 473–80.

23. Francis DP, Willson K, Thorne SA, Davies LC, Coats AJ. Oxygenation in patients with a functionally univentricular circulation and complete mixing of blood: are saturation and

flow interchangeable? *Circulation* 1999; **100**: 2198–203.

24. Hoffman GM, Ghanayem NS, Kampine JM *et al.* Venous saturation and the anaerobic threshold in neonates after the Norwood procedure for hypoplastic left heart syndrome. *Ann Thorac Surg* 2000; **70**: 1515–21.

25. Imoto Y, Kado H, Shiokawa Y, Minami K, Yasui H. Experience with the Norwood procedure without circulatory arrest. *J Thorac Cardiovasc Surg* 2001; **122**: 879–82.

26. Sano S, Ishino K, Kawada M *et al.* Right ventriclepulmonary artery shunt in first-stage palliation of hypoplastic left heart syndrome. *J Thorac Cardiovasc Surg* 2003; **126**: 504–9; discussion 509–10.

27. Pizarro C, Malec E, Maher KO *et al.* Right ventricle to pulmonary artery conduit improves outcome after stage I Norwood for hypoplastic left heart syndrome. *Circulation* 2003; **108**(Suppl 1): II155–60.

28. Maher KO, Pizarro C, Gidding SS *et al.* Hemodynamic profile after the Norwood procedure with right ventricle to pulmonary artery conduit. *Circulation* 2003; **108**: 782–4.

29. Mair R, Tulzer G, Sames E *et al.* Right ventricular to pulmonary artery conduit instead of modified Blalock–Taussig shunt improves postoperative hemodynamics in newborns after the Norwood operation. *J Thorac Cardiovasc Surg* 2003; **126**: 1378–84.

30. Hughes ML, Shekerdemian LS, Brizard CP, Penny DJ. Improved early ventricular performance with a right ventricle to pulmonary artery conduit in stage1 palliation for hypoplastic left heart syndrome: evidence from strain Doppler echocardiography. *Heart* 2004; **90**: 191–4.

31. Malec E, Januszewska K, Kolcz J, Mroczek T. Right ventricle-to-pulmonary artery shunt versus modified Blalock-Taussig shunt in the Norwood procedure for hypoplastic left heart syndrome – influence on early and late haemodynamic status. *Eur J Cardiothorac Surg* 2003; **23**: 728–34.

32. Pizarro C, Norwood WI. Right ventricle to pulmonary artery conduit has a favorable impact on postoperative physiology after Stage I Norwood: preliminary results. *Eur J Cardiothorac Surg* 2003; **23**: 991–5.

33. Jenkins PC, Flanagan MF, Jenkins KJ *et al.* Survival analysis and risk factors for mortality in transplantation and staged surgery for hypoplastic left heart syndrome. *J Am Coll Cardiol* 2000; **36**: 1178–85.

34. Gutgesell HP, Gibson J. Management of hypoplastic left heart syndrome in the 1990s. *Am J Cardiol* 2002; **89**: 842–6.

35. Ungerleider RM, Shen I, Yeh T *et al.* Routine mechanical ventricular assist following the Norwood procedure – improved neurologic outcome and excellent hospital survival. *Ann Thorac Surg* 2004; **77**: 18–22.

36. Pizarro C, Davis DA, Healy RM, Kerins PJ, Norwood WI. Is there a role for extracorporeal life support after stage I Norwood? *Eur J Cardiothorac Surg* 2001; **19**: 294–301.

37. Azakie T, Merklinger SL, McCrindle BW *et al.* Evolving strategies and improving outcomes of the modified norwood procedure: a 10-year single-institution experience. *Ann Thorac Surg* 2001; **72**: 1349–53.

38. Theilen U, Shekerdemian, L. The intensive care of infants with hypoplastic left heart syndrome. *Arch Dis Child* 2005; **90**: F97–F102.

Child with a head injury

Lisa Dyke and Peter Skippen

Introduction

In developed countries, head injury is the leading cause of death in children over 1 year of age. The goal of therapy in managing head injury is to prevent secondary injury and mitigate the cascade of events resulting in the delayed primary insult. The systemic secondary insults that have the most impact on outcome are hypotension and hypoxia, and their identification and prevention is the priority in the management of head injury.

Case history

A 5-year-old, previously healthy boy fell through the screen of a second-floor window on to concrete below. There was no initial loss of consciousness.

On arrival in the Emergency Room, he was drowsy but responsive to voice and moving all limbs purposefully and to command. Cervical spine immobilization was undertaken with an appropriately sized semi-rigid collar. His initial vital signs were respiratory rate of $24\,min^{-1}$, oxygen saturations of 96% in air, a heart rate of $76\,min^{-1}$, a blood pressure of $114/60\,mmHg$, and a GCS score of 14 (E3/V5/M6). Oxygen was administered, IV access obtained and blood sent for routine trauma panel (FBC, blood group and screen, urea and electrolytes, creatinine, glucose, liver function tests, and also serum amylase). The initial chest x-ray and cervical spine plain films were normal. The secondary survey failed to identify other significant injuries.

Approximately 60 minutes after his arrival to the hospital, the child became unresponsive with dilating sluggish pupils bilaterally. He was intubated with a size 5 cuffed oral endotracheal tube (ETT) using a rapid sequence technique. End tidal CO_2 confirmed correct ETT position. An orogastric tube was also inserted. He was placed on a transport ventilator (respiratory rate 25, tidal volume 8mls/kg, $5\,cmH_2O$ positive end expiratory pressure) and taken immediately to the Radiology Department for an urgent head CT. Hyperventilation was initiated as a rescue maneuver until a diagnosis was made. He was given $1\,g\,kg^{-1}$ mannitol during the transfer to the CT scanner. The CT scan of the head showed a skull fracture near the vault, effaced basal cisterns, evidence of diffuse axonal injury, and blood in the subarachnoid, subdural, and epidural spaces. An abdominal and pelvic CT scans was normal.

The tertiary center was contacted and management discussed. The CT scans were viewed remotely by the neurosurgeons via Picture Archival Communication System (PACS) who advised that there was no acute surgical lesion, Arrangements were made for urgent transport to the tertiary centre. The goal of management during the transfer was to support a normal for age cerebral perfusion pressure, and normalize ventilation.

Prior to transfer, the pupils had become briskly reactive. The child remained paralysed and sedated with morphine and midazolam infusions. Vital signs included arterial saturation of 98%

Case Studies in Pediatric Critical Care, ed. Peter. J. Murphy, Stephen C. Marriage, and Peter J. Davis. Published by Cambridge University Press. © Cambridge University Press 2009.

on FIO_2 0.5, MAP 75 mmHg and an $ETCO_2$ of 35 mmHg, Anticipating problems with raised intracranial pressure during the interhospital transfer, the transport team took extra mannitol, isotonoic fluids for resuscitation and a dopamine infusion for fluid unresponsive hypotension.

Progress in pediatric intensive care unit

Upon arrival at the tertiary hospital, he was taken immediately for a repeat head CT (Fig. 5.1) and xenon cerebral blood flow scan. The basal cisterns were now present. The xenon study demonstrated generous cerebral blood flow values for age ranging between 45 and 80 ml 100 g^{-1} per min with no regions of ischemia or oligemia. The child was then taken to the operating room for placement of a right frontal External Ventricular Drain (EVD). On return to the ICU, his initial ICP was 25 mmHg. He was managed according to the PICU standard head injury protocol (Table 5.1). A femoral central venous catheter was placed. He remained on infusions of midazolam and morphine at 200 and 40 mcg kg^{-1} per h, respectively and paralyzed intermittently with rocuronium as required ICP spikes or for fighting the ventilator or coughing and suctioning. An EEG was also arranged on the day of admission to exclude subclinical seizure activity. Full enteral feeds were established by day 2.

Table 5.1. *Routine therapy for children with head injury and GCS < 8*

Head in neutral position, with head of bed elevated 30 degrees
Normovolemia
Isotonic solutions for intravascular volume support (0.9% NS)
Normotension (age-related norms)
Normocarbia: $PaCO_2$ 35–40 mmHg
Normothermia: 36–36.5 °C
Requires cooling blanket for all patients
Do not cool to <36 °C
Sedation with morphine and midazolam infusions
Arterial line for blood pressure monitoring
ICP monitor – preferably EVD
EVD transducer positioned 20 cm above the tragus
Set both transducers for ICP and arterial line at the level of the tragus and calculate CPP
Target CPP >40 mmHg for children <10 years of age
Use vasopressor infusions to maintain BP: noradrenaline (norepinephrine)
Maintain ICP <20 mmHg
Fluids at 80% maintenance (maintain normovolemia)
Normal serum electrolytes: Serum sodium 140–150 mmol l^{-1} with hypertonic saline
Avoid free water infusions and rapid changes in serum sodium levels
Routine bloodwork: electrolytes and blood gases every 6 hours for the initial 48 hours
Commence enteral feeding within the first 24 hours
Repeat head CT routinely after 24–48 hours

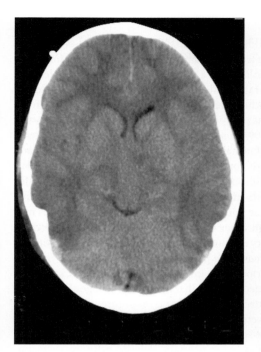

Fig. 5.1. CT scan of head showing decreased attenuation within the cortex consistent with diffuse axonal injury. A right frontal EVD has been placed.

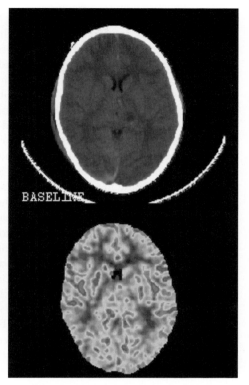

Fig. 5.2. CT scan of head and Xenon perfusion study demonstrating average cerebral blood flows in the range of 50–70 ml/100 g per min. No areas of ischemia or oligemia could be identified (see color plate section).

His ICU course was complicated by refractory raised ICP greater than 25 mmHg and seizure-like activity, despite the midazolam infusion and therapeutic phenytoin levels. Despite adequate volume resuscitation using normal saline targeting a CVP of 8–10 mmHg, an infusion of norepinephrine at 0.1. μg kg^{-1} per min was required to maintain a CPP > 40 with a MAP > 60. Normothermia was maintained and mannitol and 3% hypertonic saline were given intermittently for spikes in ICP greater than 30 mmHg.

A jugular venous bulb monitor was placed on day 2 because of ongoing spikes in ICP. The initial jugular venous saturations (SjO$_2$) as 70% giving an extraction ratio of 30%. This in combination with the initial xenon study demonstrating generous cerebral blood flow prompted careful hyperventilation, PCO$_2$'s in the low 30's. The ICP responded well to this approach, and the patient required far fewer doses of hypertonic therapies over the following 48 hours. A repeat CT scan as well as a xenon study were performed on day 4 (Fig. 5.2). The repeat CT scan demonstrated hypodense regions in the left frontal and thalamic regions. The xenon study still demonstrated generous CBF similar to the initial study despite the mild hyperventilation.

Eventually, the ICP normalized by day, sedation was weared and the child allowed to awaken. The child was extubated on day 6 and transferred to the ward for rehabilitation with ongoing right-sided weakness and an improving right facial palsy.

Discussion

Head injury differs considerably between children and adults. Diffuse cerebral swelling, as seen in this case, occurs two to five times more frequently in children than in adults following severe head trauma. On the other hand, adults have a higher incidence of mass lesions, including hemorrhagic contusions and subdural hematomas, when compared with children. In children with intracranial mass lesions, subdural hematomas occur more frequently in the younger age groups while epidural hematomas peak in incidence between 15 and 30 years of age, occurring in 5% of all head injuries and 9% of severe head injuries in this age range.[1]

Motor vehicle-related accidents account for the majority of head injuries in both children and adults. Pedestrian accidents and falls are more common in the pediatric population. Non-accidental trauma to infants and toddlers is a serious and common problem, accounting for up to one-third of head injuries admitted to pediatric intensive care units. In infants less than 1 year of age with head injuries, two-thirds of these injuries and 95% of serious head injuries may be non-accidental.[1] Clinicians must have a high index of suspicion when an infant or toddler presents with a head injury without a clear history of trauma. The most common CT scan finding is an acute interhemispheric subdural hematoma in the parietooccipital region. Other findings on CT scan include subdural hematomas of various ages, intracerebral hemorrhages, subarachnoid hemorrhages and diffuse swelling. Associated findings that are strongly suggestive of abuse are multiple skull fractures, bilateral skull fractures, fractures that cross suture lines, and retinal hemorrhages. In the past retinal hemorrhages were felt to be pathognomonic for abuse, however recent studies have shown that they may not be specific for non-accidental head trauma.[2]

Traumatic Brain Injury (TBI) is classified as either primary, delayed primary, or secondary. Primary brain injury is the damage that occurs at the moment of impact. Delayed primary injury is the biochemical and cellular response to the initial mechanical trauma, which can exacerbate the primary injury, resulting in loss of tissue not initially damaged. Secondary brain injury occurs sometime after the initial insult as a result of impaired substrate delivery (hypoxia, hypoglycemia) resulting from impaired perfusion (ischemia, hypotension) or maladaptive cellular responses to brain injury.

Severe TBI is defined by a GCS score less than or equal to 8, and guidelines for its management in infants, children and adolescents have been formulated. These are based upon expert opinion and the best available evidence.[3,4] Unfortunately, there are no high-level evidence studies (e.g. randomized controlled studies) and few studies specifically pertaining to pediatric patients.

The mainstay of managing any patient with a TBI is optimizing cerebral oxygen delivery. In the healthy child, cerebral metabolic activity is the main determinant of cerebral blood flow, and therefore oxygen delivery. Following a TBI, there are major time dependent perturbations in cerebral blood flow and oxygen delivery that are poorly understood, but maintaining cerebral perfusion pressure, controlling carbon dioxide levels and avoidance of hypoxia are all felt to be important.

Initial assessment and management in the emergency department

Initial resuscitative efforts in the emergency department, and ongoing critical care support, are aimed at the prevention and treatment of conditions likely to contribute to a secondary brain injury (Table 5.2). At the same time, the diagnosis and resuscitation of life-threatening injuries and the timely diagnosis of intracranial lesions are a priority.

Hypotension, hypovolemia, and/or hypoxia need to be identified and corrected as rapidly as possible. This can be achieved by following the standard *Airway, Breathing* and *Circulation*

Table 5.2. *Factors affecting outcome following head injury*

Severity of initial insult including GCS at scene
Type of injury
Post-resuscitation GCS
Associated injuries
Extremes of age
Secondary injuries:
Hypotension
Hypoxia
Hyperthermia
Elevated ICP
Seizures
Hypercapnea
Unknown
? Genetic

Table 5.3. *Indications for endotracheal intubation in children with head injury*

GCS ≤8
Acute increase in ICP needing hyperventilation
Hypoxia
Hypercarbia
Inability to protect airway
Severe thoracic or airway trauma
Prior to transport of patient
Combative patients prior to CT scan

approach. All children should receive 100% supplemental oxygen and bag and mask assisted ventilation as necessary. Apnea at the scene of the accident suggests a high spinal cord injury requiring further investigation. An unresponsive child with hypoventilation should be urgently intubated. Further indications for endotracheal intubation are listed in Table 5.3. Rapid sequence intubation should be used in most cases with cervical spine precautions maintained at all times. Combative patients requiring diagnostic imaging should have their airway secured and ventilation supported under general anesthesia prior to imaging. Once the airway is controlled, ventilatory management should initially be aimed at normoxia and normocarbia, monitored continuously by pulse oximetry and end-tidal CO_2 monitoring, respectively, and by serial blood gas measurement.

Immediate attention to hypovolemia and hypotension is paramount as some studies suggest that hypotension triples the mortality in pediatric brain injuries.[5] Maintenance of a normal for age mean arterial pressure is the goal in the ED. Peripheral vascular access can be difficult to obtain in children during the initial resuscitation, and intraosseous infusion of fluids and medications is indicated after two failed attempts at peripheral venous access. Isotonic crystalloid

Table 5.4. *Glasgow Coma Scale (GCS) Score*[7]

Infants	Children < 4 yr	Ages 4–15 yrs
Eye opening		
4 Spontaneous	Spontaneous	Spontaneously
3 To speech	To speech	To verbal command
2 To pain	To pain	To pain
1 No response	None	None
Verbal response		
5 Coos, babbles	Oriented – social, smiles, follows objects, converses	Oriented
4 Irritable cry	Confused, disoriented, aware of environment, consolable cries	Disoriented
3 Cries to pain	Inappropriate words, inconsolable, persistent cries	Inappropriate words
2 Moans to pain	Incomprehensible sounds, agitated, restless, inconsolable	Incomprehensible
1 No response	No response	No response
Motor response		
6 Normal spontaneous movements	Normal spontaneous movements	Obeys verbal commands
5 Withdraws to touch	Localizes pain	Localizes to painful stimuli
4 Withdraws to pain	Withdraws to pain	Withdrawal
3 Abnormal flexion	Abnormal flexion	Abnormal flexion (decorticate)
2 Abnormal extension	Abnormal extension	Extension (decerebrate)
1 No response	No response	No response

solutions are the fluids of choice (0.9% normal saline) during acute resuscitation. Free water and glucose solutions should be avoided unless hypoglycemia is demonstrated on a blood sample.

Blood pressure should be monitored in the ER every 5 minutes; however, it is important to remember that pediatric patients maintain their blood pressure despite significant hypovolemia. Shock is a late sign of hypovolemia. Clinical signs such as unexplained tachycardia and poor pulse volume indicate the need for volume resuscitation.[6] Vasopressors should not be used in the initial phase of resuscitation. If fluids alone are insufficient to maintain the patient's blood pressure or tachycardia persists, consider ongoing hemorrhage or spinal cord injury. Infants and small children can become hypovolemic from a scalp laceration due to their small circulatory blood volume.

Fluid restriction in the acute phases of resuscitation is never indicated in children with a closed head injury. Problems with salt and water balance do not occur acutely in the setting of head trauma unless free water is inadvertently administered.

The initial neurological status can be evaluated using the GCS score (Table 5.4) but then must include an ongoing assessment of the level of consciousness, pupillary size and reactivity, tone and symmetry, and regular reassessment of the GCS score.

Once the life-threatening injuries have been addressed, the secondary survey should be completed to identify all injuries and initiate their management. A complete head-to-toe examination, including front and back, is performed. The ears and nose should be inspected for signs of basilar skull fracture including hemotympanum and cerebral spinal fluid leak. Step-off deformities of the cervical and thoracolumbar spine should also be noted. Clearance of the cervical spine in the unconscious patient remains controversial and therefore immobilization should be maintained in the emergency department. Pediatric cervical spine injuries are different, and adult-specific guidelines[8] do not provide guidance for cervical spine clearance of the child with TBI.

In addition to consulting neurosurgery, the trauma team (if available at your centre) or at minimum general surgery should be consulted for all children with severe TBI, as multiple injuries are common.

Essential investigations include a complete blood count, blood glucose, serum electrolytes, group and screen, crossmatch, and coagulation profile. Liver enzymes are included in the multitrauma patient. Chest, cervical spine and pelvic X-rays are routinely obtained. Once the head CT (and abdominal CT in the multitrauma victim) has been completed, the child is transferred either to the operating room for any urgent surgical procedures, or to the PICU for stabilization and ongoing cerebral resuscitation. Specialized imaging of the vertebral column should be guided by the clinical examination and findings on routine plain radiology.

Transportation of the child with traumatic brain injury

Communication and transfer of relevant information between the referring centre, the transport physician or team and the tertiary centre is critical during the transport of a child with a TBI and improves patient outcome.

The basic approach of our transport team is to take our PICU to the patient. This approach developed because of the large distances and times required for some of our transports to the more remote areas of our country. The transport team maintains close communication with the PICU physician at all times. The use of telemedicine lends itself well to assessing and the support of critically ill children when large distances are involved, as they are in Canada and Australia. The recent introduction of PACS for radiology has made possible the rapid exchange of images that facilitate early and accurate diagnosis of intracranial lesions and allow more timely interventions and advice for the referring physician and transport team.

All patients with severe TBI require stabilization prior to transport. In certain situations particularly those involving short transport distances, such as a rapidly expanding intracranial lesion, more expeditious referral for life-saving surgery may be indicated, such as occurred in this case. A study in the UK demonstrated that the use of specialist pediatric transfer teams actually delayed rather than expedited the emergency transportation of the child to the neurosurgical service.[9] Transfer by the referring team still involves control of the airway and ventilation prior to transport. Patients should be monitored during transport using oximetry, $ETCO_2$, as well as ECG and BP monitoring. Exclusion of other life-threatening injuries prior to transport is essential (e.g. pneumothorax requiring chest drainage).

Intensive care management

Once the child is admitted to the PICU following the necessary diagnostic investigations and any urgent surgical procedures, an individualized neuroprotective strategy is applied. Controversy remains regarding many of the therapies applied to any patient with a TBI, as

Table 5.5. *Stepwise approach to the treatment of acute rises in ICP*

Step 1	Ensure the airway is secured, ventilation is appropriate, the blood pressure is in the normal range, the patient is not hyperthermic and not having a seizure.
Step 2	CSF drainage
	If a ventricular drain is in place it can be opened and allowed to drain for 5 minutes. In some patients it may be necessary to leave the drain open continuously. If this occurs it is important to turn the 3-way stopcock every 10–15 minutes to record the actual ICP. The role of CSF drainage is to reduce the intracranial fluid volume, thereby lowering ICP.
Step 3	Mannitol
	If opening the EVD fails to lower the ICP because the CSF isn't draining, administer mannitol 0.25–1 g kg^{-1}. Maintain normovolemia at all times, and follow electrolytes closely. Discontinue mannitol if hypernatremia develops.
Step 4	Hypertonic saline
	If the patient is hyponatremic (sodium <135 mmol l^{-1}), hypertonic saline should be considered as an alternative to mannitol (1–5 ml kg^{-1} 3% saline infused over 10–20 minutes). Avoid large changes in serum sodium and maintain serum osmolality <310 mmol l^{-1}
Step 5	Hyperventilation to PaCO$_2$ 30–35 mmHg only during acute resuscitation for raised intracranial pressure, or guided by JVB and cerebral flow studies.

there are no studies that clearly identify the best approach. We recommend following a standard protocol for the basic management and have included the protocol currently followed in the Pediatric Intensive Care Unit at British Columbia's Children's Hospital in Table 5.1.

The generally accepted PICU management involves maintaining normoxia, normocarbia, normovolemia, and normothermia. Cervical spine precautions should be continued until clearance is confirmed and documented in the chart by an expert in the field.

In the case of an acute neurological deterioration without an ICP monitor in place, the patient should be hyperventilated with 100% oxygen, given 1 g kg^{-1} mannitol over 20 minutes, the neurosurgeon and pediatric intensivist should be notified, and arrangements made for an urgent CT scan of the head. If an ICP monitor is in place, acute elevations in ICP are treated following the stepwise approach outlined in Table 5.5.

Neuromuscular blockade should not be used routinely, but reserved for specific indications such as intracranial hypertension and transport.[10] In the setting of raised ICP despite adequate sedation, muscle relaxants are mainly used to prevent episodes of coughing and ventilator asynchrony and thereby facilitate cerebral venous outflow. They may also be required to prevent shivering in patients who are actively cooled.

Enteral feeding should be commenced no later than 24 hours after injury. If gastric paresis persists beyond 48 hours, a jejunal feeding tube should be placed. Blood glucose levels should be monitored closely in the infant, especially if there is an unexplained acidemia or ketonuria. We recommend that electrolytes and blood gases be monitored every 6 hours during the initial 48 hours. Rapid changes in serum sodium levels should be avoided through careful monitoring of electrolytes and fluid balance, and avoiding free water infusions.

Meticulous attention is required to prevent the common ICU complications. Many of these children will have aspirated gastric contents at the time of their injury or shortly thereafter, but prophylactic antibiotics are not recommended. Expectant therapy guided by cultures is preferable. Any vascular access device inserted under less than aseptic conditions during the emergency resuscitation should be replaced within 24 hours. Pressure sore prevention for the paralyzed patient includes frequent turning from side to side.

Prophylactic anticonvulsants have not been shown to be useful in preventing late post-traumatic seizures and are not currently used routinely.[11]

Most children will require a repeat head CT within 24–48 hours, or for any unexpected or unexplained deterioration in clinical status.

Intracranial pressure/cerebral perfusion pressure management

Intracranial pressure is a reflection of the relationship between alterations in the craniospinal volume and the ability of the craniospinal axis to accommodate added volume.[12,13] The pathophysiology of raised ICP is complex. In general, elevations of ICP are due to increases in blood volume (vasodilation, venous obstruction), tissue volume (edema, clot), or increased cerebrospinal fluid volume (obstruction, increased production). Therapy of elevated ICP is aimed at one or all of these mechanisms.

The mainstay for managing these critically ill children has been monitoring of intracranial pressure and maintenance of cerebral perfusion pressure, in the hope that this will maintain adequate cerebral oxygen delivery and prevent further secondary cerebral injuries. The evidence for this is poor and it would appear that the use of ICP monitoring in children is still not universal.[14] Similarly, it is felt that intracranial hypertension is associated with increased morbidity and mortality; that elevations in ICP impact outcome through impaired cerebral perfusion and direct pressure effects on critical intracranial structures. The evidence for this is equally poor. However, if ICP is monitored, and if it is decided to treat some pre-determined level of ICP, it is important to not just treat the number, but to look at the measurement in conjunction with clinical examination, other physiologic variables such as CPP, and cranial imaging.[15]

A number of features of ICP are important to consider prior to its treatment. These include age norms for both ICP and CPP, and normal conditions that will transiently elevate ICP. ICP is normally elevated in healthy patients by such maneuvers as coughing and turning, and is usually coincident with an elevated blood pressure. An elevated ICP becomes abnormal when:

- It remains elevated and becomes a plateau rather than a spike
- Becomes elevated without a coincident rise in arterial blood pressure
- Remains elevated for less than 5 minutes, but is associated with a falling arterial BP while the ICP stays high
- Frequent and recurrent unstimulated spikes in pressure.

Current pediatric data support defining intracranial hypertension as pathologically elevated ICP greater than or equal to 20 mmHg in the setting of a normal blood pressure.[15] In our PICU, treatment is aimed at maintaining ICP <20 mmHg for children with severe TBI following the steps in Table 5.5. If these initial measures fail to lower the ICP, the following maneuvers may be considered. These are mainly experimental therapies that have been tried in the past; however, their benefits are unclear. They are not presently recommended as a general therapy, except as part of a research protocol, or in an academic centre with pediatric neurosurgeons.

1. Hypothermia.
2. Lumbar drainage may be considered as an option only in the case of refractory intracranial hypertension with a functioning ventriculostomy, open basal cisterns, and no evidence of a major mass lesion or shift on imaging studies.

3. Surgical treatment with decompressive craniectomy may be considered in pediatric patients with severe traumatic brain injury, diffuse cerebral swelling, and intracranial hypertension refractory to intensive medical management.[16,17]

Aggressive hyperventilation therapy has been used in the management of severe pediatric head injury for rapid reduction of ICP since the 1970s. Hyperventilation reduces ICP by inducing hypocapnia, which leads to cerebral vasoconstriction, reducing cerebral blood flow. However, the vasoconstrictor effect of hyperventilation lasts less than 24 hours in most patients and sustained hyperventilation may be complicated by rebound hyperemia. The management strategy of utilizing hyperventilation in children to control ICP was based on the impression that hyperemia was common after pediatric head injury. More recent studies specifically targeting the pediatric population have shown that hyperemia is uncommon and have raised concerns about the safety of hyperventilation. Routine mild or prophylactic hyperventilation ($PaCO_2$ <35 mmHg) is therefore not recommended and should be avoided.[18] In patients who show signs of cerebral herniation or acute neurologic deterioration, brief periods of hyperventilation may be considered pending a repeat CT scan and definitive therapy such as surgical decompression.[6]

Cerebral blood flow (CBF) in normal awake children is 30%–40% higher than in adults, ranging from 30–40 ml 100 g^{-1} per min during the first 6 months of life to a peak of about 110 ml 100 g^{-1} per min by age 3 to 4 years. It falls to adult levels of 50 ml 100 g^{-1} per min by about 12 years of age.[19,20] These changes in CBF mirror brain growth and development. Considering this large range, comparisons of CBF data in children are valid only when small, well-defined age ranges are selected.

Hyperemia or cerebrovascular engorgement (malignant hyperemia) has long been considered by many as the cause of diffuse swelling and raised ICP. More recent studies suggest that CBF values are relatively normal for age. Furthermore, CBF has been shown in both adults and children to fall during the initial 24 hours following a TBI, recovering to baseline levels 48–72 hours later. Regional CBF may be even more reduced in the vicinity of intracranial hematomas and contusions. Therefore, mechanisms other than excessive CBF should be considered to explain the rapid progression of brain oedema in children with traumatic brain injury.[21]

Global or regional cerebral ischemia is considered an important secondary insult to the acutely injured brain. The critical care support of these children is aimed at maintaining adequate cerebral oxygenation by early detection of situations likely to cause cerebral ischemia and preventing their occurrence. Current bedside tools for monitoring cerebral oxygenation are limited and are of a surrogate nature. For example, supporting the cerebral perfusion pressure is a common goal of the critical care management of children with a TBI, based upon the concept of normal auto regulation of cerebral blood flow and oxygen delivery.

Cerebral perfusion pressure is defined as the mean systemic arterial pressure minus intracranial pressure.

$$CPP = MAP - ICP$$

It defines the pressure gradient driving global cerebral blood flow, whereas regional flow is determined by metabolic activity. An important limitation of CPP monitoring is its inability to predict adaptation between hemodynamic profile and cerebral metabolic status.

It is unknown what is an acceptable CPP for the different ages in children. There is likely to be an age-related continuum, similar to that for CBF. A lower limit of CPP of 40 mmHg in children with TBI is generally regarded as acceptable, but the evidence for this is poor. It is unclear whether this value represents a minimal threshold or whether the optimal CPP may be above this in children,[22] although it does appear that younger children may be able to tolerate lower CPPs and still have a relatively good outcome.[23] Regardless, hypotension should be avoided at all times. Our current approach is to maintain the CPP at or above 40 mmHg for children less than 10 years of age.

Another surrogate measure of cerebral oxygenation used in some centers, and in this case, is the use of jugular venous bulb catheterization. This provides an indirect measure of global cerebral oxygenation. The lower limit for a normal jugular venous saturation (SjO_2) is 45% in normal adult subjects, but whether this applies to children is unknown.[24] There is some evidence in adult patients with TBI that episodes of cerebral desaturation are associated with a worse outcome, and preventing these episodes improves outcome. However, this has not been demonstrated prospectively nor is there a good pathophysiologic basis behind these findings. In addition, introduction of a monitor into the right internal jugular vein may actually impede venous flow from the brain.

Alternatively, cerebral blood flow can be measured, and based upon this value, certain assumptions made about the adequacy of cerebral tissue oxygenation. Xenon CT is probably the most commonly applied technique; it provides better resolution and has the ability to measure CBF in deeper brain structures as well as cortex. It can detect both regional and global ischemia but suffers from the lack of correlation to metabolic coupling.[1] The xenon study proved informative in the management of this case, demonstrating an adequate CBF despite intractable raised ICP and marginally low CPP.

More useful information is gained by using functional neuroimaging, such as Positron Emission Tomography (PET) and functional MRI. A study using PET demonstrated significant regions of ischemia using positron emission tomography despite normal SjO_2s within the first 24 hours after TBI in adult patients.[25]

Mannitol and hypertonic saline are both effective for the control of increased intracranial pressure after severe head injury, but have not been shown to improve outcome. Mannitol has been a cornerstone in the management of raised ICP in pediatric traumatic brain injury but should be reserved for euvolemic children with acute neurological deterioration to allow time for diagnostic investigations or in children with an ICP monitor demonstrating acute elevations in an elevated baseline ICP. Mannitol reduces ICP by reducing blood viscosity. CBF is maintained through reflex vasoconstriction and cerebral blood volume and ICP decrease. The effect of mannitol on blood viscosity is rapid but transient, lasting less than 75 minutes. Mannitol also reduces ICP by an osmotic effect due to the gradual movement of water from the parenchyma into the circulation. This effect develops more slowly (over 15–30 min), persists for up to 6 hours and requires an intact blood–brain barrier.[26] Serum osmolarity should be maintained below 320 mOsm l^{-1} with mannitol use.

Hyperthermia, defined as a core body temperature $> 38\,^\circ$C, is common after TBI. An extensive body of animal literature has demonstrated the harmful effects of hyperthermia in the injured brain. Hyperthermia increases the cerebral metabolic rate for oxygen and glucose that results in increased cerebral blood flow and in turn increased cerebral blood volume and raised ICP. It also potentiates secondary cellular cascade injury. Hyperthermia should be avoided in children with severe traumatic brain injury[27] as its occurrence is associated with a longer length of stay and a poorer neurological state at discharge.[28] We recommend that children with an acute neurologic insult be maintained at normothermia, using a cooling blanket if necessary.

On the other hand, hypothermia has been shown to be protective in animal models following a variety of acute neurologic insults. Unfortunately, no human clinical studies in patients with TBI have demonstrated benefit on long-term outcome, even those specifically in children such as the recent international HYP-HIT study.[29] Hypothermia is also not without risk. Possible complications include electrolyte abnormalities, cardiac arrhythmias,[30] coagulopathy and increased infections. Furthermore, rapid rewarming can exacerbate the axonal damage that results from traumatic brain injury and therefore induced hypothermia is not currently recommended as a treatment strategy for the management of traumatic brain injury, unless as a component of a research study.[31]

The use of steroids is not recommended in pediatric patients with severe traumatic brain injury, as they have not been demonstrated to show benefit. The CRASH trial, a multicentre, international, randomized placebo-controlled trial evaluated treatment with corticosteriods in 10 008 head injured adults (GCS<14). This data showed no reduction in mortality with a trend to increased mortality in the treatment arm.[32,33]

Conclusions

The management of severe head injuries must be viewed as a continuum that begins at the scene with resuscitation and the initiation of critical care, and ends with neurological rehabilitation. Protocol guided intensive care management may reduce the incidence of secondary brain injury after severe TBI, thereby improving survival and outcome. Monitoring of ICP and the control of increased intracranial pressure is a key feature of these protocols, with the goal being to maintain ICP within the normal range. This is intended to optimize cerebral perfusion pressure, oxygenation, and metabolic substrate delivery and to avoid cerebral herniation events. The future of head injury management lies in directing therapy at the biochemical and cellular responses to the trauma in an attempt to prevent the rise in intracranial pressure.

Learning points

- Head injury is a leading cause of death in children.
- Initial resuscitative efforts in the emergency department and ongoing critical care support are aimed at the detection, treatment and prevention of secondary injury.
- Hypoventilation and hypotension should be identified and corrected early.
- Maintenance of normoxia, normocarbia, normovolemia, and normothermia is the mainstay of intensive care management.
- Avoid free water administration and closely monitor serum sodium.
- Routine mild or prophylactic hyperventilation ($PaCO_2$ <35 mmHg) is not recommended and should be avoided.
- In patients who show signs of cerebral herniation or acute neurologic deterioration, brief periods of hyperventilation may be considered pending a repeat CT scan and definitive therapy such as surgical decompression.
- Mannitol therapy should be reserved for euvolemic children with acute neurological deterioration to allow time for diagnostic investigations or in children with an ICP monitor demonstrating acute elevations in an elevated baseline ICP.
- Interpretation and treatment of intracranial hypertension based on any ICP threshold should be corroborated by frequent clinical examination, monitoring of physiologic variables (e.g. CPP) and cranial imaging.

References

1. Mansfield R. Head injuries in children and adults. *Crit. Care Clinics* 1997; **13** (3): 611–26.
2. Geddes JF, Plunkett J. The evidence base for shaken baby syndrome. *Br Med J* 2004; **328**: 719–20.
3. Carney NA, Chesnut R, Kochanek PM. Guidelines for the acute medical management of severe traumatic brain injury in infants, children, and adolescents. *Pediatr Crit Care Med* 2003; **4**(3 Suppl): S1.
4. Adelson PD, Bratton SL, Carney NA *et al.* Chapter 1: Introduction. *Pediatr Crit Care Med* 2003; **4**(3 Suppl): S2–4.
5. Meyer P, Legros C, Orliaguet G. Critical care management of neurotrauma in children: new trends and perspectives. *Child Nerv System* 1999; **15**: 732–9.
6. Adelson PD, Bratton SL, Carney NA *et al.* Chapter 4: Resuscitation of blood pressure and oxygenation and prehospital brain-specific therapies for the severe pediatric traumatic brain injury patient. *Pediatr Crit Care Med* 2003; **4**(3 Suppl): S12–18.
7. James HE. Neurologic evaluation and support in the child with an acute brain insult. *Pediatr Ann* 1986; **15**: 16–22.
8. Morris CG, McCoy EP, Lavery G G. Spinal immobilization for unconscious patients with multiple injuries. *Br Med J* 2004; **329**: 495–9.
9. Tasker RC, Morris KP, Forsyth RJ *et al.* Severe head injury in children: emergency access to neurosurgery in the United Kingdom. *Emerg Med J* 2006; **23**: 519–22.
10. Adelson PD, Bratton SL, Carney NA *et al.* Chapter 9: Use of sedation and neuromuscular blockade in the treatment of severe pediatric traumatic brain injury. *Pediatr Crit Care Med* 2003; **4**(3 Suppl): S34–7.
11. Adelson PD, Bratton SL, Carney NA *et al.* Chapter 18: The role of anti-seizure prophylaxis following severe pediatric traumatic brain injury. *Pediatr Crit Care Med* 2003; **4**(3 sup): S72–75
12. Andrews PJ, Citerio G. Intracranial pressure. Part one: Historical overview and basic concepts. *Intens Care Med* 2004; **30**: 1730–3.
13. Citerio G, Andrews PJ. Intracranial pressure. Part two: Clinical applications and technology. *Intens Care Med* 2004; **30**: 1882–5.
14. Morris KP, Forsyth RJ, Parslow RC *et al.* Intracranial pressure complicating severe traumatic brain injury in children: monitoring and management. *Intens Care Med* 2006; **32**: 1606–12.
15. Adelson PD, Bratton SL, Carney NA *et al.* Chapter 6: Threshold for treatment of intracranial hypertension. *Pediatr Crit Care Med* 2003; **4**(3 Suppl): S25–7.
16. Adelson PD, Bratton SL, Carney NA *et al.* Chapter 15: Surgical treatment of pediatric intracranial hypertension. *Pediatr Crit Care Med* 2003; **4**(3 Suppl): S56–59
17. Jagannathan J, Okonkwo DO, Dumont AS *et al.* Outcome following decompressive craniectomy in children with severe traumatic brain injury: a 10-year single-center experience with long-term follow up. *J Neurosurg* 2007 **106**(4 Suppl): 268–75.
18. Adelson PD, Bratton SL, Carney NA *et al.* Chapter 12: Use of hyperventilation in the acute management of severe pediatric traumatic brain injury. *Pediatr Crit Care Med* 2003; **4**(3 Suppl): S45–8.
19. Zwienenberg M, Mulzelaar JP. Severe pediatric head injury: the role of hyperemia revisited. *J Neurotrauma* 1999; **16**: 937–43.
20. Suzuki K. The changes of regional CBF with advancing age in normal children. *Nagoya Med J* 1990; **34**: 159–70.
21. Kuluz J, McLaughlin G, Gelman B *et al.* (Abstract) Cerebral hyperemia is not common after severe head trauma in children. *Crit Care Med* 1996; **24** (1S): A135.
22. Adelson PD, Bratton SL, Carney NA *et al.* Chapter 8: Cerebral perfusion pressure. *Pediatr Crit Care Med* 2003; **4**(3 sup): S31–3.
23. Chambers IR, Jones PA, Minns RA *et al.* Which paediatric head injuries might benefit from decompression? Thresholds of ICP and CPP in the first six hours. *Acta Neurochir* 2005; **95** (suppl): 21–3.
24. Chieregato A, Calzolari F, Trasforini G *et al.* Normal jugular bulb oxygen saturation. *J Neurol Neurosurg Psychiatry* 2003; **74**: 784–6.
25. Coles J, Fryer TD, Smielewski P *et al.* Incidence and mechanisms of cerebral ischemia in early clinical head injury. *J Cereb Blood Flow Metab* 2004; **24**: 202–11.

26. Adelson PD, Bratton SL, Carney NA *et al.* Chapter 11: Use of hyperosmolar therapy in the management of severe pediatric traumatic brain injury. *Pediatr Crit Care Med* 2003; **4**(3 Suppl): S40–4.

27. Adelson PD, Bratton SL, Carney NA *et al.* Chapter 14: The role of temperature control following severe pediatric traumatic brain injury. *Ped Crit Care Med* 2003; **4**(3 Suppl): S53–5.

28. Suz P, Vavilala MS, Souter M *et al.* Clinical features of fever associated with poor outcome in severe pediatric traumatic brain injury. *J Neurosurg Anaesth* 2006; **18**: 5–10.

29. Hutchison JS, Ward RE, Lacroix J *et al.* Hypothermia therapy after traumatic brain injury in children. *N Engl J Med* 2008; **358**: 2447–56.

30. Adelson PD, Ragheb J, Kanev P *et al.* Phase II clinical trial of moderate hypothermia after severe traumatic brain injury. *Neurosurgery* 2005; **56**: 740–54.

31. Cairns CJ, Andrews P J. Management of hyperthermia in traumatic brain injury. *Curr Opin Crit Care* 2002; **8**: 106–10.

32. Roberts I, Yates D, Sandercock P *et al.* Effect of intravenous corticosteroids on death within 14 days in 10,008 adults with clinically significant head injury (MRC CRASH trial): randomized placebo-controlled trial. *Lancet* 2004; **364**: 1321–28.

33. Adelson PD, Bratton SL, Carney NA *et al.* Chapter 16: The use of corticosteroids in the treatment of severe pediatric traumatic brain injury. *Pediatr Crit Care Med* 2003; **4**(3 Suppl): S60–4.

Further reading

Guidelines for the management of severe traumatic brain injury. *J Neurotrauma* 2007; 24 Supplement 1 (can be accessed via www.braintrauma.org).

Giza CC, Mink RB, Medikians A. Pediatric traumatic brain injury: not just little adults. *Curr Opin Crit Care* 2007; **12**: 143–52.

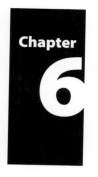

6

Management of diabetic ketoacidosis in a child

Peter J. Davis

Introduction

Diabetic Ketoacidosis (DKA) is a relatively common pediatric emergency that can occur either in children who are already known to have diabetes mellitus or as the first presentation of the condition. Cerebral edema is the major cause of morbidity and mortality in children with DKA[1] and the risk of this occurring is higher in children whose initial presentation is DKA.[2] The aim of clinical management is to rehydrate the child and to reverse the ketoacidosis using intravenous fluids and insulin, whilst prevention of any further clinical deterioration, including early recognition of cerebral oedema, is also essential.

Case history

A 7-year-old girl presented to the emergency department of her local hospital with a 2-week history of being generally unwell. Over the previous 2 days she had been vomiting and that evening she had started to become delirious. On further discussion with the mother, it was found that the girl had been drinking excessively, and unusually she had also been going to the toilet during the night. It was also thought that she had lost some weight. History, initial examination findings and investigations are shown in Table 6.1.

Examination

The child was immediately administered $15 \, l \, min^{-1}$ of oxygen by face mask. She was breathing spontaneously but shallowly and at a relatively rapid rate. Auscultation of the chest revealed bilateral air entry. She was noted to be dehydrated with sunken eyes. She was placed on an ECG monitor and intravenous access was obtained with a 22G cannula in the dorsum of the right hand. Blood was sent for FBC, U and E, glucose, venous blood gas and blood culture. A fluid bolus of 400 ml of 0.9% saline was given, following which her heart rate fell to $135 \, min^{-1}$ and her capillary refill time dropped to 3 seconds. Her Glasgow Coma Score (GCS) was assessed as 8/15 (E2, M4, V2) as she was only responsive to pain.

A calculation of her fluid requirements for the next 48 hours was made both in terms of her ongoing requirements and as replacement for her dehydration, which was estimated at 10% (ongoing requirement $= 1500 \, ml \times 2 = 3000 \, ml$ *plus* fluid deficit $= 20 \times 10 \times 10 = 2000 \, ml$; total fluid replacement over 48 hours $= 5000 \, ml \Rightarrow 104.2 \, ml \, h^{-1}$). She was commenced on an intravenous infusion of 0.9% saline with $40 \, mmol \, l^{-1}$ potassium chloride at $104 \, ml \, h^{-1}$, having already passed urine. An insulin infusion was started at $0.1 \, units \, kg^{-1} \, h^{-1}$. A second 22G cannula was inserted into the dorsum of her left hand and she was also given a dose of intravenous antibiotics (cefotaxime $50 \, mg \, kg^{-1}$). After an hour, her blood glucose, electrolytes and acid–base status were rechecked.

Case Studies in Pediatric Critical Care, ed. Peter. J. Murphy, Stephen C. Marriage, and Peter J. Davis. Published by Cambridge University Press. © Cambridge University Press 2009.

Table 6.1. *Findings on admission*

Past medical history	Fit and well Previous admission to hospital for grommets aged 2 years	
Regular medications	None	
Allergies	None known	
Examination	Awake and responsive, but slightly confused Airway clear, face mask oxygen, breath ketotic Chest clear, bilateral air entry, Sats 98% in air Respiratory rate 35 min^{-1} Normal heart sounds, pulse 150 min^{-1}, BP 95/60 Capillary refill time = 4 seconds Temperature 38 °C	
Investigations	Weight	20 kg
	FBC	Hb 16.5 g dl^{-1}, Plat 445 × 10^9 l^{-1}, WBC 34.3 × 10^9 l^{-1}
	U+Es	Na$^+$ 144 mmol l^{-1}, K$^+$ 4.1 mmol l^{-1}, Urea 13.2 mmol l^{-1}, Creatinine 117 µmol l^{-1}
	Glucose	65 mmol l^{-1}
	Venous blood gas	pH 6.82, pCO_2 11 mmHg, HCO$_3^-$ 5.7 mmol l^{-1}, BE −31.7
	Urine dip stick	Ketones ++++

The results of the repeat bloods were as shown: glucose 59 mmol l^{-1}, Na$^+$ 145 mmol l^{-1}, K$^+$ 3.5 mmol l^{-1}, pH 6.85, pCO_2 6 mmHg, HCO$_3^-$ 5.0 mmol l^{-1}, BE −31.5. After initially being somewhat combatative to procedures being performed on her, at around 2 hours after arrival in the emergency department, it was noted by the nurse looking after her that she had become unresponsive. A formal reassessment of her Glasgow Coma Score was found to be only 3/15 (E1, M1, V1). Her pupils were noted to be size 4, equal and equally reactive to light. The pediatric consultant on-call immediately contacted the local anesthetic team for airway support, and the regional pediatric intensive care unit for further advice, the concern being that the girl had severe cerebral edema. The local anesthetist performed a rapid sequence induction with propofol 60 mg and suxamethonium 25 mg, with cricoid pressure applied, after which she was successfully intubated with a size 5.5 uncuffed oral endotracheal tube, which was secured at 16 cm at the lips. After discussion of the case with the regional retrieval team, it was suggested that she should be given 1 g kg^{-1} of mannitol, and nursed head up at 30°, but that she should be transferred to the general intensive care unit rather than having a CT scan of her head performed. On further advice, the rate of her intravenous infusion of 0.9% saline with 40 mmol l^{-1} potassium chloride was also reduced to 60 ml h^{-1}. It was also advised that sodium bicarbonate should not be given. In the meantime, the regional retrieval team was activated.

On the intensive care unit the child was fully monitored with oxygen saturation, ECG and end-tidal CO_2. A nasogastric tube and urinary catheter were also inserted. She was initially ventilated on pressures of 16/5, at a rate of 25 breaths per minute, achieving an end-tidal CO_2 of approximately 25 mmHg. A 22G arterial line was inserted into her right radial artery for accurate blood pressure monitoring and for collection of hourly blood samples. A 5 FG triple lumen central line catheter was inserted into her right femoral vein under sterile conditions, using the Seldinger technique. The intracranial pressure (ICP) was estimated to be at least 20 mmHg. As her mean blood pressure was 65 mmHg, a noradrenalin infusion was started at 0.05 mcg kg^{-1} per min as an attempt to keep it above 75 mmHg, aiming for a cerebral perfusion pressure (CPP) of 55 mmHg. Throughout this time her pupils had remained size 2, equal and reactive to light.

Repeat arterial bloods performed at the time of arrival of the retrieval team were as shown: glucose 51 mmol l^{-1}, Na$^+$ 149 mmol l^{-1}, K$^+$ 3.4 mmol l^{-1}, pH 6.88, pCO_2 26 mmHg, pO_2 193 mmHg, HCO$_3^-$ 4.6 mmol l^{-1}, BE –28. Her ventilatory rate was increased to 30 breaths per minute, and her pressures were increased to 22/5 with a subsequent fall in the end-tidal CO_2 from 25 to 20 mmHg, and her oral endotracheal tube was exchanged for a nasal endotracheal tube. Intravenous fluids were continued at 60 ml h^{-1}, as were infusions of insulin at 0.1 units kg^{-1} per h. Sedation was maintained with infusions of morphine at 20 mcg kg^{-1} per h and midazolam at 100 mcg kg^{-1} per h, whilst an infusion of vecuronium 60 mcg kg^{-1} per h was started for muscle relaxation. Full monitoring, including end-tidal CO_2, and ventilation was switched to the transport equipment and another set of bloods collected before departure: glucose 49 mmol l^{-1}, Na$^+$ 150 mmol l^{-1}, K$^+$ 3.3 mmol l^{-1}, pH 6.95, pCO_2 20 mmHg, pO_2 187 mmHg, HCO$_3^-$ 4.3 mmol l^{-1}, BE –26.4.

The ambulance journey of 60 minutes was uneventful and the child remained clinically stable throughout.

Progress in pediatric intensive care unit

On arrival at the regional centre, she remained sedated on morphine and midazolam, and paralyzed using a vecuronium infusion. Paralysis was continued as normothermia could only be achieved by means of a cooling blanket. For this reason intravenous antibiotics (cefotaxime 50 mg kg^{-1}) were also continued. Ventilation was not problematic (intermittent mandatory ventilation, pressures 25/5, rate 30 breaths per minute, inspiratory time 1 second, FiO$_2$ 0.4) and her pCO_2 was kept less than 15 mmHg, with the aim of mimicking her own respiratory compensation. Hourly bloods and neurological observations were also continued.

Fluid requirements were recalculated so as to allow rehydration over 96 hours. As she had only received 2 hours of the initial calculated fluid replacement rate, to make calculations easier, it was assumed that the total deficit remained unchanged. (Ongoing requirements = 1500 ml × 4 = 6000 ml *plus* fluid deficit = 20 × 10 × 10 = 2000 ml; total fluid replacement over 96 hours = 8000 ml ⇒ 83.3 ml h^{-1}.) Insulin was continued at 0.1 units kg^{-1} h^{-1} and sucralfate was commenced for gut protection. Noradrenaline was continued at 0.05 mcg kg^{-1} per min to keep her blood pressure above 75 mmHg, and she remained cardiovascularly stable. A heparin infusion was also started at 10 units kg^{-1} h^{-1} via the femoral central venous line.

Slowly over the next few hours her acidosis began to improve, such that, at admission to PICU, her hourly bloods were as follows: glucose 37 mmol l^{-1}, Na$^+$ 151 mmol l^{-1}, K$^+$ 3.1 mmol l^{-1}, pH 7.08, pCO_2 13 mmHg, pO_2 226 mmHg, HCO$_3^-$ 3.8 mmol l^{-1}, BE –26.3. At 4 hours post-PICU admission (10 hours after her arrival at the local hospital), the glucose level was 27 mmol l^{-1} and the potassium was 2.9 mmol l^{-1}, so the intravenous fluids were changed to 0.9% saline with 60 mmol l^{-1} potassium chloride, and continued at 83 ml h^{-1}. As normothermia was being achieved, it was decided to stop cooling and paralysis. In turn, her ventilation was changed to a synchronised mode, such that she could trigger the ventilator. After 12 hours on PICU, her glucose had fallen to 13 mmol l^{-1}, so glucose was added to her fluids in the form of 5% dextrose/0.9% saline with potassium chloride. It was also noted that her serum phosphate level had fallen to less than 0.3 mmol l^{-1}, so she was given a dose of dipotassium phosphate, which brought it above 1 mmol l^{-1}. Two further doses were needed over the following 48 hours as again the levels eventually fell below 0.5 mmol l^{-1}.

By 24 hours after her initial presentation to hospital, the girl remained intubated and ventilated. She still had +2 of ketones in urine, but her biochemistry was very slowly improving with the results as shown: glucose 11 mmol l^{-1}, Na^+ 157 mmol l^{-1}, K^+ 3.9 mmol l^{-1}, Cl^- 141 mmol l^{-1}, pH 7.18, pCO_2 19.4 mmHg, pO_2 97.4 mmHg, HCO_3^- 7.0 mmol l^{-1}, BE –20. In view of her ongoing hypernatremia and hyperchloremia, the fluids were changed once more to 5% dextrose/0.45% saline with 60 mmol l^{-1} potassium chloride at 83 ml h^{-1}. Over the following 12 hours, regular nursing observation and hourly bloods continued,

At 36 hours into her hospital admission, her infusions of morphine and midazolam had been off for 6 hours, such that she was able to wake to the point that she successfully extubated. She remained somewhat tachypnoic with a respiratory rate of 25 to 30 breaths per minute, and her blood gas was still acidotic: pH 7.21, pCO_2 16.4 mmHg, pO_2 117 mmHg, HCO_3^- 6.3 mmol l^{-1}, BE –20.5. Although initially somewhat confused, over the subsequent hours her conscious level improved such that she was able to hold simple conversations with both her family and hospital staff. By 48 hours, her blood biochemistry had continued to very slowly improve and her blood cultures from the local hospital were negative, so antibiotics were stopped. Insulin was continued at 0.1 units kg^{-1} h^{-1} to reverse her ongoing ketosis.

Her bloods at 72 hours were as follows: glucose 10 mmol l^{-1}, Na^+ 150 mmol l^{-1}, K^+ 4.0 mmol l^{-1}, Cl^- 137 mmol l^{-1}, pH 7.26, pCO_2 19 mmHg, pO_2 112 mmHg, HCO_3^- 8.2 mmol l^{-1}, BE –17.1. She was still breathing at a rate of 25 to 30 breaths per minute to maintain this degree of respiratory compensation of her ongoing metabolic acidosis.

By day 4 of her PICU stay, she was fully neurologically recovered. Her insulin infusion was reduced to 0.05 units kg^{-1} per h, and she was started on oral diet. Her bloods were finally normalizing: glucose 6 mmol l^{-1}, Na^+ 145 mmol l^{-1}, K^+ 3.4 mmol l^{-1}, Cl^- 127 mmol l^{-1}, pH 7.32, pCO_2 22.5 mmHg, HCO_3^- 11.3 mmol l^{-1}, BE –13.1. Subsequently, the heparin infusion was stopped and the central line was removed. The following day she was discharged to the ward for ongoing care.

Discussion

Diabetic Ketoacidosis (DKA) is the most common cause of mortality and morbidity in children with type I diabetes mellitus. It is caused by a lack of circulating insulin, associated with increases in the counter-regulatory hormones including cortisol glucagon, growth hormone, and catecholamines. There is an increase in glycogenolysis and gluconeogenesis, whilst at the same time a reduced tissue glucose uptake, leading to hyperglycemia, plus an osmotic diuresis that results in dehydration. Increased lipolysis with ketone body production causes ketonemia, ketonuria, loss of bicarbonate and a metabolic acidosis (Fig. 6.1). The biochemical criteria for diagnosing DKA include a blood glucose >11 mmol l^{-1} with a venous pH <7.3 and/or bicarbonate <15 mmol l^{-1}. DKA with a pH<7.1 and bicarbonate <5 mmol l^{-1} is categorized as severe.

Initial assessment and management

A history of the presenting illness should be obtained. The typical presenting symptoms of diabetes mellitus include polyuria, polydipsia, significant weight loss, weakness, and

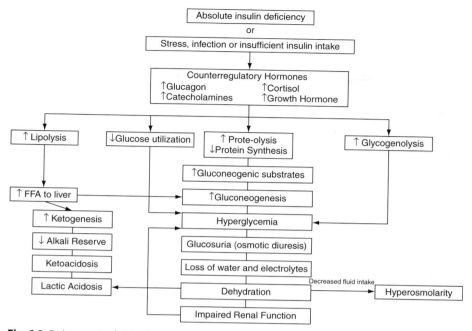

Fig. 6.1. Pathogenesis of diabetic ketoacidosis; FFA Free fatty acids (from Wolfsdorf J *et al*, 2006)

tiredness, as mentioned in the case discussed. A child may also complain of abdominal pain and may have been vomiting. These symptoms can be difficult to elucidate in a young child or infant, so potentially delaying the diagnosis, with a subsequent worsening in clinical condition. Younger children (<4 years of age) are more likely to present in DKA at the onset of their condition, as are children without a first-degree relative with type I diabetes mellitus, and those from families of lower socioeconomic status.[3]

When examining a child with DKA, it is important to estimate the degree of dehydration:

Mild (<5%)

Moderate (5–7.5%)

Severe (>7.5%)

It is easy to overestimate the degree of dehydration,[4] with consequent risks in the amount of fluid given during subsequent treatment. The maximum degree of dehydration should be assumed to be 10%. Other frequently encountered signs of DKA include tachypnea or Kussmaul breathing (sighing breathing consistent with a metabolic acidosis), hypo- or hyperthermia and ketotic breath. In this case, she was tachypnoic, severely dehydrated, and febrile.

Initial assessment and management of a child with DKA follows the ABC pattern:

A Airway

B Breathing

C Circulation

For the girl in this case, her airway was not initially problematic, but she received 100% oxygen, despite having little evidence of a primary respiratory problem. She was placed on a cardiac monitor and was noted to be shocked, with tachycardia and a prolonged capillary refill time. This was treated appropriately with 20 ml kg^{-1} of 0.9% saline, which resulted in an improvement in her circulatory status. There is no evidence for the use of colloids for treating shock in DKA. Any boluses of fluids used as part of the initial resuscitation should be subtracted in the fluid deficit calculations, even though fluid is being administered rapidly to restore the circulating volume. A brief neurological assessment should also be made at admission for subsequent reference, either using the Glasgow Coma Score for children >4 years of age or the AVPU (a = alert, v = responds to voice, p = responds to pain, u = unresponsive) score.

In children with DKA, it is important to obtain good intravenous access and collect blood samples for:

- Blood glucose
- Plasma urea and electrolytes
- Blood gas
- Full blood count
- Blood cultures

It is also essential to calculate the serum osmolality at regular intervals:

$$\text{Serum osmolality} = ([Na^+] \times 2) + [glucose] + [urea] \quad \text{(values in mmol l}^{-1}\text{)}$$

In the case presented, the initial serum osmolality was 366 mOsm l^{-1} (= 144 × 2 + 65 + 13), signifying that she was very hyperosmolar. Most children presenting with DKA are to some degree hyperosmolar, but the degree of hyperosmolality is a warning sign of the degree of illness, and rapid falls in effective osmolality are believed to be a risk factor for development of cerebral edema.[5]

The initial fluid requirement calculation needs to include the ongoing maintenance requirement plus the replacement for dehydration. Ongoing maintenance fluid values are calculated as follows:

100 ml kg^{-1} per day for first 10 kg of body weight

50 ml kg^{-1} per day for next 10 kg of body weight

20 ml kg^{-1} per day for weight above 20 kg

The fluid deficit and replacement for dehydration is calculated as follows:

$$\text{Deficit (ml)} = \text{body weight (kg)} \times \% \text{ dehydration} \times 10$$

The deficit is usually replaced over 48 hours in the first instance,[6] using 0.9% saline. Once any degree of shock has been treated appropriately, rapid intravenous fluid replacement is unnecessary and increases the risk of cerebral edema. Ongoing urinary losses are not added to the fluid calculation. Potassium should be initially included in the intravenous fluids at 40 mmol l^{-1} unless anuria is suspected, or there is evidence of peaked T waves characteristic of hyperkalemia on the ECG monitor. In DKA, anuria is very rare, as the child is usually polyuric at presentation. Potassium is a predominantly intracellular ion and is always massively depleted in DKA, whatever the serum level. Once treatment commences, the administration of insulin and the correction of acidosis drive potassium into the cells, causing serum levels to drop.

Rehydration alone will cause some decrease in blood glucose concentration, but insulin is essential to return the blood glucose level to normal, and to suppress lipolysis and ketone body production. In DKA, a continuous low-dose intravenous infusion of insulin should be administered at a rate of 0.1units kg^{-1} per h, using a solution of human soluble insulin (e.g. Actrapid) of 1 unit ml^{-1} in 0.9% saline in a 50 ml syringe, running at 0.1 ml kg^{-1} per h. There is evidence to suggest that an initial bolus of insulin is unnecessary[7] and this is now actively discouraged. The infusion rate should only be reduced to 0.05 units kg^{-1} per h if the rate of fall in blood glucose level exceeds 5 mmol l^{-1} per h. Normalization of the blood glucose concentration and resolution of ketosis invariably occur before the acidosis has corrected. An iatrogenic non-anion gap hyperchloremic acidosis occurs in almost all children with DKA during the administration of large volumes of 0.9% saline as part of the fluid resuscitation and rehydration.[8] This hyperchloremia usually slowly resolves spontaneously over a few days.

Once the serum glucose level falls below 15 mmol l^{-1}, glucose should be added to the intravenous fluids, rather than reducing the insulin. After the ketosis has fully resolved and the child is already on an adequate dose of glucose, it may be appropriate to reduce the rate of the insulin infusion before starting a subcutaneous insulin regime, especially if there is likely to be a delay in the child taking feeds, as occurred in this case. The first subcutaneous dose of insulin should be administered 30 min before stopping the insulin infusion, and should be followed by a meal.

Regular monitoring of the condition of the child is essential, including at least hourly nursing observations, with a particular emphasis on neurological findings such as headache, vomiting, a change in neurological status (e.g. restlessness, irritability, increased drowsiness) or more specific signs (e.g. pupillary responses). Blood glucose should be checked hourly, as should electrolytes, calculated osmolality, and acid–base status in the most severe cases. Other laboratory bloods should be checked at least 2–4 hourly. A raised WBC is not necessarily indicative of infection. However, DKA can be precipitated by infection, and if there are other indicators of possible sepsis such as hyperthermia, broad-spectrum antibiotics (e.g. cefotaxime 50 mg kg^{-1}) should be commenced following the collection of blood cultures, as in this case.

Assessment and management of cerebral edema in diabetic ketoacidosis

Early identification of the signs and symptoms of cerebral edema is essential when treating DKA. The risk of a child developing symptomatic cerebral oedema with raised intracranial pressure during DKA is between 0.9%[9] and 1.5%,[10] with a possible increased risk in children newly presenting with diabetes.[2] From neuroradiological studies it has been suggested that over half of all children presenting with DKA have some evidence of cerebral edema.[11] It accounts for the majority of DKA deaths in children and has a mortality rate of around 20–25%, and a similar significant morbidity rate.[2,9]

Cerebral edema typically occurs 4–12 hours after treatment is commenced, but it may even be present before treatment has started, and in patients without any clinical evidence of raised intracranial pressure.[12] The occurrence of cerebral oedema has been associated with a lower initial pCO_2, degree of acidosis at presentation,[13] and a higher initial serum urea,[9,10] which in part may reflect a greater degree of dehydration in children affected. The risk of developing cerebral oedema may also be related to falls in serum osmolality during therapy,[5,14] as seen by a fall in glucose without a concomitant rise in sodium. It has been suggested that the pathophysiology of cerebral oedema in diabetic ketoacidosis may involve a transient loss of cerebral autoregulation, leading to paradoxical cerebral hyperaemia and the development of vasogenic cerebral edema.[15]

There is also evidence that treatment of DKA may precipitate cerebral oedema, particularly commencement of insulin infusions within the first hour and larger amounts of fluid volumes within the first 4 hours of treatment.[10] In view of this, it is now recommended that as rehydration alone will to some extent reverse the initial acidosis, that the insulin infusion is not started until 1 hour of fluid treatment has been completed.

There is some evidence to support an association between the use of sodium bicarbonate for correction of acidosis and an increased risk of cerebral edema.[9] For this reason, as there is no evidence to show that use of bicarbonate confers any clinical benefit, it is no longer recommended in the treatment of DKA, especially as even severe acidosis is reversible by fluid and insulin replacement. Insulin administration stops further ketoacid production, and results in the metabolism of keto-anion and the regeneration of bicarbonate. The only roles for bicarbonate adminsitration in DKA may be to affect the action of adrenalin during cardiopulmonary resuscitation in profound acidosis, or in potentially life-threatening hyperkalemia.

It has been suggested that treatment of cerebral edema in diabetic ketoacidosis has been associated with worsened outcome if extreme hyperventilation is continued following intubation and ventilation.[16] Other variables found to be associated with a poor outcome were greater neurological depression at the time of diagnosis of cerebral edema. This may just reflect the degree of illness. Use of hyperventilation certainly decreases cerebral blood flow and may contribute to cerebral ischaemia, potentially worsening any ongoing brain injury. Although statistical analysis has suggested a mean pCO_2 <22 mmHg during the first 3 hours of ventilation for cerebral edema secondary to DKA as a cut-off level for poor outcome,[16] it remains unclear what level of pCO_2 is actually optimal. It has been suggested that, to maintain CSF pH within a range that is recoverable and compatible with survival, hyperventilation may need to be undertaken to levels similar to that managed by the patient when spontaneously breathing.[17] For full control of ventilation to be effective in this context, the child should at least initially be sedated and muscle relaxed.

Treatment for cerebral oedema should be started as soon as the condition is suspected. A dose of 1 g kg^{-1} of intravenous mannitol is part of the first-line therapy, although there is no definitive evidence as to any beneficial or detrimental effect of its use, or the optimal dosage.[16] Repeated doses may also be given if there is no initial response. The successful use of hypertonic saline for altered mental status associated with DKA has also been reported,[18] and, although there is no evidence for its use in established cerebral edema secondary to DKA, it has been shown to be effective in other causes of raised intracranial pressure and indeed may be advantageous physiologically in DKA as unlike mannitol, it does not cause an osmotic diuresis. The rate of fluid administration should also be reduced to maintenance levels only and once the child has been stabilised, rehydration should proceed slowly over 72 to 96 hours. Other simple neuroprotective measures should be instituted, including nursing head up at 30°, and aiming to keep the child in the midline and normothermic.

CT scanning is not particularly reliable at estimating intracranial pressure in children with generalized cerebral edema[19] but may exclude other causes of deterioration in mental status that may occur with DKA, such as cerebral venous thrombosis[20] or cerebral hemorrhage,[21] or infarction. This should not delay the institution of emergency treatment. Maintenance of a presumed cerebral perfusion pressure (CPP) may also require the introduction of noradrenalin to appropriately raise the blood pressure and the insertion of a central venous catheter. The use of femoral central venous catheters in children with DKA has been associated with an increased risk of deep venous thrombosis,[22] possibly secondary to degree of dehydration. The use of low-dose heparin (10 units kg^{-1} per h) via the central line may reduce this risk, particularly in smaller children, although if there are concerns related to the possibility of intracerebral hemorrhage, this should be excluded radiologically before heparin is administered.

Throughout the ongoing intensive care stay, general clinical measures to prevent intracranial hypertension should be continued. These include: maintenance of adequate ventilation and oxygenation; maintenance of adequate CPP; sedation, and when necessary, paralysis; control of body temperature; serial neurological examination.

Learning points

- The aim of clinical management is to rehydrate and to reverse the ketoacidosis initially using intravenous 0.9% saline with 40 mmol l^{-1} potassium chloride and an insulin infusion.

- Dehydration should not be over-estimated (maximum 10%) and rehydration should occur over at least 48 hours. Fluid boluses should be limited to 30 ml kg^{-1} in total.

- The insulin infusion should not be started until after the first hour of fluid treatment and remain at 0.1 units kg^{-1} per h, unless the fall in glucose concentration exceeds 5 mmol h^{-1}, in which case it should be reduced to 0.05 units kg^{-1} h^{-1}. The insulin infusion should never be stopped.

- When the glucose concentration falls below 15 mmol l^{-1}, glucose should be added to the intravenous fluids.

- Sodium bicarbonate should not be used to treat DKA, as its use has been associated with an increased risk of cerebral edema.

- Hourly monitoring of blood glucose, electrolytes, calculated osmolality, and blood gases should be performed in severe cases (pH<7.1 and bicarbonate <5 mmol l^{-1}).

- Symptomatic cerebral oedema occurs in approximately 1% of all cases of DKA and is the major cause of morbidity and mortality in children with DKA.

- Deteriorating level of consciousness should be assumed to be due to cerebral oedema and treated aggressively.

- Initial management of cerebral edema should include 1 g kg^{-1} of intravenous mannitol or hypertonic saline, reduction of intravenous fluid infusion rate to maintenance level, plus intubation and ventilation aiming for a pCO_2 of similar to that achieved by the patient pre-intubation if airway protection is deemed necessary.

- A cranial CT with contrast is not required to confirm cerebral edema, but may exclude other causes of a decreased conscious level.

References

1. Edge JA, Ford-Adams M, Dunger DB. Causes of death in children with insulin dependent diabetes 1990–96. *Arch Dis Child* 1999; **81**: 318–23.

2. Edge JA, Hawkins MM, Winter DL, Dunger DB. The risk and outcome of cerebral oedema developing during diabetic ketoacidosis. *Arch Dis Child* 2001; **85**: 16–22.

3. Pinkey JH, Bingley PJ, Sawtell PA, Dunger DB, Gale EA. Presentation and progress of childhood diabetes mellitus: a prospective population-based study. The

Bart's–Oxford Study Group. *Diabetologia* 1994; **37**: 70–4.

4. Mackenzie A, Barnes G, Shann F. Clinical signs of dehydration in children. *Lancet* 1989; 2(8663): 605–7.

5. Carlotti AP, Bohn D, Halperin ML. Importance of timing of risk factors for cerebral oedema during therapy for diabetic ketoacidosis. *Arch Dis Child* 2003; **88**: 170–3.

6. Harris GD. Fiordalisi. I. Physiologic management of diabetic ketoacidemia. A 5-year prospective pediatric experience in 231 episodes. *Arch Pediatr Adolesc Med* 1994; **148**: 1046–52.

7. Fort P, Waters SM, Lifshitz F. Low-dose insulin infusion in the treatment of diabetic ketoacidosis: bolus versus no bolus. *J Pediatr* 1980; **96**: 36–40.

8. Taylor D, Durward A, Tibby SM *et al.* The influence of hyperchloraemia on acid base interpretation in diabetic ketoacidosis. *Intensive Care Med* 2006; **32**: 295–301.

9. Glaser N, Barnett P, McCaslin I *et al.* Risk factors for cerebral edema in children with diabetic ketoacidosis. *N Engl J Med* 2001; **344**: 264–9.

10. Edge JA, Jakes RW, Roy Y *et al.* The UK case-control study of cerebral oedema complicating diabetic ketoacidosis in children. *Diabetologia* 2006; **49**: 2002–9.

11. Glaser NS, Wootton-Gorges SL, Buonocore MH *et al.* Frequency of cub-clinical cerebral oedema in children with diabetic ketoacidosis. *Pediatr Diabetes* 2006; **7**: 73–4.

12. Krane EJ, Rockoff MA, Wallman JK, Wolfsdorf JI. Subclinical brain swelling in children during treatment of diabetic ketoacidosis. *N Engl J Med* 1985; **312**: 1147–51.

13. Edge JA, Roy Y, Bergomi A *et al.* Conscious level in children with diabetic ketoacidosis is related to severity of acidosis and not to blood glucose concentrations. *Pediatr Diabetes* 2006; **7**: 11–15.

14. Hale PM, Rezvani I, Braunstein AW, Lipman TH, Martinez N, Garibaldi L. Factors predicting cerebral edema in young children with diabetic ketoacidosis and new onset type I diabetes. *Acta Paediatrica* 1997; **86**: 626–31.

15. Roberts JS, Vavilala MS, Shaw KA *et al.* Cerebral hyperemia and impaired cerebral autoregulation associated with diabetic ketoacidosis in critically ill children. *Crit Care Med* 2006; **34**: 2258–9.

16. Marcin JP, Glaser N, Barnett P *et al.* Factors associated with adverse outcomes in children with diabetic ketoacidosis-related cerebral edema. *J Pediat* 2002; **14**: 793–7.

17. Tasker RC, Lutman D, Peters MJ. Hyperventilation in severe diabetic ketoacidosis. *Pediatr Crit Care Med* 2005; **6**: 405–11.

18. Kamat P, Vats A, Gross M, Checchia PA. Use of hypertonic saline for the treatment of altered mental status associated with diabetic ketoacidosis. *Pediatr Crit Care Med* 2003; **4**: 239–42.

19. Hirsch W, Beck R. Behrmann C, Schobess A, Spielmann RP. Reliability of cranial CT versus intracerebral pressure measurement for the evaluation of generalised cerebral oedema in children. *Pediatr Radiolog* 2000; **30**: 439–43.

20. Keane S, Gallagher A, Ackroyd S, McShane MA, Edge JA. Cerebral venous thrombosis during diabetic ketoacidosis. *Arch Dis Child* 2002; **86**: 204–5.

21. Mahmud FH, Ramsay DA, Levin SD *et al.* Coma with diffuse white matter haemorrhages in juvenile diabetic ketoacidosis. *Pediatrics* 2007; **120**; e1540–6.

22. Gutierres JA, Bagatell R, Samson MP, Theodorou AA, Berg RA. Femoral central venous catheter-associated deep venous thrombosis in children with diabetic ketoacidosis. *Crit Care Med* 2003: **31**: 80–3.

Further reading

Dunger DB, Sperling MA, Acerini CL *et al.* ESPE/LWPES consensus statement on diabetic ketoacidosis in children and adolescents. *Arch Dis Child* 2004; **89**: 188–94.

Wolfsdorf J, Glaser N, Sperling MA. American Diabetes Association. Diabetic ketoacidosis in infants, children, and adolescents: a consensus statement from the American Diabetes Association. *Diabetes Care* 2006; **29**: 1150–9.

Wolfsdorf J, Craig ME, Daneman D *et al.* International Society for Pediatric and Adolescent Diabetes. Diabetic ketoacidosis. *Pediatr Diabetes* 2007; **8**: 28–43.

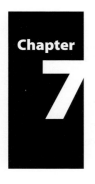

Chapter 7

Tricyclic antidepressant poisoning in children

Ian A. Jenkins

Introduction

Cyclic (tri- or tetra-) antidepressant poisoning in children has been becoming less common in the last few years (Fig. 7.1).[1]

This may be due to the switch in emphasis in the pharmacological treatment of depression from the tri- or tetra-cyclic antidepressant drugs (TCA) to the Selective Serotonin Re-uptake Inhibitors (SSRIs), such as fluoxetine; however, the amount of TCAs prescribed does not seem to be decreasing (Fig. 7.2).[2]

TCAs are used not only in the treatment of depression, where they are still suited to various conditions, but also in the treatment of chronic pain, particularly the neuralgias, and in nocturnal enuresis in older children.

In poisoning, which can be deliberate or accidental, these drugs produce a characteristic clinical picture, which is important to recognize as this leads to specific life-saving treatment. It is for this reason that, despite the diminishing incidence of TCA poisoning, it is important to be aware of the features of this particular type of poisoning.

Case history

Day 1 – Emergency department.

A 16-month-old girl was admitted to the emergency department (ED) at 10.00 h with a 40-minute history of fitting. After making an unusual cry, she had been found by her parents at about 09.00 h. She then had a fit and they called an ambulance. As she appeared to have continuous fits, the paramedic crew gave her two diazepam suppositories (2.5 mg each) during the transfer. However, she continued to fit.

On arrival in the ED, she was noted to be unconscious and unresponsive to pain. There was brief myoclonic jerking and periods of apnea. The airway was patent but breathing inadequate. Manual ventilation via face mask and self-inflating bag was commenced and her color and saturations improved with good air entry on auscultation. She felt hot centrally and cool peripherally, pulse rate 120 b min^{-1}, regular but with poor volume, capillary refill time 4–5 seconds, tympanic temperature 35.8 °C.

Intravenous access was established. Glucose (bedside stick test) 8.9 mmol l^{-1}; venous blood gas showed a metabolic acidosis (pH 7.07, Base deficit –11.7 mmol l^{-1}, lactate 4.7 mmol l^{-1}, K 4.7 mmol l^{-1}).

A working weight of 10 kg was estimated and further treatment given; lorazepam 1 mg intravenously (IV) and 200 ml 0.9% saline IV. With little effect seen on the convulsive activity, a further 1 mg lorazepam was given IV.

She became bradycardic and the saturations dropped. Another operator took over the ventilation and the saturations and color improved. However, it was noted that the QRS morphology on the ECG had changed. A further 200 ml bolus of 0.9% saline was commenced.

Case Studies in Pediatric Critical Care, ed. Peter. J. Murphy, Stephen C. Marriage, and Peter J. Davis. Published by Cambridge University Press. © Cambridge University Press 2009.

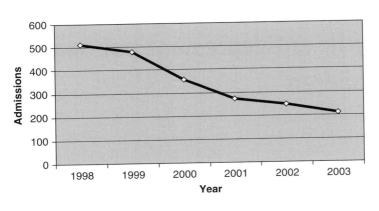

Fig. 7.1. Hospital admissions in England with tricyclic poisoning in children under 14 years old.

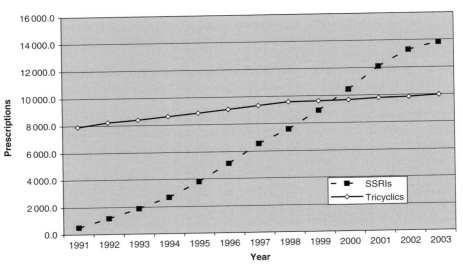

Fig. 7.2. Antidepressant prescriptions 1991–2003 in England.

With this last development the pediatric intensive care unit (PICU) team were summoned. It was decided to secure the patient's airway by intubation. At 10.20 h, the child was given 50 mg of thiopental and 20 mg suxamethonium. A 4.5 mm oral endotracheal tube was passed and, on auscultation, there was good air entry on both sides of the chest. The saturations were 96%. In view of the resistant fit activity, paraldehyde 2 ml in olive oil was given rectally.

At this point another episode of bradycardia ensued, 47 b min^{-1}, and so cardiac compressions were commenced. Atropine 200 micrograms was given IV, followed by two doses of adrenaline 100 mcg, with 240 ml of human albumin solution (HAS) and bicarbonate (0.5 ml kg^{-1}). This period of cardiopulmonary resuscitation (CPR) lasted approximately 6 minutes before return of an easily palpable pulse. Given the presentation, convulsions combined with wide complex polymorphic arrhythmia, a diagnosis of tricyclic ingestion was considered. Bicarbonate 2 mmol kg^{-1} and phenytoin 18 mg kg^{-1} were given while femoral arterial and venous catheters were inserted.

Table 7.1. *Summary of initial clinical findings*

Past medical history	Healthy. No known medical conditions	
Regular medications	None	
Allergies	None	
Presenting history	Found drowsy and with abnormal cry. Started to fit at 0900 till admitted to ED. Given two 2.5 mg diazepam suppositories by paramedic ambulance crew with no apparent effect	
Examination	Airway patent. Breathing poor, apneas caused by convulsions. Saturations not recorded. CRT 4–5 seconds, pulse 120 but poor volume. Peripheries cool, central temperature 35.8 °C. Unresponsive to voice and pain. No rash, no neck stiffness	
Investigations	Weight	10 kg (estimate)
	FBC	Hb 10.9 g dl^{-1}, WCC 16 × 10^9 l^{-1}, Plats 369 × 10^9 l^{-1}
	Electrolytes	Urea 6.5 mmol l^{-1}, Creatinine 50 mcg l^{-1}, Na$^+$ 144 mmol l^{-1}, Cl$^-$ 108 mmol l^{-1}, K 3.3 mmol l^{-1}
	Liver & Bone Chemistry	CRP <10 mg l^{-1}, Mg^{2+} 0.72 mmol l^{-1}, Ca^{2+} 1.83 mmol l^{-1}, ALT 14I U l^{-1}
	Coagulation	Normal
	Venous Blood Gas	pH 7.07, pO$_2$ 24.3 mmHg, pCO$_2$ 70.3 mmHg, base deficit −11.7, MetHb 0.5%, COHb 0.5%
	Glucose	10 mmol l^{-1}
	ECG	Rate 111, PR 246 ms, Qtc 549 ms, QRS 132 ms

During insertion of the catheters, another episode of pulseless electrical activity (PEA) occurred, responding to further 2 minutes of CPR and 1 bolus of 100 mcg of adrenaline. Another episode of PEA occurred immediately afterwards, requiring further basic life support and another two boluses of 100 mcg adrenaline.

Blood was taken for full blood count, electrolytes, glucose, C-reactive protein, liver and bone chemistry, blood culture and a toxicology screen for paracetamol, salicylates, opioids, amphetamines and TCAs. An adrenaline infusion was now started at 0.1 mcg kg^{-1} per min.

At this point, the parents, upon questioning by other staff, indicated that there were tablets of dosulepin in the house (previous British Approved Name – dothiepin), the mother having taken them up to 1 month before this episode. However, she was sure that her daughter could not have either taken them herself or the other children had access to them.

The patient was now in a somewhat more stable condition, with an arterial saturation of 97 and mean arterial pressure of 45 mmHg, and so she was transferred to the PICU (Table 7.1).

Progress in paediatric intensive care unit

Day 1 – PICU

She arrived on PICU at 1140 h. She was ventilating adequately on pressure controlled ventilation: rate of 20, pressures 20/5 cmH$_2$O, FiO$_2$ 0.6. Her SpO$_2$ was 100% and her arterial blood results: pH 7.39, pCO$_2$ 30 mmHg, pO$_2$ 194 mmHg, Bicarbonate 18 mmol l^{-1}, base deficit −5.4, Na 139 mmol l^{-1}, K 3.4 mmol l^{-1}, Ca 1.21 mmol l^{-1}, lactate 3.2 mmol l^{-1}, Hb10.4 g dl^{-1}.

Her heart rate was 90–120, irregular in rate and volume. The QRS was broadened and there was still a tendency to polymorphism. The QRS duration was 0.12–0.132 seconds and the QTc 0.549s (Fig. 7.3).

The abdomen was soft with a 2 cm liver edge and a nasogastric tube and a urinary catheter were present. Rather unexpectedly, she was passing urine at this stage.

Her pupils were dilated but the pupils responded to light. She was unconscious and unresponsive, but no sedative or muscle relaxant had been given since intubation in the ED.

She was started on cefotaxime and high dose aciclovir with IV fluids of 80% of normal maintenance allowance for her weight. Since the working differential diagnosis at this stage included TCA poisoning, she was given further bicarbonate (20 mmol and later 23 mmol), to treat the current acidosis and cardiac arrhythmia. Pediatric cardiological advice had been sought and amiodarone 5 mg kg^{-1} was given IV as a loading dose at 12.00 h.

Table 7.1 gives the results of the preliminary investigations. For the hypomagnesemia and the hypokalemia, she was given potassium 2 mmol and magnesium 3 mmol at 13.00 h.

At 12.30 h, the senior pediatric cardiologist on duty reviewed the situation. An echocardiogram was performed showing a normal structural heart, but with impaired ventricular function. Adenosine was given in three doses, 50, 100 then 200 mcg kg^{-1} to elucidate the arrhythmia. It appeared to be either junctional or ventricular in origin. In view of the fact that the etiology of her presentation was still not clear, a long QT syndrome was still a possibility. An attempt to place an atrial pacing wire under echo control to attempt overdrive atrial pacing was unsuccessful. As the inherent rhythm was ventricular with atrioventricular block, it was decided that, in view of the danger of amiodarone causing heart block and lowering cardiac output, a ventricular wire should be inserted and plans were made to take her to the cardiac catheter room to achieve this. During the period (12.00 h. to 14.00 h.) there were three episodes of VT preceded by increasingly polymorphous QRS complexes (Fig. 7.4).

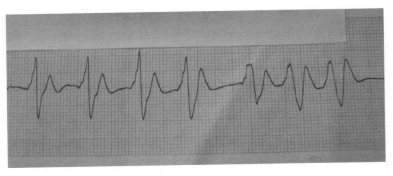

Fig. 7.3. ECG on arrival in PICU. Rate 90–120, QRS 0.12–0.132 s, QTc 0.549 s (normal <0.45) (see color plate section).

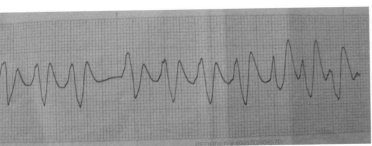

Fig. 7.4. ECG 1 hour later showing polymorphous QRS complexes leading to ventricular tachycardia (see color plate section).

The first was treated with CPR immediately, quickly followed by DC shocks – 2 J kg^{-1} twice, then 4 J kg^{-1} with a good result. The subsequent two episodes were treated with given 4J/kg directly with good results.

During this period, advice from the Regional Poisons Service had been sought. This was:

- To keep the arterial pH between 7.45 and 7.5 with bicarbonate and hypertonic saline;
- Give enteral charcoal 1 g kg^{-1} 4 hourly;
- To avoid Class 1a antiarrhythmic drugs (quinidine, procainamide, and disopyramide);
- If arrhythmias become troublesome, consider the use of phenytoin, β-blockers and magnesium sulphate (the latter having been shown to be of benefit in rats);
- Glucagon may be of benefit for resistant hypotension;
- Physostigmine was no longer recommended for treatment of fits or arrhythmias due to occurrence of asystole and worsening seizures.

At 14.30 h, 30 ml of 5% saline was given IV, bringing the sodium concentration up from 140 to 149 mmol l^{-1}. Many of the other measures, outlined above, were already in place.

An EEG at 15.40 h showed an electroclinical seizure of 5 seconds' duration, with spike and slow waves that indicated a liability to generalized seizures. Her heart rhythm remained unstable, but there were no further episodes of VT, but the rate was relatively slow, varying from 55 to 75 b min^{-1}. At 17.00 h, she was taken to the cardiac catheterization room to have a ventricular pacing wire inserted.

During the procedure, it was reported that the serum screening had proved positive for TCAs. The wire was successfully placed and ventricular pacing was set at 120 b min^{-1} with an immediate increase in the arterial blood pressure from 120/80 to 140/80. The amiodarone dosage was held at 5 mcg kg^{-1} per min and the adrenaline infusion was rapidly reduced in the next few hours. The aciclovir was stopped. The cefotaxime, however, was retained, as there were secretions aspirated from the chest and there was a gas exchange deficit, causation for both yet to be elucidated. A nasopharyngeal aspirate, taken in the morning was reported as showing no evidence of respiratory syncytial virus, adenovirus, parainfluenza, or influenza A or B.

On return to the PICU she was hyperpyrexial, 39 °C centrally, soon reaching 41.4 °C and 37 ° C peripherally despite cooling measures, she was treated with paracetamol, a cooling mattress and ice packs. Two hours later, her temperatures were 36.5 °C centrally and 35.5 °C peripherally.

Her condition stabilized and, over the course of the night, her mean blood pressure was maintained at 55–65 mmHg and the adrenaline infusion weaned to 0.06 mcg kg^{-1} per min. Her heart rate rose from the set 120 to 160. The rhythm was still thought to be ventricular in origin, so the amiodarone infusion was increased to 10 mcg kg^{-1} per min and a bolus of magnesium was given (0.3 mmol kg^{-1}), the pacing rate increased to 140 and capture was obtained, holding the heart rate at that level. During this period the pH was maintained at 7.45–7.5 with sodium bicarbonate 2 mmol kg^{-1} per h. The lactate dropped from 4 to 1.8 mmol kg^{-1} and the CVP from 11 to 6 mmHg. At 04.00 h the heart rate increased to 145 b min^{-1} and the morphology indicated sinus rhythm. The pacing and the sodium bicarbonate infusion were turned off and, in view of apparent lightening of the conscious state, a midazolam infusion was started at 100 mcg kg^{-1} per h.

Day 2

At 07.00 h, the heart was in sinus rhythm, 145 b min^{-1}. The amiodarone infusion was stopped. The ECG markers were, in seconds: QRS 0.12, PR 0.12, QTc 0.469. Thus, although a normal rhythm had appeared, conduction, and repolarization were still abnormal. Arterial blood gas, 6 hours after the bicarbonate infusion stopped was: pH 7.4, pO_2 109 mmHg (FiO_2 0.5, PEEP 5), CO_2 41 mmHg (ventilation pressures 18/5, rate 20), Base excess +0.1, bicarbonate 24 mmol l^{-1}, Na 157 mmol l^{-1}, K 4.6 mmol l^{-1}, ionized Ca 1.01 mmol l^{-1}. Urine output was good (4.8 ml kg^{-1} per h), the lactate 1.6 mmol l^{-1} and the temperatures 36.5 °C central, 36 °C peripheral.

Over the course of the day, the FiO_2 could be dropped to 0.4 and spontaneous respiratory efforts were such that the SIMV rate was turned down to 5 breaths min^{-1}. There was no return of acidosis and no more bicarbonate was administered. All cooling measures were removed and the adrenaline infusion finally ceased at 1500. The lactate was 1.2 mmol l^{-1}, sodium 152 mmol l^{-1}, potassium 3.8 mmol l^{-1}, Ca 2.11 mmol l^{-1}, Mg 1.6 mmol l^{-1}, urea 8.4 mmol l^{-1}, creatinine 66 μmol l^{-1}, urine output 2.5 ml kg^{-1} per h, ALT 1883 IU l^{-1}, CRP <10, WCC 36.3 × 10^9 l^{-1} (neutrophils 27.0), platelets 325 × 10^9 l^{-1}, coagulation normal. She was on midazolam 150 mcg kg^{-1} per h but woke during this second night, moving all limbs and reaching for the endotracheal tube appropriately, pupils 3 mm bilaterally.

Day 3

The ventilator was now down to a rate of 5 breaths min^{-1} as SIMV, with pressures of 17/6 with 40% O_2. There was no acidosis. The ECG showed sinus rhythm 130/minute and the following intervals: PR 127 s, QRS 124 s, QTc 484 s. The sedation was turned off and she was extubated at 1500 h to nasal CPAP. Her blood tests at this stage; Na 153 mmol l^{-1}, Urea 8 mmol l^{-1}, creatinine 62 mcg l^{-1}, ALT 8069 IU l^{-1}, INR 1.55, APTR 1.08, WCC 17 × 10^9 l^{-1} (neutrophils 12).

At this juncture a case conference was held to try and establish the mechanism by which this girl had gained access to the dosulepin and this is referred to later.

Day 4 and 5

Over the next 24 hours she was weaned from the nasal CPAP with physiotherapy directed to a consolidation at the base of the right lung. Nasogastric feeds were increased to 125 ml kg^{-1} per day and the serum sodium dropped slowly to 149 mmol l^{-1}. She remained apyrexial but exhibited some irritability and showed uncoordinated movements. During Day 5 she was discharged to the medical ward.

Day 6 to Day 20

Day by day there was a gradual improvement in her ataxia, both fine and gross motor activity. There was also a gradual diminution in her irritability and improvement in her general affect. By discharge, she possessed normal fine motor movements with good coordination, was interested in surroundings and toys and, in particular, interacting with family in a happy manner.

Social history

The parents were interviewed on Day 2 to try and establish the circumstances in which this child had ingested the TCA. She was the youngest of two siblings of her mother's present union, her elder daughter aged 2 years 9 months. Her mother also had a son aged 5 years 9 months by a previous union, who also lived with her, her new partner and the two girls. On the day of presentation, the two older children woke at about 07.00 h and played in various rooms. The parents heard an unusual cry and went to her room at 09.00 h. The child then had a fit and they called the ambulance. The mother had been under treatment for depression, taking dosulepin until month before. They were kept on the top shelf of a kitchen cupboard, thought to be unreachable by any of the children (even if standing on a chair). On return from his daughter's admission to the hospital, the father found the dosulepin in the normal place. There was one strip present in the box with six tablets removed. The mother thought that this should have been an intact strip but could not be certain. No tablets or foil strips were found in the bedrooms. Their friends' daughter was babysitting the night before 20.30–22.30 h. There had been no problems with the children reported during that period, the children having been put to bed before the parents went out. The other children were seen and examined and there were no cause for concern detectable. In view of the ongoing uncertainty regarding the mechanism of administration of the drug, the matter was referred to the Child Protection Team, including Police and Social Services, for further investigation and management.

Five months later

She was reviewed by the Community Pediatric Service and was behaving and developing normally. In the intervening period she had undergone both a hearing test and an MRI of her brain. Both investigations were reported as normal.

Discussion

A rational approach to treatment depends on an accurate appreciation of the pharmacology of this class of drug (the pharmacokinetic properties and pharmacodynamic actions), the clinical features of toxicity and the pathophysiology behind them.

Pharmacology

There are four main pharmacodynamic actions:

(a) Anticholinergic actions (muscarinic). This is exploited in the treatment of enuresis but, at toxic levels, the features resemble overdose of atropine or hyoscine with pronounced anticholinergic blockade, namely; peripheral – tachycardia, decreased sweating (anhidrosis); and central – decreased conscious state (drowsiness, disorientation delerium and convulsions), disturbed hypothalamic thermoregulation (pyrexia) and dilated pupils (mydriasis).

(b) Inhibition of noradrenaline (and serotonin) reuptake at nerve terminals. This is the main therapeutic action centrally in the treatment of endogenous depression. In toxicity, any transient rise in blood pressure is superseded by the catecholamine depletion that ensues with resultant hypotension.

(c) Direct alpha-adrenergic blockade. Reduction in peripheral vascular resistance and further hypotension.

(d) Inhibition of fast myocardial sodium channels by membrane stabilizing/local anesthetic effect – similar to Class 1 drugs of Vaughan Williams' classification of anti-arrhythmic drugs. Sasynuik has delineated the pathophysiology of poisoning thus: decreased conduction velocity with prolongation of action potential and depolarization; the refractory period is shortened but the net effect on the QT interval, due to the grossly widened QRS in more severe cases, is prolongation; depression of contractility.[3]

Tricyclics are rapidly absorbed from the gastrointestinal tract despite the anticholinergic effects. Tricyclics are bases and are ionized in the gastric lumen. However, once in the alkaline medium of the small bowel, they are less ionized and cross the gut wall. In the plasma they are highly protein bound but the free fraction increases when the plasma pH decreases. Therefore, under conditions of acidosis, more is available to be redistributed into the tissues and exert greater effects. Plasma levels do not reflect the total load as the drug is highly protein bound and the free (ionised) fraction will decrease with a rise in the plasma pH. Generally, this class of drug has a long elimination half-life (e.g. amitryptiline = 31–46 hours) and first-pass metabolites often have intrinsic activity as well. Slowing of the intestinal transit will increase entero-hepatic circulation, exacerbating these effects. Final elimination is via hepatic conjugation and renal excretion.

Clinical presentation

The principal clinical features are:

- Neurological – decreased conscious state, confusion, respiratory depression and convulsions;
- Cardiovascular – tachycardia, hypotension, vasodilatation, decreased contractility, prolonged QRS, heart block, ventricular tachyarrhythmias, and metabolic acidosis.

Features of poisoning may range from isolated drowsiness and/or ataxia to a combination of the more severe manifestations listed above. With a positive history but in the absence of symptoms, the child should be observed for 6 hours. A history of the amount taken may be helpful, but usually in children it is hard to be certain of this and other features should be considered. Any signs of toxicity will have appeared in this time.

Seizures are associated with a QRS >0.1 seconds[4] and, in a group of such patients, Boehnert reported that 34% of these developed seizures and 14% ventricular arrhythmias.[4] However, no ventricular arrhythmias were seen in this series unless the QRS ≥0.16 seconds. When the ECG lead aVR was examined, the amplitude of the terminal R wave appeared to be a better predictor of both seizures and arrhythmias, independently of age, but these authors note that the Receiver Operating Curve (ROC) analysis for this aVR derivative did not differ significantly from that for simple QRS interval measurement.[5]

The genesis of the acidosis in TCA poisoning needs to be explained. Early in the presentation, before appropriate supportive measures are undertaken, there may well be a respiratory acidosis due to the neurological effects of the drug causing a decreased conscious level and respiratory depression. There is often a metabolic component that dominates and this can be quite severe. The etiology of this is multifactorial:

- Direct α-blockade action produces vasodilatation and hypotension.
- Direct peripheral anticholinergic action increases the heart rate and decreases diastolic filling time.
- Direct binding of TCA to fast sodium channels produces conduction defects throughout the myocardium. Where heart block ensues, this affects coordinated filling of the heart and, when the His–Purkinje conduction mechanism is affected (wider QRS), then systolic efficiency is reduced.
- Inhibition of voltage dependent calcium channels that impairs myocardial contractility.[6]
- Central anticholinergic actions increase metabolic activity, disrupt temperature homeostasis and impair sweating. These actions generate pyrexia, which will be exacerbated markedly by seizure activity.

Thus, increased demands, coupled with diminished cardiac output, generate the metabolic acidosis. However, it is important to note that TCA poisoning can exist without an acidosis.

It is therefore important to realize that an acidosis does not need to be present for the patient to receive the specific treatment of alkalinization. Sodium bicarbonate is effective even in the absence of acidosis.[3]

Treatment strategies

General

As with all emergency cases, life support should be commenced with rapid assessment and management of basic functions; ensuring integrity of the airway, adequate ventilation and oxygenation and volume support of the circulation. Initiation of baseline investigations should be undertaken early to assess blood chemistry and gases, glucose level, blood cultures and, where poisoning suspected, plasma and urine assays for either immediate screening or storage until the history is more clear. It is, however, important to realize that blood levels of TCA will not reflect the load of ingested drug nor the clinical severity. This is due to delayed absorption and variability in protein binding. There has been some debate as to the place of gastric lavage and instillation of charcoal. The rationale for gastric lavage was partly based on the fact that TCAs would slow gastric emptying due to their anticholinergic action. However, the consensus appears to be that it is only effective if carried out within 1 hour of the ingestion and the rationale for charcoal is, again, somewhat theoretical. In practice, there is equipoise amongst studies either supporting or refuting the benefits of charcoal.[7]

Specific treatment for TCA poisoning

Alkalinization

Original studies from France in the 1960s reported benefits of administration of sodium bicarbonate. In 1973, Brown reported benefits of sodium bicarbonate administration in five children together with experimental work in dogs exploring these actions.[8] The beneficial effects of sodium bicarbonate have been confirmed by other workers and the place of sodium bicarbonate in tricyclic poisoning is well established. Brown also found that administering trishydroxyaminomethane (THAM), where this corrected the acidosis, also reversed arrhythmias.[8]

In experimental intoxication with TCA in dogs, sodium bicarbonate reverses the impairment of conduction by raising the pH, as previously shown, but also by increasing extracellular fluid sodium, which also diminishes the local anesthetic action and reverses the channel blockade.[3] The mechanism for the local effect of alkalinization is thought to be an uncoupling of the TCA molecule from the sodium channel[9] and this may be associated with a decreased "protonation" of the drug-receptor complex.[3] Additionally, alkalinization will lower ECF potassium, thus reducing the hyperpolarization across the myocyte and this is thought to be of benefit.[3]

Although the ECG in TCA poisoning shows lengthening of both the QRS and the QT intervals, experimentally repolarization is shortened. This is explained by a biphasic phenomenon: in mild toxicity the QT is shortened but with larger doses the QT is lengthened.[3] The QRS interval is a component of and so will affect the QT interval; this is particularly true at higher heart rates, when it has been observed that the QRS will lengthen in a rate-dependent manner.[10] When the heart rate is artificially controlled (by crushing the sinus node in an animal model), then the QTc does not lengthen and none of those animals developed ventricular tachycardia (VT).[10] However, when sinus tachycardia was allowed to occur, then the QTc did lengthen significantly and most of those animals developed VT. When atrially paced at a higher rate, all the animals developed VT. A case was therefore made for the administration of beta blocking agents; however, the clinical context of hypotension and poor myocardial function does not usually permit this.

Hyperventilation has been proposed as a means of alkalinization, but this may lower the seizure threshold due to further reducing cerebral blood flow where there may already be decreased cardiac output.[10] In an experimental model, raising pH by lowering the partial pressure of CO_2 was not as effective as administration of bicarbonate[3] and Brown found the effects of hyperventilation partial and transient.[8]

The optimal degree of alkalinization is not yet clear. In a study of 58 regional poison centre directors in the United States, Seger found that the commonest criterion for starting bicarbonate was a QRS width of ≥ 0.1 seconds and the most often quoted range for target pH was 7.45 to 7.55. In the absence of robust data, she concluded that such centers should collaborate to produce a consensus document on such treatment criteria.[6]

Inotropic support

As mentioned above, a high heart rate will increase the degree of conduction delay and increases the QRS width. Therefore, it might be expected that inotropes would exacerbate this. Knudsen and Abrahamsson studied TCA poisoning in rats examining the effects of adrenaline, noradrenaline and sodium bicarbonate separately and then combining bicarbonate with one or other of the two inotropes.[9] They found that there was no evidence that inotropes made the conduction deficit worse over controls. However, the time to developing arrhythmias compared to controls was shortened by use of noradrenaline alone or noradrenaline and sodium bicarbonate, very slightly lengthened with adrenaline alone, and lengthened more by administration of sodium bicarbonate. The Adrenaline–bicarbonate combination not only provided the most delay of arrhythmia development, but was associated with the most effective shortening of the QRS as well as the greatest number of survivors.

In analysis of Kaplan–Meier survival plots, they found that, in terms of numbers of survivors, the control group – with no added therapy – fared worse, then, in order of increasing survival, bicarbonate alone, noradrenaline alone, noradrenaline combined with bicarbonate, adrenaline alone and then, as the treatment giving most survivors, adrenaline in combination with sodium bicarbonate.

They noted that the use of adrenaline and bicarbonate seemed to be associated with a drop in the serum potassium concentration and they postulated that this might be one mechanism for the beneficial actions seen. The possible benefits of the relative drop in the potassium concentration was also noted by Sasynuik.[3]

Hypertonic saline

There is some debate regarding the benefit of intravenous hypertonic saline in the management of TCA poisoning. Clearly, there is a theoretical basis for this, as has been stated above.[3,9] Although there have been case reports of beneficial effects in humans[13] and in experimental animal models, no consistent pattern has emerged.[11] In an *in vitro* preparation of amitryptiline–toxic canine myocardium, Sasynuik examined the effects of three different solutions on restoring conduction velocity: a high sodium solution, a low pCO_2/high pH/ normal sodium solution (*quasi* respiratory alkalosis) and a high sodium/high pH solution, attempting to simulate the conditions that would apply with therapeutic administration of hypertonic saline, hyperventilation, and sodium bicarbonate, respectively. The sodium bicarbonate had most effect, followed by the respiratory alkalosis, with the high sodium solution having least effect. In his *in vivo* experiments in amitryptiline – toxic dogs, Brown detected no effect with a high sodium bolus dose (approx. 4 ml kg^{-1} of 6N saline).[8]

Antiarrhythmics

TCAs impede fast myocyte sodium channels affecting the rapid phase 0 of the action potential cycle. This decreases conduction velocity, increases the duration of the action potential, and decreases conduction through the His–Purkinje system. The resultant effects are a lengthening of the QRS and a predisposition to re-entry arrhythmias, heart block and asystole.[3] The degree of impairment of conduction is heart rate dependent.[3,10] Any arrhythmic agent that decreases conduction velocity, the duration of the action potential and the refractory period should be avoided. In the Vaughan Williams classification, this would include Class 1a (quinidine, procainamide, disopyramide), Class 1c (flecanide), and Class 3 (amiodarone, propafenone, sotalol).

However, Class 1b (lidocaine, phenytoin, mexilitene), although slowing phase 0, reduce total action potential duration. Phenytoin appears to selectively increase conduction in Purkinje fibres[12] and so has potential theoretical benefits in TCA poisoning. However, there are no clinical data to support its use in this context.

In view of their characteristics, only Class 1b drugs should be used in refractory arrhythmias, but only after other measures such as alkalinization, electrolyte correction and cardiovascular support with volume and inotropes have already been undertaken.

In the case reported here, no specific advice regarding the disadvantages of amiodarone were received from the Poisons Advice Service. It is likely, though conjectural, that the conduction defect already apparent in this case was exacerbated by the use of this agent and may have contributed to the need for pacing intervention.

Other therapies

Although it is recognized that any ingested TCA will be highly protein bound, hemoperfusion has been proposed as a means of clearing the body of ingested drug particularly by removing what free fraction exists and so enabling diffusion of TCA away from active sites such as the myocardium. The amount of drug actually removed appears to be disappointing.[7] However, this technique will only extract what free drug there is in the intravascular compartment and may distract the treating team from ensuring that other, simpler measures are employed to the full. For example, in a recent case report in a 17-month-old child, alkalinization was never achieved before the procedure started and there were six episodes of ventricular fibrillation during the 2-hour hemoperfusion.[14]

Magnesium has been used with apparent success and, although some supportive experimental work has been performed,[15] there are as yet not enough data regarding this treatment to inform routine practice. It may be an alternative to lidocaine in arrhythmias refractory to more established treatment as outlined above.

Glucagon has been proposed as a treatment for both arrhythmias and hypotension refractory to catecholamine infusions in various case reports,[16] but it is questionable again whether more standard treatment, for example, alkalinization, had been carried out in line with what is already known and generally accepted.[17] A recent review failed to show any convincing evidence for recommending the use of glucagon in this setting.[18]

Antigen-binding fragments (Fab) have been in use for some years in the treatment of digoxin overdose and have been developed to bind with TCAs. These substances have half-lives of 12–20 hours and so relatively similar to those of TCAs. However, the amount (in milligrams) of these polyclonal antibodies required is many times the drug burden and there is a cost implication in developing these commercially as well as contending with their known potential for renal toxicity.[19,7]

Learning points

- The mainstay of treatment at all times will be to ensure there is a clear airway, efficient ventilation, and gas exchange and the addressing of any circulatory failure.

- If there is any respiratory depression, given the delayed progression of these TCA poisonings, then intubation and ventilation to ensure control of gas exchange should be undertaken early, with a view to ensure that the patient is well oxygenated and normocarbic.

- The circulation should be supported with volume initially and, if hypotension or under perfusion are refractory to this, then an adrenalin infusion should be commenced, remembering that its effects may be beneficial and additive to those sodium bicarbonate.[9] It can be administered peripherally while central access is secured.

- Monitoring of ECG, peripheral saturations, and end-expired CO_2 should be established early and the QRS interval should be assessed. If this is 0.1 seconds or greater, then sodium bicarbonate should be administered with a view to alkalinizing the patient (e.g. to a pH of 7.45–7.55), *even in the absence of an initial acidosis.*[3]

- If arrhythmias occur and do not respond to these measures, then consider giving lidocaine or phenytoin. It should be remembered that any antiarrhythmic agent other than these two is likely to cause more problems than it is likely to solve and this is borne out by the clinical course of our patient where the administration of amiodarone was ill-advised.

- Seizures should be treated with benzodiazepines (lorazepam) and this can be followed by an infusion of midazolam if the patient is ventilated. Phenytoin *may* be of benefit in treating both seizures and arrhythmias but the evidence does not exist to support this.

- Pyrexia will exacerbate the acidosis, especially where the cardiac output is poor, and should be treated actively. This may require ongoing muscle relaxation as part of the ventilation strategy to facilitate cooling. If muscle relaxants are used, then prophylactic anticonvulsants should be given and the EEG monitored.

- At all stages of this process, the team should seek and follow the advice of their local Poisons Centre to ensure timely and up-to-date practice. Consequently, Poisons Centres must ensure that the advice they give is consistent with the most recent evidence.

Acknowledgments

The author would like to thank Dr. James Fraser, Dr. Heather Duncan, Dr. Nigel Humphreys, Dr. Andrew Tometzki, and the Nurses of the Paediatric Intensive Care Unit in Bristol for their help in treating this patient, and Ms. Elizabeth Jordan, Librarian of the Learning Resources Centre, United Bristol Healthcare Trust, for her help in locating the older references.

References

1. http://www.dh.gov.uk/ PublicationsAndStatistics/Publications/fs/en. Department of Health, England, 2005.

2. http://www.publications.doh.gov.uk/ prescriptionstatistics/index.htm Department of Health, England, 2005.

3. Sasynuik BI, Jhamandas V, Valois M. *Ann Emerg Med* 1986; **15**: 1052–9.

4. Boehnert MT, Lovejoy FH. Value of the QRS duration versus the serum drug level in predicting seizures and ventricular arrhythmias after an acute overdose of tricyclic antidepressants. *N Engl J Med* 1985; **313**: 474–9.

5. Liebelt EL, Francis PD, Woolf AD. ECG lead aVR versus QRS interval in predicting seizures and arrhythmias in acute tricyclic antidepressant toxicity. *Ann Emerg Med* 1995; **26**: 195–201.

6. Seger DL, Hantsch C, Zavoral T *et al.* Variability of recommendations for serum alkalinisation in tricyclic antidepressant overdose: a survey of US poison center medical directors. *J Toxicol Clin Toxicol* 2003; **41**(4): 331–8.

7. Kerr GW, McGuffie AC, Wilkie S. Tricyclic antidepressant overdose: a review. *Emerg Med J*; **18**: 234–41.

8. Brown TCK, Barker GA, Dunlop ME *et al.* The use of sodium bicarbonate in the treatment of tricyclic antidepressant induced arrhythmias. *Anaest Intens Care* 1973; **1**(3): 203–10.

9. Knudsen K, Abrahamsson J. Epinephrine and sodium bicarbonate independently and additively increase survival in experimental amitryptiline poisoning. *Crit Care Med* 1997; **25**(4): 669–74.

10. Ansel GM, Coyne K, Arnold S *et al.* Mechanisms of ventricular arrhythmia during amitryptiline toxicity. *J Cardiovasc Pharmacol* 1993; **22**(6): 798–803.

11. Seger D. Tricyclic antidepressant treatment ambiguities. *Ann Emerg Med* 2004; **43**(6): 785–6.

12. Opie LH. Drugs and the heart. *Lancet,* 1980: 39–57.

13. McKinney P, Rasmussen R. Reversal of severe tricyclic antidepressant-induced cardiotoxicity with intravenous hypertonic saline solution. *Ann Emerg Med* 2003; **42**: 20–4.

14. Dönmez O, Cetinkaya M, Rahmiye C. Hemoperfusion in a child with amitryptiline intoxication. *Pediatr Nephrol* 2005; **20**: 105–7.

15. Knudsen K, Abrahamsson J. Magnesium sulphate in the treatment of ventricular fibrillation in amitryptiline poisoning. *Eur Heart J* 1997; **18**: 881–2.

16. Sensky PR, Olczak SA. High-dose intravenous glucagons in severe tricyclic poisoning. *Postgrad Med J* 1999; **75**: 611–12.

17. Schuster-Bruce MJL. High dose intravenous glucagon in severe tricyclic poisoning. *Postgrad Med J* 2000; **76**: 453.

18. Teece S, Hogg K. Glucagon in tricyclic overdose. *Emerg Med J* 2003; **20**: 264–5.

19. Flanagan RJ, Jones AL. Fab antibody fragments: some applications in clinical toxicology. *Drug Saf* 2004; **27**(14): 1115–33.

Chapter 8

Management of hemolytic uremic syndrome

Gabrielle A. Nuthall

Introduction

Hemolytic uremic syndrome (HUS) is an important cause of acute renal failure in children. The majority of cases are diarrhea-associated HUS, which occurs sporadically and, less commonly, in outbreaks. Atypical cases, which are not associated with diarrhea, also occur. Treatment is mainly supportive and designed to support renal function until there is spontaneous recovery.

Case history

A previously well 19-month-old boy presented with a 4-day history of bloody diarrhoea. He had been seen by his primary care physician on day 2 of the illness and started on amoxycillin. On the day of admission, his mother was not sure when he had last passed any urine and he was lethargic and floppy. He was again seen by his primary care physician and referred to the local hospital.

Examination

On arrival in the emergency department, he looked unwell with a decreased level of responsiveness and was irritable. He was breathing spontaneously with good bilateral air entry, a respiratory rate of 32 and saturations of 99% in $4\,l\,min^{-1}$ of oxygen via face mask. His heart rate was 166 with normal heart sounds, blood pressure of 80/42 mmHg and a delayed capillary refill time of 4 seconds. His abdominal examination was unremarkable. Glasgow Coma Score (GCS) was assessed as 13/15 (eyes-4, verbal-4, motor-5). Pupils were equal and reactive. He was placed on a cardiac monitor, intravenous access was obtained, and blood was sent for FBC, U and Es, glucose and a blood culture. An arterial blood gas was also obtained. He was given a 240 ml bolus of normal saline ($20\,ml\,kg^{-1}$) and started on maintenance fluids. He had a stat dose of a third-generation cephalosporin and a Chest X-Ray (CXR), which was normal. For results, see Table 8.1.

After discussion with the pediatrician on call, it was felt most likely that he had HUS and the paediatric intensive care unit (PICU) were contacted and elected to organise to retrieve the patient by air ambulance with their transport team. His blood film was then reported as having fragmented red blood cells, supporting the initial diagnosis of HUS.

When the PICU transport team arrived at the referring hospital, his vital signs were HR 141, sinus rhythm, BP 80/45, spontaneously breathing with a respiratory rate of 32 breaths $min^{-1}$and saturations of 99% in $4\,l\,min^{-1}$ of oxygen. His capillary refill had improved to 2 seconds following his initial bolus of normal saline. However, his GCS had decreased to 10/15 (eyes-3, verbal-3, motor-4) and it was decided to intubate him for the transfer. His pupils remained equal and reactive. For a rapid sequence induction, he was given

Case Studies in Pediatric Critical Care, ed. Peter. J. Murphy, Stephen C. Marriage, and Peter J. Davis. Published by Cambridge University Press. © Cambridge University Press 2009.

Table 8.1. *Findings on admission*

Past medical history	Fit and well	
Regular medications	None	
Allergies	None known	
Examination	Decreased level of responsiveness	
	Airway clear, face mask oxygen	
	Spontaneous respirations, RR 32	
	Chest clear with bilateral air entry, Sats 99% in O_2	
	Normal heart sounds, HR 161, BP 80/42	
	Capillary refill time = 4 seconds	
	Temperature 36.8°C	
Investigations	Weight 12 kg	
	FBC	WCC 23.9×10^9 l^{-1}, Hb 86 g l^{-1}
		platelet 56×10^9 l^{-1}
	U + E's	Na 119 mmol l^{-1}, K 5.4 mmol l^{-1},
		Urea 31 mmol l^{-1},
		Creatinine 0.43 mmol l^{-1}, Ca total
		1.84 mmol l^{-1}
	Glucose	6.9 mmol l^{-1}
	Arterial blood	pH 7.23, O_2 15.4 kPa, CO_2 3.9 kPa
	Gas (ABG)	HCO_3 12 mmol l^{-1}

propofol 25 mg and suxamethonium 25 mg and intubated uneventfully with a size 4.5 uncuffed endotracheal tube, initially orally and then changed to a nasal tube, secured at 15 cm at the nares, for the transport. A nasogastric (NG) tube and urinary catheter were also inserted along with a second intravenous line. His ventilatory settings were as follows: rate of 20 with a peak inspiratory pressure (PIP) of 18 mmHg and a positive end expiratory pressure (PEEP) of 5 mmHg. He had saturations of 100% in 40% oxygen.

Repeat electrolytes showed that his K^+ had risen to 6.8 and he was given stat doses of Resonium A (6 g via NG), 1.2 units of insulin and 120 ml of 10% dextrose intravenously (IV). Following this, his K^+ fell to 5.2, in view of his low HCO_3 he was also given a dose of bicarbonate of 15 mmol over half an hour.

He was then transferred to PICU via air ambulance. He had a non-eventful transfer, his sedation was managed with a morphine infusion of 20 mcg kg^{-1} per h and intermittent doses of diazepam, and he had stable vital signs and ventilation.

Progress in the intensive care unit

On arrival in the pediatric intensive care unit, his vital signs and ventilation remained stable. He had a 22G arterial line inserted into his left radial artery, for blood sampling and continuous blood pressure monitoring. He had repeat FBC, U and Es, coagulation screen and arterial blood gas (ABG) sent. The results of these were Hb 100 g l^{-1}, platelets 79×10^9 l^{-1}, white cell count $18.0 \times 10^9\,l^{-1}$, Na^+ 120 mmol l^{-1}, K^+ 4.4 mmol l^{-1}, glucose 5.6 mmol l^{-1}, urea 30 mmol l^{-1}, creatinine 0.47 mmol l^{-1} and anion gap 19.9, pH 7.27, O_2 31.1 kPa, CO_2 4.3 kPa, HCO_3 14.6 mmol l^{-1}. The coagulation screen was normal. He was given a second dose of HCO_3 of 15 mmol over half an hour.

He had not passed any urine since the time of his arrival in the presenting hospital and, upon further questioning of his mother, may not have passed urine for up to 48 hours before admission.

After review of his clinical and laboratory findings, the intensive care specialist and pediatric renal physician decided he needed renal replacement therapy. Soon after arrival, he went to the operating room for insertion of a Tenkhoff catheter and subsequently started on peritoneal dialysis that evening. Peritoneal Dialysis (PD) was started with hourly dwell cycles with a volume of 10 mls kg per 1 and 1.5% dialyslate fluid.

He remained hemodynamically stable overnight with minimal ventilatory requirements. PD worked well overnight and the repeat bloods in the morning were improved: Na^+ 132 mmol l^{-1}, K^+ 4.2 mmol l^{-1}, urea 30.8 mmol l^{-1}, creatinine 0.45 mmol l^{-1}, Hb 82 g l^{-1}, platelets $91 \times 10^9\,l^{-1}$ and WCC $17.4 \times 10^9\,l^{-1}$, the blood film was reported as having thrombocytopenia with the presence of spherocytes, cell fragments, and polychromatic cells, consistent with a microangiopathic hemolytic anemia. ABG was also improved, pH 7.28, O_2 13.3 kPa, CO_2 5.2 kPa, HCO_3 18 mmol l^{-1}.

In view of his abnormal GCS at presentation, a CT scan of his brain was organized the morning following admission. This was normal, with no evidence of cerebral edema or focal lesions. His sedation was stopped and over the day he slowly woke up and was able to be extubated in the afternoon following admission. His peritoneal dialysis was successfully increased to a volume of 20 ml kg^{-1} and to 2-hourly cycles. He was tolerating a small amount of enteral feed and, while still not completely his normal self, had a GCS of 15/15. He was therefore transferred to the ward the following morning to continue his peritoneal dialysis and while grading up on his enteral feeds. The third-generation cephalosporin started at presentation was continued for 48 h then stopped as his blood culture was negative.

Over the next 36 hours on the ward, he again became increasingly drowsy and when reassessed by the PICU team had a GCS fluctuating between 5 (E = 3, M = 2, V = 1) and 11 (E = 4, M = 4, V = 3) with at times an irregular breathing pattern. He was intubated with a rapid sequence induction, using propofol 25 mg, suxamethonium 25 mg, and an oral 4.5 uncuffed endotracheal tube. He had a repeat CT scan of his head, which was normal. He was taken back to the PICU and ventilated overnight. The following morning he was again able to be extubated but remained in the PICU for a further 3 days with a fluctuating level of consciousness. By the time of discharge to the ward he had a GCS of 15. The fluctuating level of consciousness since his presentation was attributed to HUS encephalopathy.

Over this time his PD continued with 2-hourly cycles of 300 ml of 1.5% diasylate. At the time of transfer to the ward his urea was stable at 19 mmol l^{-1} and his creatinine at 0.4 mmol l^{-1}. He was fully enterally fed and his fluid balance status was stable. He remained anuric.

He spent a further 2 weeks on the ward receiving PD, over which time his renal function gradually improved. By 17 days following his second PICU discharge, his renal function was recovered enough to allow removal of the Tenkhoff catheter and he was discharged the same day. At the time of discharge, his urea was 9.2 mmol l^{-1}, his creatinine was 0.11 mmol l^{-1} and his electrolytes were normal. His neurological examination at this point was entirely normal.

He was seen in clinic 1 week after discharge where he was entirely well, with his renal function continuing to improve. His local hospital were asked to continue his follow-up, with a 2-monthly creatinine, urine analysis, and blood pressure check, until they were all normal. Following this, the recommendation was for a yearly creatinine, urine analysis, and blood pressure check.

Discussion

Hemolytic uremic syndrome (HUS) is a major cause of acute renal failure in children. In one series 60% of children presenting to a PICU with acute renal failure requiring renal replacement therapy had diarrhea associated HUS.[1] HUS is characterized by microangiopathic hemolytic anemia (anemia secondary to red blood cell fragmentation), thrombocytopenia and acute renal impairment (see Fig. 8.1). There are two distinct subgroups of HUS. The majority (~90%) of cases are associated with a diarrheal illness and is called typical or D+HUS. A smaller subgroup, usually called atypical cases (aHUS), are associated with a variety of causes (idiopathic, inherited complement regulatory defects, autoimmune disease, drugs, neuraminidase producing *Strep. pneumoniae* infection, HIV, pregnancy, inherited metabolic disease, and tumors).

The incidence of HUS varies between countries from 0.51–2.0 per 100 000 in the <5-year-old group and 0.25–1.5 per 100 000 in those <15 years old,[2–6] see Table 8.2 for details. Despite increasing awareness of food-borne diseases and measures undertaken for prevention, the worldwide incidence of diarrheal-associated HUS is largely unchanged.

Diarrhea-positive cases are associated with Shiga toxin producing *Escherichia coli* (STEC) in the majority of cases (70–80%), also known as verotoxins. In North America, New Zealand, and Japan STEC 0157:H7 is the predominant serotype.[7] Europe previously experienced the same predominance of STEC 0157:H7, but recent reports show that the number of cases associated with this serotype is falling[3] and in Australia the predominant serotype is 0111:H-.[7] Other infectious agents have also been implicated, especially enterohemorrhagic *E. coli* and *Shigella dysenteriae* type 1.[8] Diarrhea-associated HUS may occur sporadically, or in outbreaks, with reports that the outbreak-associated HUS has higher morbidity and mortality with up to 80% having anuric renal failure, compared to ~50% in sporadic cases.[4,8] There is also a seasonal variation in most reports with summer predominance.[4,9] There has been some suggestion that the risk of developing HUS after a gastrointestinal illness is increased if antibiotic therapy was instituted for the diarrheal illness.[10]

Mortality for childhood HUS is most recently reported at between 2% and 6.6%.[3,4,8,9,10] A spectrum of extra renal manifestations, such as central nervous system (CNS) involvement,

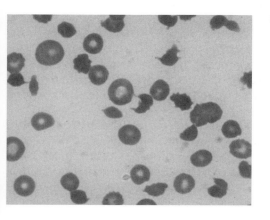

Fig. 8.1. Blood smear showing schistocytes (red blood cell fragmentation) (see color plate section).

Table 8.2. *Incidence of HUS across continents*

	Incidence per 100 000
New York [2]	
<5	2.0
5–14	0.4
Austria [3]	
<5	0.51
<15	0.36
Germany [3]	
<5	1.71
<15	0.71
Australia [4]	
<5	1.35
<15	0.64
Great Britain [5]	
<15	1.5
Italy [6]	
<15	0.25

[2] Chang
[3] Gerber
[4] Elliot
[5] Eriksson
[6] Tozzi.

colitis with colonic perforation, pancreatitis, and cardiac failure have all been reported. In places where renal support is available for acute renal failure, these extra renal manifestations are now the major determinants of mortality. The pathophysiology of these is multifactorial, but widespread thrombotic microangiopathy is consistently found in autopsy specimens[11] and is thought to play a large part in the acute renal failure seen with HUS. Predictors of severity and increased risk of mortality are an elevated white cell count ($>20 \times 10^9$ l^{-1}), a severe gastrointestinal prodrome, anuria early in the course, prolonged anuria and neurological involvement.[3,4,8,9,12]

The majority require a hospital stay with some requiring intensive care support. In one Australian study 115 children with diarrheal-associated HUS had a median duration of hospital stay of 13 days (2–87 days), with 41% (47) children requiring intensive care for a median of 4 days (1–18 days).[7]

Atypical HUS is less common, reported as being between 15% and 35% of total cases.[7,13] Again, it is most common in those under 5 years of age, but tends to have a higher mortality (reported as being as high as 26%) and morbidity than that of diarrhea-associated HUS. The incidence of extra renal manifestations is as high as 50%, and these patients more commonly need acute renal replacement therapy (up to 75% of cases) and go on to develop chronic and end-stage renal failure (up to 50% of cases), especially those with recurrent episodes of

HUS.[13] Recently, it has been found that aHUS is a disease of complement dysregulation with 50% of cases involving complement regualatory gene mutations.[14]

Initial assessment and management

A history of the presenting illness should be acquired. Of those with the typical and outbreak HUS, almost all will have a diarrheal illness, with the rest having some gastrointestinal symptoms. Approximately half of those with diarrhea will have blood in their stools. It is important to obtain a history of urine output, not only for fluid balance status, but also as an indicator of anuric renal failure. A history of CNS involvement, altered level of consciousness or seizures, is also important as it increases the likelihood of mortality and morbidity. A family history and history of recent medications may provide information helpful to diagnosis in those with atypical disease.

As with all critically ill children initial assessment should start with the ABCs (airway, breathing and circulation). For any child with a gastrointestinal illness, assessment of fluid status and degree of dehydration is always important. Dehydration is usually described as being:

MILD =   <5%

MODERATE =   5–7.5%

SEVERE =   >7.5%

A recent weight is one of the most useful ways to assess the degree of dehydration. Clinical assessment of the degree of dehydration uses the signs and symptoms of decreased urine output, dry mouth, decreased skin turgor, sunken eyes and or fontanelle, tachycardia, and changes in CNS status.

A useful formula to remember to manage replacement of fluids in dehydration is:

Percentage dehydration × weight in kg × 10 = fluid deficit (in ml)

Fluid given for resuscitation should always be isotonic and patients should be reassessed immediately after fluid boluses have been given and a close eye kept on electrolytes.

For the child in this case, his airway was clear and he was breathing spontaneously with good saturations. He was receiving oxygen via face mask as is appropriate for any acutely unwell child. He was tachycardic and had some mild decrease in his peripheral perfusion. He was assessed as being between 5% and 7.5% dehydrated and for this he received a fluid bolus of 20 ml per kg of crystalloid. He responded to this bolus by decreasing his heart rate and improving his capillary refill time and required no further boluses of fluid.

Following the assessment of the ABCs, a neurological assessment should also be made using either the Glasgow Coma Score (GCS) see Table 8.3, or the AVPU score (a = alert, v = responds to voice, p = responds to pain, u = unresponsive).

In this case the child had a GCS that was falling and a decision was made to intubate him for the air transport to ensure safety of his airway. Any child with an acute GCS <8 should be intubated for airway protection. This is especially important during transportation of sick children where access to the airway is not as readily available as in a hospital setting. This child continued having a fluctuating level of consciousness after his transfer to the ward which necessitated a second ICU admission. He had two CT scans of his head, both of which were normal. The CNS symptoms were attributed to having an HUS encephalopathy. He had no long-term neurological sequalae.

Table 8.3. *Glasgow Coma Scale*

Glasgow Coma Scale (4–15 years)		Children's Coma Scale (<4 years)		
Response	Score	Response		Score
Eyes		Eyes		
Open spontaneously	4	Open spontaneously		4
Verbal command	3	React to speech		3
Pain	2	React to pain		2
No response	1	No response		1
Best motor response		Best motor response		
Verbal command:		Spontaneous or obeys verbal command		6
Obeys	6	*Painful stimulus:*		
Pain stimulus:		Localises pain		5
Localises pain	5	Withdraws in response to pain		4
Flexion with pain	4	Abnormal flexion to pain (decorticate posture)		3
Flexion abnormal	3	Abnormal extension to pain (decerebrate posture)		2
Extension	2	No response		1
No response	1	Best verbal response		
Best verbal response		Smiles, oriented to sounds, follows objects, interacts		5
Orientated and converses	5	*Crying*	*Interacts*	
Disorientated and converses	4	Consolable	Inappropriate	4
Inappropriate words	3	Inconsistently consolable	Moaning	3
Incomprehensible sounds	2	Inconsolable	Irritable	2
No response	1	No response	No response	1

Neurological involvement in the acute phase of HUS occurs in about a third to a fifth of all cases. The forms of acute neurology seen include seizures, altered level of consciousness, irritability, or focal neurology (e.g. hemiparesis or aphasia). The mortality of those with neurological involvement has been reported to be as high as 23%[5] and in most series the majority of those who die have some form of CNS involvement.[4,5,11] Those with seizures have a higher incidence of long-term neurological sequelae.[5] Electroencephalograms (EEGs) tend to show a picture of generalized slowing consistent with an encephalopathic picture, those with seizures may have additional findings, some of which have a worse prognosis for long-term neurological sequalae.[5] The exact pathophysiology of the neurology seen in HUS is not known. It has been suggested that it may be metabolic in origin,[11] related to focal toxin mediated mechanisms resulting in focal vascular endothelial injury or to the widespread thrombotic microangiopathy that is associated with the acute real failure and colitis.[16]

Once a child with HUS has been resuscitated and has stable electrolytes, the aim should always be to provide adequate nutrition with enteral feeding, or parenterally if the gut is not able to be used.

The incidence of pancreatitis is poorly defined, as an amylase is not always checked in the acute illness. It has been reported to occur as frequently as in 20% of cases.[11] It does not appear to be clinically apparent in the majority of cases, but endocrine pancreatic insufficiency does occur, both acutely and permanently, with reports of long-term insulin-dependent diabetes mellitus occurring[4,11] so it should be considered both in the acute phase and in the follow-up of patients with HUS. In this case his glucose was normal on presentation and pancreatic insufficiency was not a problem.

Hypertension is present in ~50% of cases of HUS. If hypertension occurs, it typically does so as renal blood flow is increasing, and is usually transient, but treatment is indicated if it persists for more than 24–36 hours.

Although this patient did not require a blood transfusion for his anemia, a number of patients with HUS do require transfusions. It is unusual for these patients to require platelets, despite thrombocytopenia, but their use should be considered in those with active bleeding or a platelet count below 20×10^9 l^{-1}.

In classic diarrhea-associated HUS, antibiotic use has been implicated in precipitating HUS.[17,18] Diarrhea caused by *Escherichia coli* should therefore not automatically be treated with antibiotics. However, patients who present with a clinical picture of sepsis should be treated with clinically appropriate antibiotics, even if a case of atypical HUS is part of the differential diagnosis.[19]

Assessment and management of renal failure in HUS

In those with diarrhea-associated HUS, the incidence of those requiring renal replacement therapy of some kind is 50–70%.[4,8,9,13] In this group recurrence of HUS is uncommon and, while most have renal recovery, there are reports of up to 20% progressing on to chronic renal failure or end stage renal disease (ESRD).[4,8,9,13,15] The risk of HUS recurrence post-renal transplant is <1% in typical HUS but is approximately 50% in aHUS.[14]

There is no international consensus on the level of metabolic derangement or oliguria at which renal replacement therapy should be instituted. If a patient is completely anuric and has a moderately to severely raised urea and creatinine, most clinicians would advocate starting renal replacement therapy. The younger the patient, the lower the threshold should be for early institution of renal replacement therapy. Younger patients tolerate acute uremia poorly and it enables the implementation of adequate nutrition in a catabolic child. Peritoneal dialysis (PD) is the preferred method of renal replacement therapy when there is isolated failure of the kidneys, such as in HUS. Occasionally in a very unstable patient continuous venoveno hemofiltration (CVVH) may be required. The main advantages of PD is that it is a continuous therapy that requires neither anticoagulation nor vascular access. It is relatively simple to use and effective in children of all ages. A PD catheter needs to be inserted, the catheter type and place of insertion (operating room vs. ICU) differs between centers and should be decided upon by the surgical, nephrology and intensive care staff. The PD prescription needs to be individualized according to patient size and condition and this should be done in conjunction with a nephrologist. The general principle is to start with the solutions with the lowest concentration of glucose available, at an initial volume of 10 ml kg^{-1} and 1 hour dwell times. This can be then be altered as needed.

The child in this case was anuric on presentation to the PICU and had significant metabolic derangement with a urea of 30 mmol l^{-1} and a creatinine of 0.447 mmol l^{-1}. He was hemodynamically stable and a decision was therefore made to send him to the operating room for insertion of a Tenkhoff catheter. He was started on PD with hourly dwell cycles, a volume of 10 ml kg^{-1} and 1.5% diasylate. PD was straightforward and continued for 23 days until his own renal function had improved enough for his Tenkhoff catheter to be removed.

Role of plasma exchange

The role of plasma exchange in HUS is not established. There is some overlap between HUS and thrombotic thrombocytopenic purpura (TTP) and discriminating aHUS from TTP can present a major diagnostic challenge. TTP is a disorder primarily of adults, but is also characterized by microangiopathic hemolytic anemia, thrombocytopenia and impairment of multiple organ systems. Typically, TTP is diagnosed when neurological features predominate and aHUS when renal failure predominates.[14] The role of plasma exchange in some forms of TTP is reported as being useful.[8,20,21] There are also successful reports of the use of plasma exchange in high-risk adult HUS patients, more particularly in those cases associated with outbreaks or with aHUS.[14,22,23] In cases that are difficult to manage, those with severe extra renal manifestations and those in whom there is an overlap with TTP, its use may be considered. There is also discussion in the literature about the use of plasma infusion ($30–40$ ml kg^{-1} initial dose, then 20 ml kg^{-1} daily) in both aHUS and TTP.[14]

Learning points

- The management of any acutely unwell child should always start with the basics – Airway, Breathing and Circulation followed by a neurological assessment.

- The management of HUS is mainly supportive.

- Any fluid balance and electrolyte problems should be recognized and addressed.

- Risk factors for severe disease and mortality should be assessed and taken into account when making management decisions: elevated white cell count, severe gastrointestinal prodrome, prolonged anuria, neurological symptoms, and atypical disease.

- Renal replacement therapy is required in ~50% of these children, and intensive care support in up to 40%. Consideration of transfer to a hospital setting where this is possible should therefore be considered early on in their presentation.

- Plasma exchange and or plasma infusion may have a role in the management of a minority of these patients.

- With rapid diagnosis and good supportive management the majority of cases with typical HUS do well and have no long-term morbidity.

References

1. Wong W, McCall E, Anderson B, Segedin E, Morris M. Acute renal failure in the paediatric intensive care unit. *NZ Med J* 1996; **109**: 459–61.

2. Chang H, Tserenpuntsag B, Kacica M, Smith P, Morse D. Hemolytic uremic syndrome incidence in New York. *Emerg Infect Dis* 2004; **10**: 928–31.

3. Gerber A, Karch H, Allerberger F, Verweyen HM, Zimmerhackl LB. Clinical course and the role of Shiga toxin-producing *Escherichia coli* infection in the haemolytic–uremic syndrome in pediatric patients, 1997–2000, in Germany and Austria: a prospective study. *JID* 2002; **186**: 493–500.

4. Elliott EJ, Robins-Browne RM, O'Loughlin EV *et al*. Nationwide study of haemolytic uraemic syndrome: clinical, microbiological, and epidemiological features. *Arch Dis Child* 2001; **85**: 125–31.

5. Eriksson KJ, Boyd SG, Tasker RC. Acute neurology and neurophysiology of haemolytic-uraemic syndrome. *Arch Dis Child* 2001; **84**: 434–5.

6. Tozzi AE, Caprioli A, Minelli F *et al*. Shiga toxin-producing *Escherichia coli* infections assoicated with hemolytic uremic syndrome, Italy, 1988–2000. *Emerg Infect Dis* 2003; **9**: 106–8.

7. Elliot E, Williams K, Ridley G *et al. Ninth Annual Report.* Australian Paediatric Surveillance Unit. 2001; 9–11.

8. Corrigan JJ, Boineau FG. Hemolytic–uremic syndrome. *Pediatr Rev* 2001; **22**: 365–369

9. Boyce TG, Swerdlow DL, Griffin PM. Current Concepts: Escherichia coli O157: H7 and the Hemolytic-Uremic Syndrome. *N Engl J Med* 1995; **333**: 364–8 (abstr).

10. Wong C, Jelacic S, Habeed RL, Watkins SL, Tarr PI. The risk of the haemolytic-uremic syndrome after antibiotic treatment of *Escherichia coli* O157:H7 infections. *N Engl J Med* 2000; **342**: 1930–6.

11. Siegler RL. Spectrum of extrarenal involvement in postdiarrheal haemolytic-uremic syndrome. *J Pediatr* 1994; **125**: 511–18 (abstr)

12. Banatvala N, Griffin PM, Greene KD *et al.* The United States National Prospective Hemolytic Uremic Syndrome Study: microbiologic, serologic, clinical and epidemiologic findings. *JID* 2001; **183**: 1063–70.

13. Neuhaus TJ, Calonder S, Leumann EP. Heterogeneity of atypical haemolytic uraemic syndromes. *Arch Dis Child* 1997; **76**: 518–21 (abstr).

14. Kavanagh D, Goodship T, Richards A. Atypical haemolytic uraemic syndrome. *Br Med Bull* 2006; 77–78: 5–22.

15. Amirlak I, Amirlak B. Haemolytic uraemic syndrome: an overview. *Nephrology* 2006; **11**: 213–18.

16. Gallo GE, Gianantonio CA. Extrarenal involvement in diarrhoea – associated haemolytic–uremic syndrome, *Pediatr Nephrol* 1995; **9**: 117–19.

17. Wong CS, Jelacic S, Habeeb RL, Watkins SL, Tarr PI. The risk of the haemolytic–uraemic syndrome after antibiotic treatment of *Escherichia coli* O157:H7 infections. *N Engl J Med* 2000; **342**: 1930–6.

18. Safdar N, Said A, Gangnon RE, Maki DG. Risk of haemolytic uremic syndrome after antibiotic treatment of *Escherichia coli* O157: H7 enteritis: a meta-analysis. *J Am Med Assoc.* 2002; **288**: 996–1001.

19. Phillips B, Yyerman K, Whiteley SM. Use of antibiotics in suspected haemolytic-uraemic syndrome. *Br Med J* 2005; **330**: 409–410

20. Hollenbeck M, Kutkuhn B, Aul C, Leschke M, Willers R, Grabensee B. Haemolytic-uraemic syndrome and thrombotic-thrombocytopenic purpura in adults: clinical findings and prognostic factors for death and end-stage renal disease. *Nephrol Dial Transpl* 1998; **13**: 76–81.

21. Andersohn F, Hagmann FG, Garbe E. Thrombotic thrombocytopenic purpura/ haemolytic uraemic syndrome associated with clopidogrel: report of two new cases. *Heart* 2004; **90**: e57 (abstr).

22. Ruggenenti P, Noris M, Remuzzi G. Thrombotic microangiopathy, haemolytic uremic syndrome, and thrombotic thrombocytopenic purpura. *Kidney Int* 2001; **60**: 831–846 (abstr).

23. Dundas S, Murphy J, Soutar RL, Jones GA, Hutchinson SJ, Todd WTA. Effectiveness of therapeutic plasma exchange in the 1996 Lanarkshire *Escherichia coli* O157:H7 outbreak. *Lancet Infect Dis* 1999; **354**: 1327–30.

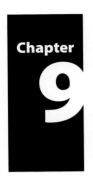

Chapter 9

Management of severe acute asthma in children

Christian Stocker and Mike South

Introduction

Asthma is a highly prevalent disease in children, and is associated with substantial morbidity. Acute exacerbations of asthma range in severity from mild, manageable with outpatient care, to life-threatening, requiring intensive care and mechanical ventilation (MV). Severe acute asthma (SAA) refers to acute life-threatening asthma – or status asthmaticus – if the lower airway obstruction causing severe respiratory distress and/or respiratory failure persists despite treatment with inhaled bronchodilators.[1] Both acute life-threatening asthma and SAA bear an increased risk of mortality if not treated early and adequately. Most children admitted to the hospital with SAA improve with supplemental oxygen, inhaled β2-agonists, and systemic corticosteroids. However, some of these children fail to respond to the initial therapy.

Case history

A 13-year-old girl with a history of recurrent exacerbations of asthma was brought to hospital with a sudden onset of severe respiratory distress 2 hours earlier. She had not improved, despite repeated doses of aerosolised salbutamol. In the ambulance, she had been treated with continuous nebulized salbutamol 0.5%, diluted 1:4 with saline, oxygen, and peripheral venous access was established.

Examination and initial management

On arrival in the emergency department, the child was conscious, mildly agitated, sitting upright, and her saturations were 92% in $6 \, l \, min^{-1}$ oxygen flow via the nebulizing mask. Her respiratory rate was $45 \, min^{-1}$, she was able to talk in sentences of three to four words, there was distinct nasal flaring and marked retractions, barely visible chest excursion, and the breath sounds were decreased with moderate wheezing over all lung fields. The ECG monitor revealed a regular sinus rhythm at a rate of $140 \, min^{-1}$, and she was warm and well perfused.

Nebulization was continued non-stop with undiluted salbutamol solution (0.5%), and a dose of 250 mcg ipratropium bromide added to the nebulizer. Oxygen flow was increased to $8 \, l \, min^{-1}$, and a dose of $1 \, mg \, kg^{-1}$ of methylprednisolone given intravenously. Additional peripheral intravenous access was established, and a salbutamol infusion with a loading dose of $5 \, mcg \, kg^{-1}$ per min for 60 minutes was started.

Upon completion of the loading dose the salbutamol infusion was continued at a dose of $1 \, mcg \, kg^{-1}$ per min. Clinical reassessment revealed a conscious patient who seemed more agitated with increasing respiratory effort. The percutaneous oxygen saturation was 88% in $10 \, l \, min^{-1}$ oxygen, the respiratory rate had increased to $55 \, min^{-1}$, and there seemed to be more intercostal and suprasternal retraction and nasal flaring. The wheezing was unchanged, air entry and chest movement continued to be poor, the heart rate had increased

Case Studies in Pediatric Critical Care, ed. Peter. J. Murphy, Stephen C. Marriage, and Peter J. Davis. Published by Cambridge University Press. © Cambridge University Press 2009.

to 165 min^{-1}, whilst her skin was still warm and well perfused. Because of the deteriorating clinical state, the girl was transferred to the pediatric intensive care unit.

Progress in the pediatric intensive care unit

A loading dose of 10 mg kg^{-1} aminophylline was given intravenously over 1 hour, after which she seemed to stabilize with improved oxygen saturations; the aminophylline was continued at a dose of 0.7 mg kg^{-1}per h. Over the following hour her condition again deteriorated with inability to speak, a decrease in chest movement and air entry, and a drop in oxygen saturations to 85%. A pneumothorax was excluded by chest radiograph, and she was placed on non-invasive assisted ventilation using triggered full-face mask biphasic positive airway pressure (BiPAP) at 5 and 20 cmH$_2$0. An arterial blood gas revealed a pH of 7.1, pCO$_2$ 65 mmHg, pO$_2$ 75 mmHg, BE –8, lactate 8 mmol l^{-1}, and a potassium of 2.3 mmol l^{-1}.

Over the next hour, despite mask BiPAP there was no significant improvement in ventilation and oxygenation, whilst at the same time she had an increasingly fluctuating conscious state and markedly decreased peripheral perfusion. It was decided that she should be invasively ventilated so she underwent a rapid sequence induction with ketamine 2 mg kg^{-1}, suxamethonium 1.5 mg kg^{-1} followed by orotracheal intubation. Initially, the ventilator was set at a rate of 30 min^{-1}, I:E ratio 1:4, PIP 40 cmH$_2$O, and PEEP 0 cmH$_2$O. Considering a rise in arterial pCO$_2$ from 110 to 130 mmHg, the PEEP was increased to 8 cmH$_2$O. Anesthesia was maintained with infusions of ketamine, midazolam, and paralysis with a vecuronium infusion, nebulization therapy was stopped, and magnesium sulphate at a dose of 30 mg kg^{-1}per h was added to the continuous intravenous treatment with salbutamol and aminophylline.

After 12 hours, permissive hypercarbia ventilation, tolerating a pH of 7.15 and arterial saturations of 85%, there was significant improvement in her tidal volumes. Muscle relaxation was discontinued after 24 hours, and the ventilator parameters were at physiological levels by 36 hours. However, further weaning was delayed due to muscle weakness secondary to critical illness myopathy such that, by the fifth day in the intensive care unit, she was still no nearer to extubation. An elective tracheotomy was performed and she was finally weaned off mechanical ventilation 10 days after her admission to PICU.

Discussion

Initial assessment and management

The objective assessment of the child with SAA is difficult. Obtaining spirometry data such as the FEV$_1$ in the young and the sick patient is impracticable. Also, even in compliant patients with SAA spirometry data is of disputable clinical, therapeutic, and predictive value.[2] The existing pediatric asthma scores do not unequivocally comply with the clinical standards of validity, prediction of outcome, description of severity, and evaluation of response to therapy.[3]

Given the current lack of useful objective assessment tools, careful clinical evaluation of the three vital organs systems, following the ABC pattern, including disciplined separation of signs for respiratory distress, from signs for respiratory failure, remains the most reliable tool in assessing severity, and for decision making on management of the SAA. Signs of respiratory distress include tachypnoea, retractions, nasal flaring and respiratory noises. However, the signs of respiratory distress are neither specific, nor sensitive for severity of status asthmaticus, since anxiety of the patient, and effects of the anti-asthmatic drugs can severely confound these findings. In our experience, there is often over-reliance on the amount of wheezing heard on auscultation in the assessment of severity.

Signs of respiratory failure are more useful for assessment of severity of the asthma, and for guidance of management of the patient. The diagnosis of respiratory failure is based on the clinical signs for poor oxygenation *and* poor ventilation, *and* the sequelae of global respiratory insufficiency on the two other vital organ systems, the central nervous and the cardiovascular system. The cardinal sign of poor oxygenation is central cyanosis. Signs of poor ventilation are inadequate respiratory rate, poor chest movement on inspection, and poor air entry on auscultation; talking and coughing rely on generation of an appropriate tidal volume (tidal volume ~ chest movement *and* air entry). From a hemodynamic viewpoint, the signs of low cardiac output state (LCOS) such as tachycardia, prolonged capillary refill time, cold and mottled skin, and peripheral cyanosis should be sought. Regarding the central nervous system, both *decreased* and *increased* (agitation) level of consciousness occur in the context of respiratory failure.

First-line treatment for SAA in children includes high-dose inhaled bronchodilators – aerosolized or nebulized β2-agonists and anticholinergics – and oral or intravenous corticosteroids.[4,5] While administration of the drug by meter-dose inhaler (MDI) with a holding chamber (spacer) is generally recommended, wet nebulization using oxygen flow may be the more appropriate delivery system for the oxygen dependent child with SAA. All patients with SAA have hypoxemia and hypoxia causes death. Administration of high concentrations of oxygen is therefore mandatory. The suppression of the hypoxic drive in children is never a problem.

In the fully oxygen-dependent child, continuous nebulized, undiluted salbutamol solution (0.5%) should be started immediately, and 250 mcg ipratropium bromide added to the nebuliser every 20 minutes for the first hour, then 4 hourly (diluted to 4 ml solution if no longer on continuous nebulization). Recommended oxygen flows to drive the nebulizer are 10–$12 \, l \, min^{-1}$ in the child younger than 2 years, and $8 \, l \, min^{-1}$ in children 2 years or older. Delivery of aerosolized bronchodilator therapy in the mechanically ventilated patient remains controversial. To date there is little evidence regarding clinical efficacy of inhaled medications delivered through an endotracheal tube.[6] Inhalational therapy is usually discontinued with initiation of invasive mechanical ventilation, since intravenous administration of bronchodilators is considered more efficient in comparison. There is even less data regarding the use of inhaled medication during Non-Invasive Mechanical Ventilation (NIMV).

Corticosteroids are very effective, and most beneficial if given early in children with SAA[7]. Children appear to respond well to oral steroids (prednisolone $1 \, mg \, kg^{-1}$), but given gastric stasis and poor absorption in the really sick patient treated with bronchodilators, a primary or additional intravenous dose of $1 \, mg \, kg^{-1}$ methylprednisolone, continued every 6 hours, is advisable.

Most children admitted to hospital with SAA will improve with the first-line treatment. If they are unresponsive, what should come next? Most physicians will reach next for either intravenous salbutamol or aminophylline. Salbutamol and aminophylline have been shown to be individually better than placebo in SAA.[8,9] Aminophylline seems to have advantages for efficacy at the cost of more adverse effects when compared to salbutamol.[10] Although common practice, there is only very limited evidence about the efficacy of using salbutamol and aminophylline together.[11] Whatever the choice between these two agents, the use in an optimal and safe fashion is crucial, and parallel continuation of the first-line therapy recommended. It is suggested to infuse salbutamol at $5 \, \text{mcg} \, \text{kg}^{-1} \, \text{min}^{-1}$ for the first hour and then continuing the infusion at $1 \, \text{mcg} \, \text{kg}^{-1}$ per min. [12] For aminophylline the recommended intravenous loading dose is $10 \, \text{mg} \, \text{kg}^{-1}$ over 1 hour followed by an infusion of $1.1 \, \text{mg} \, \text{kg}^{-1}$ per h (children 1–9 years of age) or $0.7 \, \text{mg} \, \text{kg}^{-1}$ per h (children 10–16 years of age). Strict monitoring of plasma levels of theophylline, aiming at concentrations between 60 to 110 $\mu \text{mol} \, \text{l}^{-1}$, is mandatory. If used in combination, it is important to infuse the two drugs by separate intravenous access lines.

Intravenous magnesium sulphate appears to be beneficial in patients who present with SAA.[13] Although the clinical benefit is not convincing, and despite poor data on its use in very young children, the known safety and low cost of the agent make magnesium sulphate therapy a reasonable addition in patients who do not respond to first- and second-line treatment as outlined above. It is recommended to infuse $50 \, \text{mg} \, \text{kg}^{-1}$ magnesium sulphate 50% over 20 minutes and then continuing the infusion at $30 \, \text{mg} \, \text{kg}^{-1}$ per h; the serum level of Mg^{2+} should reach 1.5–$2.5 \, \text{mmol} \, \text{l}^{-1}$.

Other proposed second-line drug therapies include alternative β2-agonists such as adrenaline, ketamine, inhalational anesthetic agents such as halothane, or inhaled helium-oxygen mixtures (Heliox^{tm}). Despite the presence of Heliox in respiratory medicine for more than 60 years, and an intriguing theoretical basis for its use, at this time, it does not seem to have a role in the initial treatment of the non-intubated or ventilated patient with SAA.[14] Similarly, there are no useful comparative studies demonstrating the efficacy of adrenaline, ketamine or halothane, although these are quite commonly administered in children with SAA.

Children with SAA are commonly dehydrated on admission, and may require fluid resuscitation with boluses of $10 \, \text{ml} \, \text{kg}^{-1}$ 0.9% normal saline if dehydration is associated with hypotension or low cardiac output. However, while a sufficient degree of hydration is considered beneficial for mucociliary clearance in the lung, overhydration should be strictly avoided because of the risk of pulmonary edema in association with the simultaneously increased activity of anti-diuretic hormone in these patients. Fluid management therefore includes mild fluid restriction, to 70%–80% of the calculated maintenance, or to 50%–60% if the patient is ventilated with humidified gases, usually using a solution of 5% dextrose in 0.45% of saline.

Ventilatory support for the child with severe acute asthma

Non-Invasive Mechanical Ventilation (NIMV)

The most common methods of NIMV are continuous positive airway pressure ventilation (CPAP) and non-invasive positive pressure ventilation by a face mask. NIMV finds increasing use for various forms of respiratory failure, and also in children with SAA.[15] NIMV may be indicated in conjunction with second-line drug therapies, or as an alternative to invasive MV. Conditional are the compliance of the patient, and appropriate monitoring equipment, including arterial blood gas analysis. A possible approach would be to start NIMV with CPAP at a positive end-expiratory pressure (PEEP) level of $5 \, \text{cmH}_2\text{O}$. The second PEEP level – or pressure support level given a trigger sensitivity of $0.5 \, \text{cmH}_2\text{O}$ – is then titrated in steps of 2–$3 \, \text{cmH}_2\text{O}$ to achieve a tidal volume of 4–$6 \, \text{ml} \, \text{kg}^{-1}$ (if this can be measured). Although NIMV has been successfully used in an increasing number of patients with SAA, may be well tolerated and may reduce PICU admissions if used in the emergency department,[16] there is insufficient data to recommend its routine use in conjunction with first- or second-line drug therapy.[17]

Intubation and Mechanical Ventilation (MV)

The decision for endotracheal intubation and MV of patients with SAA should be carefully evaluated. Intubation of children with SAA may be detrimental by worsening of hypoxemia and acidosis, and of bronchospasms due to vagal stimulation. Also, whatever the mode of MV in SAA, there is a greater risk of acute air leaks by barotrauma, and permanent lung damage by volutrauma and hyperoxia. MV may also aggravate hemodynamic impairment, and increase the risk for infection.

The guiding principle for the indication of MV is continuing clinical deterioration despite maximal medical therapy. More specifically, MV is indicated in the presence of signs of respiratory failure, including low cardiac output and decreased level of consciousness. It should not be delayed by absence of hypoxemia, or attempts to obtain an arterial pCO_2, a FEV_1 or peak expiratory flow rate, or a measured fall in systolic blood pressure on inspiration (pulsus paradoxus).

For intubation, fast and safe airway access is imperative. Therefore, a rapid sequence induction technique is mandatory: sufficient preoxygenation with 100% oxygen, application of cricoid pressure, administration of an adequate hypnotic agent such as ketamine 2–3 mg kg^{-1}, which has sedative, analgesic, and reportedly bronchodilatory effects, a fast-acting neuro muscular blocking agent such as suxamethonium (2 mg kg^{-1} <1 year of age, 1.5 mg kg^{-1} >1 year of age), and orotracheal intubation with a guide-wired and preferably cuffed endotracheal tube. Premedication with an anticholinergic drug such as glycopyrrolate 0.01 mg kg^{-1} or atropine 0.02 mg kg^{-1} can be considered but is not absolutely indicated. The use of opiates for induction should be discouraged for their ability to worsen bronchospasm by systemic histamine release, and chest rigidity when administered as a fast bolus.

Conventional MV using a pressure-limited ventilation mode, combined with a controlled hypoventilation strategy (permissive hypercarbia, peak inspiratory pressure 35 cmH$_2$O or less, pH >7.15), may be most appropriate for MV of the patient with SAA. If possible, bearing in mind the ventilatory rate necessary to achieve a pH >7.15, expiratory times should be lengthened such that as much expiration as possible can take place, and reduce the degree of "breath stacking."

The patient should initially be fully sedated and muscle relaxed. Proposed drugs for sedation are morphine 20–60 mcg kg^{-1}per h, midazolam 1–4 mcg kg^{-1}per min and/or ketamine 10–20 mcg kg^{-1}per min infusion, and for paralysis a vecuronium 1–10 mcg kg^{-1}per min infusion; pancuronium for paralysis may be disadvantageous because of its higher incidence of cardiovascular and autonomic side effects.

The use of PEEP is controversial because of the potential to further elevate the lung volume and contribute to barotrauma of the lung and to low cardiac output. When initially ventilating a child with SAA who is sedated and paralyzed appropriately, the general consensus worldwide is to set no PEEP or minimal PEEP. In selected patients where conventional settings fail to improve gas exchange, PEEP in incremental steps and under close monitoring of the arterial pCO_2, the intrinsic PEEP and trapped gas volume, may be beneficial, perhaps by maintaining patency of airways proximal to the "asthmatic" obstruction during expiration. The intrinsic PEEP and the trapped gas volume can be estimated by stopping the ventilator at end-expiration for 15 seconds; the intrinsic PEEP equals the PEEP measured at the end of a usual breath minus the PEEP at the end of the prolonged expiration, and the trapped gas volume equals the tidal volume to end-expiration minus the usual tidal volume. If gas trapping with severe hemodynamic compromise is suspected, expiratory time should be prolonged, or even more aggressively, the patient pre-oxygenated and then disconnected from the ventilator every hour for 30–60 seconds, or even forced manual expiration of the chest.

Every effort should be made to discontinue the neuro muscular blocking agents within 12–24 hours because of the association of their use, especially in combination with corticosteroids, with critical illness myopathy.[18] Heavy sedation may facilitate the cessation of the muscle relaxants.

For most patients, the duration of MV is a matter of 1 or 2 days. During the weaning process, the patient can be allowed to breathe spontaneously. Synchronized intermittent mandatory and pressure-support ventilation modes are helpful in facilitating the patient's cooperation with MV and reduction of sedation at the same time. Precipitation of bronchospasms due to increasing awareness and the presence of the endotracheal tube around the time of extubation can be overcome by the use of short-acting sedative agents such as propofol.

Although there is a case report of the use of high frequency oscillatory ventilation (HFOV) in a young child with SAA,[19] there is a general lack of evidence to support the use of high frequency ventilation modes, either HFOV or high frequency jet ventilation (HFJV), in patients with SAA. It is believed that high frequency modes may worsen alveolar distension, or that vibration may trigger further bronchospasm, and their use has therefore been generally discouraged. Similarly, given the relatively favorable outcomes and low mortality of children with SAA managed in intensive care, the additional survival rate provided by extracorporeal membrane oxygenation (ECMO) is most likely marginal, and considering the potential complications possibly harmful. However, there certainly is a role for ECMO as rescue treatment in patients who cannot be stabilized when mechanically ventilated.

Complications of severe acute asthma

Failure to recognize the seriousness of respiratory failure, or to treat the episode early and appropriately, remains the chief contributing cause of poor outcome in SAA. Efforts should be made to avoid MV in SAA, since intubation and ventilation of these patients are associated with a higher incidence of complications compared to patients ventilated for other causes of respiratory failure.[20] Causes of mortality in the ventilated child with SAA are acute air leaks, sepsis, and the low cardiac output syndrome.

Barotrauma is responsible for acute air leaks such as pneumothorax, interstitial, mediastinal, or subcutaneous emphysema, and can occur in the ventilated and non-ventilated patient, although rarely in younger children.[21]

In addition to the direct, mechanical heart–lung interaction, arterial hypotension and low cardiac output syndrome can also arise from hypoxemia, acidosis, and arrhythmias. The latter may be triggered by a combination of predisposition, catecholaminergic drug stimulation, hypokalemia, hypoxemia, and acidosis. In children treated for SAA, supraventricular trachycardia (SVT) is probably the most commonly observed arrhythmia. If hemodynamically unstable, or not self-limited, the SVT can reportedly be converted using intravenous adenosine despite continuation of the anti-asthmatic pharmacotherapy. Also, there is a theoretical risk of ventricular tachyarrhythmias triggered by bronchodilator induced prolongation of the QT_c time, which underlines the importance of ECG and potassium monitoring.

Critical illness myopathy (CIM) is a rare complication which presents as difficulty in weaning from MV, and is most often reported in patients with SAA, sepsis, or post-transplant, in association with exposure to corticosteroids and/or neuromuscular blocking agents.[18] It seems that the duration of administration rather than the type of muscle relaxant is the main factor for development of the myopathy. Upon clinical suspicion, CIM is diagnosed based on electromyographic and biopsy findings. Most patients fully recover within 3 months, but morbidity from other complicating illnesses is not insignificant. If the SAA leads to cardio-respiratory collapse requiring resuscitation and intubation, the hypoxic–ischemic encephal-opathy should be sought and assessed by imaging and electrophysiologic means for prognostic purposes as soon as the patient has stabilised.

The intensive care mortality of SAA is relatively low: 1%–2% of children with SAA admitted to the intensive care unit at the Royal Children's Hospital in Melbourne, Australia, die (unpublished data 2004). However, despite a continuously decreasing prevalence of asthma over the last decade, the absolute number of patients with SAA admitted to our unit, as well of those needing mechanical ventilation, and of asthma-related deaths, has remained unchanged in 20 years.[22] This would suggest a relative increase in severity and mortality of childhood asthma overall.

Learning points

- Clinical evaluation is the most important tool for assessment of the child with SAA, and for guidance of therapy.

- It is the signs of respiratory failure that should predominantly guide second-line therapy and more advanced interventions.

- Consider over-treatment with bronchodilators in a child who has ongoing respiratory distress, but without features of severe airway obstruction (such as chest wall retraction) or features of respiratory failure.

- In general, first-line treatment in the child with SAA is purely pharmacological.

- Second-line treatment is mainly pharmacological, but non-invasive MV may be considered in the cooperative child.

- Invasive MV is third-line treatment, and usually only after exhaustion of pharmacological resources.

- The patients requiring MV are likely to do well with meticulous attention to detail in ventilator care. A small percentage of ventilated asthmatics will die; the causes are barotrauma, sepsis, hypotension, and cardiac arrhythmias.

- The risk of death or an adverse outcome from SAA is small once the child has reached a high-quality care facility.[11]

- Improved asthma management in inpatient and outpatient care, use of inhaled cortico-steroids, and fast access to a high-quality care facility, seem to be the key elements in the decrease of asthma morbidity and mortality worldwide over the last decade.[23]

References

1. Phelan POA, Robertson C. Asthma: clinical patterns and management. *Respiratory Illness in Children*. Oxford, Blackwell, 1994; 149.
2. Bacharier LB, Strunk RC, Mauger D, White D, Lemanske RF Jr, Sorkness CA. Classifying asthma severity in children: mismatch

between symptoms, medication use, and lung function. *Am J Respir Crit Care Med* 2004; **170**: 426–32.
3. Mitra AD, Ogston S, Crighton A, Mukhopadhyay S. Lung function and asthma symptoms in children: relationships and

response to treatment. *Acta Paediatr* 2002; **91**: 789–92.

4. Plotnick LH, Ducharme FM. Combined inhaled anticholinergics and beta2-agonists for initial treatment of acute asthma in children. *Cochrane Database Syst Rev* 2000: CD000060.

5. Rowe BH, Spooner CH, Ducharme FM, Bretzlaff JA, Bota GW. Corticosteroids for preventing relapse following acute exacerbations of asthma. *Cochrane Database Syst Rev* 2000: CD000195.

6. Jones A, Rowe B, Peters J, Camargo C, Hammarquist C. Inhaled beta-agonists for asthma in mechanically ventilated patients. *Cochrane Database Syst Rev* 2001: CD001493.

7. Rowe BH, Spooner C, Ducharme FM, Bretzlaff JA, Bota GW. Early emergency department treatment of acute asthma with systemic corticosteroids. *Cochrane Database Syst Rev* 2000: CD002178.

8. Yung M, South M. Randomised controlled trial of aminophylline for severe acute asthma. *Arch Dis Child* 1998; **79**: 405–10.

9. Browne GJ, Penna AS, Phung X, Soo M. Randomised trial of intravenous salbutamol in early management of acute severe asthma in children. *Lancet* 1997; **349**: 301–5.

10. Roberts G, Newsom D, Gomez K, et al. Intravenous salbutamol bolus compared with an aminophylline infusion in children with severe asthma: a randomised controlled trial. *Thorax* 2003; **58**: 306–10.

11. South M. Second line treatment for severe acute childhood asthma. *Thorax* 2003; **58**: 284–5.

12. Shann F. Dose of intravenous infusions of terbutaline and salbutamol. *Crit Care Med* 2000; **28**: 2179–80.

13. Rowe BH, Bretzlaff JA, Bourdon C, Bota GW, Camargo CA Jr. Magnesium sulfate for treating exacerbations of acute asthma in the emergency department. *Cochrane Database Syst Rev* 2000: CD001490.

14. Rodrigo G, Pollack C, Rodrigo C, Rowe BH. Heliox for nonintubated acute asthma patients[update of Cochrane Database Syst Rev 2003:CD002884]. *Cochrane Database Syst Rev* 2006: CD002884.

15. Thill PJ, McGuire JK, Baden HP, Green TP, Checchia PA. Noninvasive positive-pressure ventilation in children with lower airway obstruction. *Pediatr Crit Care Med* 2004; **5**: 337–42.

16. Beers SL, Abramo TJ, Bracken A, Wiebe RA. Bilevel positive airway pressure in the treatment of status asthmaticus in pediatrics. *Am J Emerg Med.* 2007; **25**: 6–9.

17. Non-invasive ventilation in acute respiratory failure. *Thorax* 2002; **57**: 192–211.

18. Marinelli WA, Leatherman JW. Neuromuscular disorders in the intensive care unit. *Crit Care Clin* 2002; **18**: 915–29.

19. Duval EL. van Vught AJ. Status asthmaticus treated by high-frequency oscillatory ventilation. *Pediatric Pulmonology* 2000; **30**: 350–3.

20. Sydow M. Ventilating the patient with severe asthma: nonconventional therapy. *Minerva Anestesiol* 2003; **69**: 333–7.

21. Davis AM, Wensley DF, Phelan PD. Spontaneous pneumothorax in paediatric patients. *Respir Med* 1993; **87**: 531–4.

22. Robertson CF, Roberts MF, Kappers JH. Asthma prevalence in Melbourne schoolchildren: have we reached the peak? *Med J Aust* 2004; **180**: 273–6.

23. Sly RM. Optimal management improves asthma morbidity and mortality. *Ann Allergy Asthma Immunol* 2003; **90**: 10–12.

Further Reading

McFadden ER Jr. Acute severe asthma. *Am J Respir Crit Care Med* 2003; **168**: 740–59.

The neonate with total anomalous pulmonary venous connection

Robert Mazor, Gordon Cohen, and Lynn D. Martin

Introduction

Patients with total anomalous venous connection (TAPVC) account for 1%–5% of all cases of congenital heart disease. Anomalous pulmonary venous drainage is frequently part of a constellation of abnormalities seen in heterotaxy syndrome, but is most commonly seen as an isolated lesion in patients with otherwise normal intracardiac connections.[1] Broadly defined, TAPVC is the anomalous drainage of well-oxygenated pulmonary venous blood into the deoxygenated systemic venous circulation. The anatomy of the pulmonary-to-systemic venous connections is quite variable. The heterogeneity of these connections leads to differential physiology, with a wide spectrum of presenting symptoms, clinical course, and surgical outcome.

Perhaps the most critical factor influencing the presenting symptoms and clinical course is the presence of obstruction to pulmonary venous blood flow along the pathway. Obstructed TAPVC remains one of the true congenital heart surgical emergencies. Medical therapies are only temporizing measures and do not allow for lasting stabilization. However, it seems that poorer pre-operative clinical condition is a risk factor for worse post-operative outcome. A study looking at a single institution's surgical outcome over a 30-year period demonstrated an improvement in outcome during a period marked by a more aggressive approach to pre-operative medical stabilization.[2] Patients with obstructed TAPVC are occasionally misdiagnosed as having persistent pulmonary hypertension (PPHN) because the underlying physiology and clinical presentation are similar. This leads to a delay in diagnosis and treatment, which may adversely affect morbidity. Therefore, a thorough interrogation of the pulmonary venous anatomy is essential as part of the evaluation of any newborn with severe PPHN regardless of the presumed etiology. These issues emphasize the importance of making an accurate and timely diagnosis.

The presence of TAPVC is an absolute indication for surgical repair. The timing of surgery is dependent upon the clinical situation at the time the diagnosis is made. Following surgery, even the sickest pre-operative patients generally demonstrate marked improvement. The short- and long-term outcome of patients with TAPVC in the current era is generally good. Acute mortality seems to be related to the presence of pulmonary hypertension. However, long-term outcome is tied to the development of recurrent pulmonary venous stenosis, which may be related to the adequacy of the initial repair.

Case history

A 3.5 kg, term infant female was born at a local institution to an 18-year-old gravida 1 para 1 woman. The mother was Group B Strep positive. Therefore, she received 3 doses of ampicillin prior to delivery. Shortly after birth, the infant developed respiratory distress and had a temperature of 38 °C. She was taken to the Neonatal Intensive Care Unit (NICU),

Case Studies in Pediatric Critical Care, ed. Peter. J. Murphy, Stephen C. Marriage, and Peter J. Davis. Published by Cambridge University Press. © Cambridge University Press 2009.

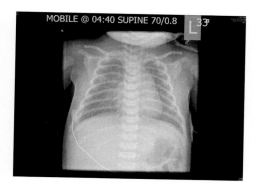

Fig. 10.1. Chest X-ray.

where her condition quickly deteriorated. She was intubated for progressive hypoxemia and required rapid escalation of inotropic infusions consisting of dopamine, dobutamine, and adrenaline (epinephrine) to maintain marginal hemodynamics. A complete septic workup was performed and antibiotics ampicillin and gentamicin were started. Chest X-ray demonstrated bilateral parenchymal opacity (Fig. 10.1). An echocardiogram revealed normal intracardiac connections. However, the anatomy of the pulmonary veins was not commented upon. There was suprasystemic pulmonary arterial pressure, right to left shunting via a patent foramen ovale (PFO), and the left side of the heart appeared under filled. A presumptive diagnosis of PPHN secondary to sepsis was made; therefore, inhaled nitric oxide was initiated at 20 ppm. On day 2 of life her condition continued to deteriorate; therefore, referral was made for transport to the local tertiary care center due to the possible need for extracorporeal membranous oxygenation (ECMO).

Clinical course in the IICU

Upon arrival to the Infant Intensive Care Unit (IICU), she was afebrile. Her heart rhythm was sinus tachycardia with occasional premature atrial contractions, and her heart rate was 170 b min^{-1}. Her respiratory rate was 40 breaths min^{-1}. Her mean arterial blood pressure was 40 mmHg. Her systemic oxygen saturation was 93% with a FiO$_2$ of 1.0. She was pharmacologically muscle relaxed and ventilated using conventional ventilation in a pressure-control mode. Her peak airway pressure was set at 28 cm H$_2$O with positive end-expiratory pressure (PEEP) of 6 cmH$_2$O. She was on inhaled nitric oxide at 20 ppm. She had reasonable chest rise and air entry. Her chest X-ray demonstrated diffuse bilateral patchy parenchymal opacity with a normal cardiac silhouette. Cardiac examination revealed a regular rhythm with occasional ectopy, and a loud second heart sound. There was a 2/6 systolic murmur heard loudest in the left parasternal position. Ongoing inotropic support consisted of: dopamine 30 mcg kg^{-1} per min^{-1}, dobutamine 20 mcg kg^{-1} per min, adrenaline 0.2 mcg kg^{-1} per min. Her distal extremities were cool with a prolonged capillary refill time. Her abdomen was full with the liver edge palpable 4 cm below the right costal margin. Her admission data is summarized in Table 10.1.

Over the next 24 hours, she received several boluses of crystalloid to maintain adequate perfusion. Despite marginal hemodynamics, she continued to produce urine at a rate of 2 ml kg^{-1} per h. Her systemic oxygen saturations remained in the low 90s with frequent spontaneous systemic desaturation episodes despite escalation of PEEP to 10 cmH$_2$O. Her

Table 10.1. *Admission data*

Examination:	
	Vital signs: afebrile, HR-170, RR-40 BPM, MAP-40 mmHg, O_2 saturation 93%
	Intubated, muscle relaxed
	Reasonable chest rise and aeration
	Loud second heart sound, 2/6 systolic murmur
	Full abdomen, liver edge 4 cm below costal margin
	Cool distal extremities
Investigations:	
Serum	Na^+ 133 meq l^{-1}, K^+ 2.5 meq l^{-1}, HCO_3^- 22 meq l^{-1} Cl^- 106 meq l^{-1}, BUN 22 mg dl^{-1}, Cr 1.0 mg dl^{-1}, Glu 168 mg dl^{-1}
CBC	WBC 17 000 mm^{-3}, Hct 51%, Plat 219 000 mm^{-3}
Coag. panel	PT 14.4s, INR 1.3, PTT 53s, Fibrinogen 209 mg dl^{-1}, TT 29s, D-dimer <5 mcg dl^{-1}
Arterial blood gas	pH 7.38, pCO_2 33 mmHg, pO_2 50 mmHg, BD −6
Infectious	Viral respiratory FA nasal wash-negative
	Bacterial cultures (mother pretreated) from referring hospital:
	Blood – negative 48 hours
	Urine – negative 48 hours
	CSF – negative 48 hours

chest X-ray demonstrated worsening of the diffuse parenchymal opacification. Because she continued to have significant isolated atrial ectopy, the cardiology service was consulted. A repeat echocardiogram demonstrated a confluence of all four pulmonary veins behind the left atrium. There was a single venous channel arising from the confluence that traveled caudally through the diaphragm and connected to the ductus venosus, where there was significant obstruction to flow. The markedly enlarged right ventricle appeared hypokinetic. The left ventricle appeared compressed, but with normal systolic function. Right ventricular pressure was estimated to be suprasystemic. Flow through the PFO was entirely right to left (Fig. 10.2). Given these findings, the patient was taken urgently to the cardiac operating room for surgical repair.

Operative course

Owing to the delay in diagnosis and the patient's poor clinical condition, it was felt by the surgeons that the risk of an operative mortality was extremely high. As a result, the surgical plan included the use of post-operative Venoarterial (VA)-ECMO support. Initially, an incision in the right neck was made and the right carotid and right jugular veins were exposed. Heparin was then given and the right carotid was cannulated and connected to the arterial limb of the bypass circuit. The sternum was then opened, thymus removed, pericardium opened, and the right atrium was cannulated and connected to the venous limb of the bypass circuit. The patient was placed on cardiopulmonary bypass and cooled down to 18 °C. Once the target temperature was reached, the bypass flow was stopped, the patient was exsanguanated, and the right atrial cannula removed. The heart was then retracted superiorly and rightward. The descending vein was identified and ligated. An incision was made in the pulmonary venous confluence and carried out into the branches of the left and right pulmonary veins. An

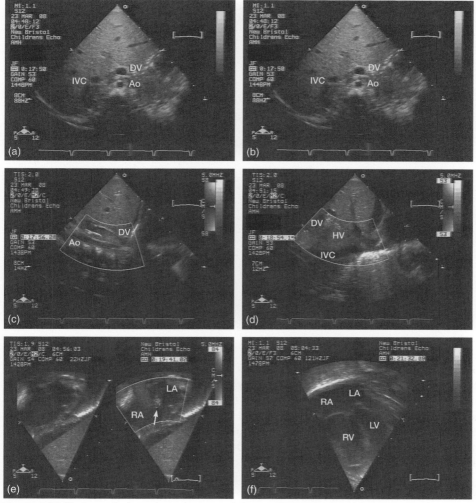

Fig. 10.2 (a)-(j). Series of echocardiograph images of obstructed TAPVC. RV = Right Ventricle, LV = Left Ventricle, IVC = Inferior Vena Cava, Ao = Aorta, DV = Descending Vein, LPV = Left Pulmonary Vein, HV = Hepatic Vein, PVS = Pulmonary Veins (for (c), (d), (h), and (j), see color plate section).

incision was then made in the left atrium, along the left atrial appendage extending right-ward, nearly to the intratrial groove. An intraatrial communication was created by removing the tissue in the fossa ovalis. Creation of a wide-open atrial septal defect would allow adequate decompression of the left heart while on VA-ECMO and would provide a source of right-to-left shunting in the event of a pulmonary hypertensive crisis after separating from ECMO. The pulmonary venous confluence was then anastamosed to the left atrium. Once the anastamosis was complete, the patient was placed back on cardiopulmonary bypass and rewarmed. The intra-operative transosophageal echocardiography confirmed a widely pat-ent surgical anastamosis with a reassuring flow pattern in the pulmonary veins. Following rewarming, no attempt was made to wean from cardiopulmonary bypass. The right internal jugular vein was cannulated and connected to the venous limb of the ECMO circuit. The

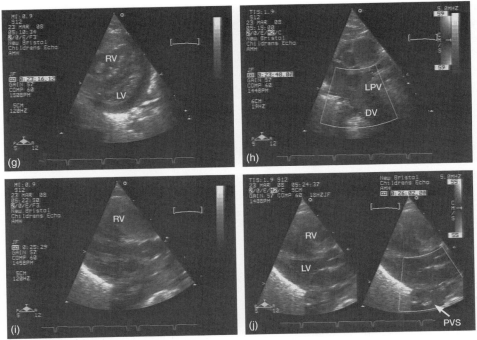

Fig. 10.2 (a)-(j). (cont.)

patient was briefly taken off cardiopulmonary bypass, and the arterial cannula was then connected to the arterial side of the VA-ECMO circuit. ECMO flow was then commenced. The right atrium was decannulated, hemostasis was obtained, a chest tube was placed in the mediastinum and the chest was closed. The patient was transferred to the Cardiac Intensive Care Unit (CICU) on inhaled nitric oxide 20 ppm, dopamine 5 mcg kg^{-1} per min, and milrinone 0.7 mcg kg^{-1} per min.

Clinical course in the CICU

Over the next several days, the patient showed gradual improvement of her biventricular function with decrease in estimated pulmonary artery pressures as determined by serial echocardiogram. She was successfully weaned from ECMO support on post-operative day 6. She was started on sildenafil 0.5 mg kg^{-1} every 4 hours and weaned off inhaled nitric oxide on post-operative day 9. She was weaned from mechanical ventilatory support and the trachea was extubated on post-operative day 11. She remained in the CICU for 3 additional days for respiratory monitoring, advancement of feeds, and weaning of sedation. She was ultimately discharged from the hospital on post-operative day 20. Her discharge echocardiogram revealed good biventricular pressure. There was mild turbulence in the area of the surgical anastamosis with an estimated pressure gradient of 5 mmHg across that area.

Outpatient course

She was asymptomatic at her initial 1-month follow-up visit. Her hemodynamics, as assessed by echocardiography, were essentially unchanged from discharge. Routine follow-up was scheduled for 2 months. One month later, she was seen in the emergency department with moderate respiratory distress and fever. A CXR revealed asymmetry of her pulmonary vascular markings, with pulmonary vascular congestion of the left lung. An echocardiogram revealed low velocity, non-phasic flow in the left pulmonary veins with significant turbulence at the anastamotic site. She was admitted and a cardiac catheterization was performed, revealing 2/3 systemic-level pulmonary artery pressures. There was an estimated 20 mmHg pressure gradient noted across the surgical anastamosis of the pulmonary vein confluence and left atrium. The interventional cardiologists were unable to gain access to the left pulmonary veins. Pulmonary angiography confirmed the diagnosis of significant, diffuse stenosis of the left pulmonary venous system. She was taken to the cardiac operating room the following day, where visual inspection revealed extensive stenosis of the left pulmonary venous system and a mild narrowing at the anastaomtic site. A "suture-less" repair using an *in situ* pericardial patch was performed, and the patient recovered uneventfully.

Discussion

Embryology

Although the exact developmental aberration involved in the pathogenesis of TAPVC remains in question, a review of normal venous embryology is important to any discussion of the topic. The human lungs develop from the embryologic foregut. As such, their blood supply derives from the splanchnic plexus. Early in development, there is no direct pulmonary venous connection to the heart. Rather, these vessels drain via the primitive systemic venous system: the umbilicovitelline and the right and left cardinal veins. Soon, there is an out pouching from the left atrium, called the common pulmonary vein. The common pulmonary vein meets the primitive pulmonary venous system to establish the typical connection between the pulmonary veins and the heart. It is believed that a mishap in the formation of this connection is at the root of this disorder. Without a direct connection to the left atrium, the pulmonary veins must drain via one or more of the primitive venous pathways, which ultimately differentiate into the systemic venous system. The factor(s) involved in the persistence of one or another venous pathway is not known.

Morphology

A wide range of anomalous pulmonary to systemic venous connections occurs. The complex forms of anomalous venous drainage that occur in the context of visceral heterotaxy syndromes are beyond the scope of this chapter. Rather, we will focus on the more "typical" forms of TAPVC seen as isolated lesions. Several classification systems of TAPVC have been suggested. The most commonly used scheme details the anatomic position of the anomalous venous drainage relative to the heart, with some authors assigning a number to each major category: supracardiac (type 1), cardiac (type 2), infracardiac (type 3), mixed type (type 4). Each of these groups can be further subdivided into obstructed and non-obstructed. Although obstruction is described in all four types of TAPVC, it is seen most commonly in infracardiac (type 3) and rarely seen in cardiac (type 2) TAPVC (Fig. 10.3).

Supracardiac (type 1)

This anatomy accounts for approximately 50% of cases of TAPVC. Roughly 50% of these patients have pulmonary venous obstruction at presentation.[3] In this situation, the pulmonary veins join a confluence behind the left atrium with a vertical vein ascending from the

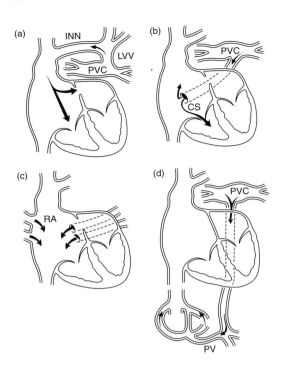

Fig. 10.3. The four most common anatomical defects in TAPVC. From Nichols *et al.* (1995).

confluence to join the systemic venous system, typically the innominate vein (Fig. 10.3(a)). The vertical vein usually ascends anterior to the left pulmonary artery and left bronchus and remains unobstructed. However, the vertical vein can become compressed if it passes between the left pulmonary artery (anterior) and the left bronchus (posterior).

Cardiac (type 2)
These patients represent approximately 25% of TAPVC. The pulmonary veins enter a dilated confluence behind the heart and either enter the coronary sinus (Fig. 10.3(b)) or drain directly into the right atrium (Fig. 10.3(c)). Although this pathway is occasionally narrowed, usually at the point of entrance to the coronary sinus, a significant physiologic obstruction is uncommon. A restrictive atrial communication may also occur with this type of defect.

Infracardiac (type 3)
This situation accounts for around 15% of patients with TAPVC. The distal site of connection occurs below the diaphragm. The pulmonary veins form a confluence behind the left atrium. A common vessel descends anterior to the esophagus and passes through the diaphragm via the esophageal hiatus. This vessel most frequently enters the portal vein, but may drain via the ductus venosus, hepatic veins, or inferior vena cava (Fig. 10.3(d)). Obstruction to venous flow occurs in roughly 85% of patients, most commonly occurring in the intrahepatic portions of the venous pathway due to progressive restriction of the ductus venosus.

Mixed (type 4)
As the name implies, patients with this lesion have a mixture of anomalous and/or normal drainage patterns. These patients account for approximately 10%–15% of patients with

TAPVC. The resultant physiology is quite variable, and is dependent on the combination of the venous drainage patterns.

Physiologic considerations

Because both systemic and pulmonary venous blood returns to the right atrium and ventricular level communications are uncommon, the majority of systemic output is dependent upon an atrial level communication. The adequacy of this communication is of paramount importance in determining the early clinical course. As pulmonary vascular resistance decreases after birth, pulmonary blood flow increases. With increasing anomalous pulmonary venous return to the right atrium and a restrictive atrial level communication, right atrial pressure rises. This leads to an increased volume load delivered to the right ventricle, which is necessarily ejected into the pulmonary circulation. The elevated "downstream" right atrial pressure is transmitted to both the systemic and pulmonary venous systems. The effect on the pulmonary venous system is an elevated pulmonary capillary pressure and finally elevated pulmonary artery pressure. The elevated pulmonary artery pressure adds a significant pressure load to the already volume loaded right ventricular, leading to right ventricular failure. Additionally, restriction to trans-atrial flow may lead to limitation of left ventricular filling and systemic cardiac output.

Just as a restrictive atrial communication leads to elevated downstream pressure, so too do areas of obstruction along the anomalous venous pathways. The elevated pressure is transmitted to the pulmonary capillary bed, leading to pulmonary vascular congestion. As pulmonary capillary hydrostatic pressure rises, there is an increase in the transudation of fluid into the pulmonary interstitium. Pulmonary lymphatic drainage via the thoracic duct may be limited due to the associated elevation of systemic venous pressure, leading to significant pulmonary edema formation. Additionally, obstruction of pulmonary venous return to the heart may lead to significant compromise of systemic cardiac output due to inadequate preload.

In the setting of severely elevated pulmonary artery pressures, a patent ductus arteriosus allows for a "pop-off" of pulmonary blood flow, preventing suprasystemic pulmonary artery pressures. The decrease in pulmonary blood flow may lead to a beneficial decrease in pulmonary edema formation, at the expense of systemic hypoxemia. However, in the face of low systemic cardiac output, systemic hypoxemia may lead to inadequate oxygen delivery and worsened clinical condition.

Treatment

Pre-operative

TAPVC is an absolute indication for surgical repair. The pre-operative management strategy, including the timing of surgery, depends on several factors. Most important of these is the presence of pulmonary venous obstruction. Obstructed TAPVC is one of the few congenital cardiac surgical emergencies. Despite this, it seems that a period of attempted stabilization prior to surgery results in improved outcome.[2] Even in the best situations, the intensivist frequently finds himself faced with pre-operative management decisions while the operative team is mobilized. Controlled mechanical ventilation should be provided. Judicious use of PEEP to maintain the lung's functional residual capacity in the face of significant pulmonary edema is often beneficial. However, extreme elevations of intrathoracic pressure should be avoided to prevent excessive afterload on the failing right ventricle.

Although oxygen is beneficial in patients with hypoxemia caused by pulmonary edema, indiscriminate administration should be avoided due to its significant pulmonary vasodilatory effects.

Administration of prostaglandin E_1 (PGE_1) in this setting remains controversial and its use should be considered on a case-by-case basis. In situations where there is low systemic cardiac output and a small patent ductus arteriosus, ductal dilatation by PGE1 may afford an increase in right to left flow with improved overall oxygen delivery, despite increasing systemic desaturation. An additional benefit of decreased blood flow into an obstructed pulmonary vascular system may also be seen. However, due to its pulmonary vasodilatory properties, PGE1 may lead to a decrease in pulmonary vascular resistance with consequent increase in pulmonary blood flow and worsening of pulmonary edema. An additional purported benefit of PGE1 is dilation of the ductus venosus. Thus PGE1 may be of benefit in cases of infracardiac TAPVC where obstruction is present at the level of the ductus venosus.

Use of inotropic agents and judicious fluid administration are also frequently used as temporizing measures in the setting of severe systemic hypoperfusion, especially with severely depressed ventricular function. In the most extreme cases, ECMO can be considered to achieve hemodynamic and metabolic stabilization prior to operative intervention.

Operative

Typically, repair of TAPVC involves the use of circulatory arrest as part of the cardiopulmonary bypass strategy.[4] The reasons for this are twofold. First, the venous cannula limits the ability to move the heart and expose the venous confluence and thus needs to be removed in order to achieve optimal exposure to ensure a perfect anastamosis. Second, the amount of venous return that enters the field from the bronchial circulation is excessive and interferes with the visualization of the reconstruction. Hence, the use of circulatory arrest is the preferred strategy. It should be noted that it is possible to do the repair without circulatory arrest and this is a strategy employed by some centers, but is less commonly used.

The typical repair involves placing the patient on cardiopulmonary bypass with a single arterial cannula in the aorta and a single venous cannula placed in the right atrium. Once bypass is commenced, the patient is cooled down to 18 °C. The cooling usually is done over a period of 20–25 minutes. Once the target temperature is reached, the aorta is cross-clamped and antegrade cardioplegia is given down the aortic root to stop the heart. Once the cardioplegia is delivered, the pump is turned off and the patient is drained of blood. The venous cannula is then removed from the heart. The heart is then retracted up (there are a variety of maneuvers to do this) and the venous confluence, which usually lies outside the pericardial space, is dissected out along its length. An incision is then made in the venous confluence and can be extended just to the very beginning of the branches. A counter-incision is then made in the left atrium. A connection is then created between the left atrium and the venous confluence. The suture line is running and usually performed with either prolene or PDS suture. We choose to remove the tissue from the fossa ovalis so that there is a patent atrial level communication. This allows for right-to-left shunting of blood at the atrial level in the event of a pulmonary hypertensive crisis and will allow maintenance of cardiac output at the expense of cyanosis. Once the pulmonary arterial pressures drop, there is usually bi-directional shunting and later left-to-right shunting across the atrial communication. The hole is usually small and does not create a problem for the growing child and can be closed in the cardiac catheter laboratory later in life if a problem persists.

Once the reconstruction is complete, the atrial cannula is replaced, the bypass machine is turned back on, the cross-clamp is removed from the aorta and the patient is rewarmed. When the patient is warm, they are weaned from cardiopulmonary bypass. We employ a post-bypass strategy of modified ultrafiltration. When ultrafiltration is complete, protamine is given, hemostasis obtained, chest drains placed and the chest closed.

Post-operative

The vast majority of patients show significant improvement following operative repair. However, many patients will have significant residual biventricular dysfunction and pulmonary hypertension in the immediate post-operative period depending on their pre-operative condition. Strategies aimed at optimizing biventricular function and preventing pulmonary hypertension are the cornerstones of post-operative management. Monitoring central venous, right atrial, pulmonary artery, and/or left atrial pressure monitoring is frequently useful.

There have been several reports of the use of ECMO in patients with TAPVC, in the pre- and post-operative setting. In many circumstances the pre-operative ECMO patients represent patients who were emergently cannulated and later diagnosed with TAPVC once on ECMO.[5-7] A review of the Extracorporeal Life Support Organization (ELSO) data from 1976–1992 demonstrated discouraging results with respect to mortality and neurological outcome in patients with TAPVC who required ECMO either pre-, intra-, or post-operatively[7]; however, a review from the current era is not available. Despite these data, ECMO is a valuable modality in patients with significant post-operative ventricular dysfunction by promoting myocardial recovery via unloading of the ventricles.

Inhaled nitric oxide, a selective pulmonary vasodilator, has been used in the management of post-operative pulmonary hypertension in congenital heart disease.[8] As such, it has a prominent place in the intensivist's armamentarium in the management of pulmonary hypertensive crisis after TAPVC repair. The occurrence of post-operative pulmonary hypertensive events is a significant risk factor for early death following repair of TAPVC.[2] This suggests that strategies targeting prevention of pulmonary hypertensive events might have an impact on outcome. There have been no investigations designed to specifically examine the beneficial use of post-operative nitric oxide with respect to mortality or the development of post-repair pulmonary venous obstruction. However, a recent study demonstrated a trend toward improved early mortality in patients with pre-operative pulmonary venous obstruction who were treated with inhaled NO in the post-operative period.[1] On the other hand, Rosales et al. described a patient who had adverse hemodynamic sequelae during the use of nitric oxide in this setting.[9] In most cases, the patient can be weaned from NO within a few days. Sildenafil, a potent, selective inhibitor of phosphodiesterase type 5 should be considered in cases where it is difficult to wean from nitric oxide.[10]

Outcome

The natural history of TAPVC is characterized by progressive heart failure and invariably death. The time course of decompensation depends upon such variables as the presence of pulmonary venous obstruction, associated cardiac and non-cardiac lesions, and ventricular morphology. The morbidity and mortality of TAPVC have improved over time.[2] This improvement is likely to be due to better operative technique and advances in pre-operative and post-operative care. In the current era, the vast majority of patients who undergo operative repair have excellent short and long-term outcome.[1-3,11,12] Multiple investigators have demonstrated that neither the presence of pre-operative obstruction, nor the anatomical classification is a predictor of outcome.[1,2] The presence of single ventricular physiology, however, remains a predictor of poor outcome.[1]

Perhaps the most important determinant of outcome beyond the acute post-operative period is the occurrence of recurrent pulmonary vein obstruction (RPVO). The pathophysiologic mechanisms responsible for the development of this disorder remain unknown. There seem to be three patterns of re-stenosis: intra-atrial thickening leading to ostial stenosis, obstruction of the anastamotic site, and diffuse intrinsic pulmonary vein stenosis. These can occur in isolation or, more commonly, in combination. In some patients, there appears to be an association between the presence of turbulence in the initial pulmonary vein repair and the development of RPVO, leading some to hypothesize that RPVO occurs as a byproduct of imperfect hemodynamics after initial repair. However, the same authors acknowledge that RPVO also occurs after a seemingly satisfactory repair.[14] Early occurrence of re-stenosis is more common with intrinsic pulmonary vein stenosis, with such patients having a worse outcome than those patients who present remote from their initial operation.[3,11,13] Multiple case series have been published without a unifying predictive risk factor for PVOS, suggesting the likelihood that its cause is multifactorial. Most centers agree that the development of RPVO is associated with poor prognosis. A "suture-less" surgical procedure has been developed in an attempt to alter this outcome with promising initial results.[15]

Conclusions

Total anomalous pulmonary venous connection is a relatively uncommon form of congenital heart disease. However, in the presence of pulmonary venous obstruction, these patients are often quite unstable at the time of presentation. Obstructed TAPVC remains one of the true congenital cardiac surgical emergencies. Despite this, the short- and long-term outcomes of these patients have improved over the past several years. At least in part, this is a byproduct of improved pre-operative and post-operative intensive care management.

Learning points

- A thorough interrogation of the pulmonary venous anatomy is essential as part of the evaluation of any newborn with severe PPHN, regardless of the presumed etiology.
- The most critical factor influencing the presenting symptoms and clinical course is the presence of obstruction to pulmonary venous blood flow along the pathway. Although obstruction is described in all four types of TAPVC, it is seen most commonly in infracardiac (type 3) and rarely seen in cardiac (type 2) TAPVC.
- The presence of TAPVC is an absolute indication for surgical repair. The timing of surgery is dependent upon the clinical situation at the time the diagnosis is made.
- Strategies aimed at optimizing biventricular function and preventing pulmonary hypertension are the corner-stones of post-operative management. The occurrence of post-operative pulmonary hypertensive events is a significant risk factor for early death status post-repair of TAPVC.
- Improved early mortality has been noted in patients with pre-operative pulmonary venous obstruction who were treated with inhaled NO in the post-operative period.
- The most important determinant of outcome beyond the acute post-operative period is the occurrence of recurrent pulmonary vein obstruction (RPVO).

Acknowledgments

The authors are grateful to Dr. Rob Martin, Bristol Royal Hospital for Children for providing the echocardiograms in Fig. 10.2.

References

1. Hancock Friesen CL, Zurakowski D, Thiagarajan R *et al*. Total anomalous venous connection: an analysis of current management strategies in a single institution. *Ann Thorac Surg* 2005; **79**: 596–606.
2. Bando K, Turrentine M, Ensing G *et al*. Surgical management of total anomalous pulmonary venous connection: thirty year trends. *Circulation* 1996; **94** (suppl II): II-12–II-16.
3. Hyde JAJ, Stumper O, Barth M.J *et al*. Total anomalous pulmonary venous connection: outcome of surgical correction and management of recurrent venous obstruction. *Eur J Cardiothorac Surg* 1999; **15**: 735–41.
4. Stark J. F, de Leval MR. Anomalous pulmonary venous return and cor triatriatum. In Stark JF, de Leval MR eds. *Surgery for Congenital Heart Defects*. Saunders 1994; Chapter 21, 329–42
5. Ishino K, Alexi-Meskishvili V, Hetzer R. Myocardial recovery through ECMO after repair of total anomalous pulmonary venous connection: the importance of left heart unloading. *Eur J Cardiothorac Surg* 1997; **11**: 585–7.
6. Ishino K, Alexi-Meskishvili V, Hetzer R. Preoperative extracorporeal membrane oxygenation in newborn with total anomalous pulmonary venous connection. *Cardiovasc Surg* 1999; **7**: 473–5.
7. Stewart DL, Mendoza JC, Winston S. Use of extracorporeal life support in total anomalous pulmonary venous drainage. *J Perinatol* 1996; **16**: 186–90.
8. Curran R, Mavroudis C, Backer C *et al*. Inhaled nitric oxide for children with congenital heart disease and pulmonary hypertension. *Ann Thorac Surg* 1995; **60**: 1765–71.
9. Rosales AM, Bolivar J, Burke RP *et al*. Adverse hemodynamic effects observed with inhaled nitric oxide after surgical repair of total anomalous pulmonary venous return. *Pediatr Cardiol* 1999; **20**: 224–6.
10. Atz AM, Wessel DL. Sidenafil ameliorates effects of inhaled nitric oxide withdrawl. *Anesthesiology* 1999; **91**: 307–10.
11. Michielon G, Di Donato RM, Pasquini L *et al*. Total anomalous pulmonary venous connection: long-term appraisal with evolving technical solutions. *Eur J Cardiothorac Surg* 2002; **22**: 184–91.
12. Bogers AJJC, Baak R, Lee PC *et al*. Early results and long-term follow-up after corrective surgery for total anomalous pulmonary venous return. *Eur J Cardiothorac Surg* 1999; **16**: 296–9.
13. Caldarone C, Najm H, Kadletz M *et al*. Relentless pulmonary vein stenosis after repair of total anomalous pulmonary venous drainage. *Ann Thorac Surg* 1998; **66**: 1514–20.
14. Ricci M, Elliott M, Cohen GA *et al*. Management of pulmonary venous obstruction after correction of TAPVC: risk factors for adverse outcome *Eur J Cardiothorac Surg* 2003; **24**: 28–36.
15. Lacour-Gayet F, Zoghbi J, Serraf AE *et al*. Surgical management of progressive pulmonary venous obstruction after repair of total anomalous pulmonary venous connection *J Thorac Cardiovasc Surg* 1999; **117**: 679–87.

Further reading

Critical Heart Disease in Infants and Children. Nichols DG, Camerron DE, Greely WJ, Lappe DG, Upgerleider RM, Wetzel RC. Mosby-Year Book Inc, 1995.

11 Critical care for a child with 80% burns

Heather Duncan

Introduction

Children who sustain burns to more than 80% of total body surface have a high mortality. Burn shock, sepsis and respiratory failure are major causes of death in severe burns.[1–4] The key to reducing mortality and morbidity is adequate fluid resuscitation, early burn excision and dedicated multidisciplinary team care for these complex patients.[2] In dedicated burns centers, if the patient survives, the long-term outlook is good for physical disability and quality of life.[2]

Case history

A previously well 2-year-old girl was trapped in her room during a house fire. She presented to the local accident and emergency department with stridor, a hoarse cry and moaning with pain. Pulse oximetry was normal with $15\,l\,min^{-1}$ face mask oxygen. She was assessed to have 80% partial and full thickness total body surface area (TBSA) burns, including her face and hands, and circumferential burns to her trunk and limbs. No other signs of trauma were evident. She was shocked, tachycardic, with a slightly elevated blood pressure. History, initial examination and findings and investigations are summarized in Table 11.1.

Emergency treatment

An intra-osseous needle was inserted into the right tibia followed by a femoral venous line (there were no visible veins). Blood samples taken and fluid resuscitation initiated at 300 ml kg^{-1} per h (based on 4 ml kg^{-1} per %TBSA). She was pre-oxygenated and her airway secured via a rapid sequence induction, using an uncut nasal 4.5 endotracheal tube (ETT), secured at 16 cm at the nostril. Carbonaceous sputum below her swollen vocal cords confirmed an inhalation burn injury. Morphine 0.3 mg kg^{-1} was administered intravenously for pain and a morphine infusion started at 60 mcg kg^{-1} per h. Further intravenous access was not immediately possible, so another intra-osseous line was inserted and 5% dextrose and 0.45% saline maintenance fluid was started at 50 ml kg^{-1} per h. A femoral arterial line was sited for invasive blood pressure monitoring.

Two hours after admission, the regional retrieval team arrived at the district general hospital. On their arrival, she was sedated (midazolam 150 mcg kg^{-1} per h), and muscle relaxed with intermittent boluses (atracurium 0.5 mg kg^{-1}) and she was pressure-cycle ventilated on pressures of $20/2\,cmH_2O$, at a rate of $20\,min^{-1}$ in 100% oxygen. SaO$_2$ was 90% and there was good air entry bilaterally with no added sounds on auscultation. Chest X-ray showed clear lung fields and the slightly long endotracheal tube had been repositioned. Pulmonary edema had been suspected and a dose of furosemide (0.5 mg kg^{-1}) had been given intravenously. Positive end expiratory pressure (PEEP) was increased, in increments, to $8\,cmH_2O$ with an improvement in SaO$_2$ to 95%. Arterial blood gas analysis confirmed adequate ventilation, oxygenation and that the carboxyhemaglobin (COHb) had decreased from 3.6% to 1%.

Case Studies in Pediatric Critical Care, ed. Peter. J. Murphy, Stephen C. Marriage, and Peter J. Davis. Published by Cambridge University Press. © Cambridge University Press 2009.

Table 11.1. *Summary of clinical examination and initial investigations at admission to accident and emergency department*

Past medical history	Fit and well Fully vaccinated
Regular medications	None
Allergies	None known
Examination	Severe burns, estimated 80% Stridor, moaning with pain Adequate oxygenation with face mask oxygen Respiratory rate 48 min^{-1} Heart rate 156 min^{-1} Blood pressure 120/60 mmHg Capillary refill time >5 seconds Temperature 35.8 °C Decreased level of consciousness; responding only to pain
Investigations	Weight	15 kg
	Height	100 cm
	FBC	Hb 9.4 g dl^{-1}, WBC × 10^9 l^{-1}, Platelets × 10^9 l^{-1}
	U+Es	Na$^+$ 140 mmol l^{-1}, K$^+$ 4.3 mmol l^{-1}, Urea 8.7 mmol l^{-1}, Creatinine 72 µmol l^{-1}
	Glucose	20.9 mmol l^{-1}
	Venous blood gas	pH 7.03, PaCO$_2$ 5.0 kPa, PaO$_2$ 53.6 kPa, COHb 3.6%, BE −19, Lactate 12.7
	CXR	Normal lung fields, endotracheal tube at carina
	Trauma XR series	No fractures

Hemodynamically, she was unstable, requiring ongoing fluid boluses for tachycardia (180 beats min^{-1}) and hypotension (65/35 mmHg), in addition to the resuscitation and maintenance fluids. Urine output was <0.5 ml kg^{-1} per h. An adrenal infusion 0.1 mcg kg^{-1} per min was started and blood products ordered. The burns were cleaned, dressed with Flamazine and covered with gauze dressings.

Prior to transfer, the femoral venous line was rewired and replaced with a triple lumen central line, a second right internal jugular triple lumen line was inserted and the intra-osseous lines removed. The 60-minute road ambulance transfer, back to the regional burn centre, was uneventful. Fluid resuscitation continued and she was transfused with a unit of packed red cells.

Progress in pediatric intensive care unit (PICU)

Shortly after arriving at the regional PICU, she was reassessed by the burns surgeon before undergoing a 3-hour procedure in theater, which involved escharotomy of both arms, both legs, and partial excision of the burn. The TBSA was reassessed to 88% full thickness burns

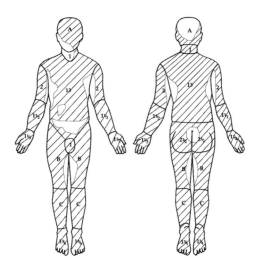

Fig. 11.1. Distribution of burns based on a Lund–Browder type body map. The hatched area represents full thickness burn.

(Fig. 11.1). Her facial burns were dressed with Polyfax and the burns on her limbs and trunk were dressed with Flamazine and gauze.

Ventilatory compliance deteriorated in the first 12 hours but, following excision of the burn, both the systemic inflammatory response and respiratory failure improved. Her maximum ventilatory requirements during the period on pressure regulated volume control were tidal volume 130 ml, delivering pressures of 30/8 cmH$_2$O at a rate of 25 min^{-1} in 100% oxygen. Gas exchange was satisfactory with arterial blood gas measurements of pH 7.20, PaCO$_2$ 6.3 kPa, PaO$_2$ 12.1 kPa, COHb 0.3%, BE −12.5, and lactate 2.2. Chest X-ray showed a gradual clearing of bilateral homogenous shadowing suggestive of an acute respiratory distress syndrome picture. In keeping with a mild inhalation injury, within 10 days she was on synchronized volume-controlled ventilation with pressure support. The same tidal volumes were delivering pressures of 17/7 and she was well oxygenated in 30% oxygen. Gradual weaning of ventilatory support was interrupted by an episode of line sepsis on day 15 post-burn. Despite the need for frequent anesthetics she was extubated 23 days after the burn injury, and, 3 days later, discharged to the burns high dependency unit.

Hemodynamically, she stabilized over the first 24 hours, the adrenaline infusion was stopped within 12 hours. She had high fluid requirements (Table 11.2) to maintain normal blood pressure, central venous pressure at 10 cmH$_2$O and adequate urine output of >1 ml kg^{-1} per h.

Enteral feeds were started at 8 hours post-burn. Nasogastric feeds were initially poorly tolerated so a nasojejunal feeding tube was inserted to achieve the target of 75 ml h^{-1} of Nutrini High Energy supplement. Energy requirements were calculated to deliver 165 kcal kg^{-1} per day and protein 3.4 g kg^{-1} per day. In an attempt to achieve full daily energy requirements, parenteral nutrition was used to supplement the initial reduced enteral intake, as well as during the episodes of sepsis and when the nasojejunal tube was temporarily displaced. The hyperglycemia, present at admission, did not resolve and an insulin infusion (0.05–0.2 units kg^{-1} per h) was needed for most of her PICU admission to maintain normoglycemia. Trace elements

Table 11.2. *Volumes of fluid in ml administered during the first 4 days post-burn excluding blood products administered for blood loss during surgical procedures. Resuscitation volumes were calculated on 80% TBSA burns*

Time from burn	0–1 h	1–8 h	8–24 h	24 h	Day 2	Day 3	Day 4
Intravenous fluid	600	4645	5225	10 470	2295	1940	1030
Oral feed			550	550	690	1430	1725
Total	600	4645	5575	11 020	2990	3370	2755
Balance	600	4585	5210		2540	2624	2156
Expected from Parkland formula	350	2450	3200	6000			
	170%	189%	163%	183%			

(selenium, zinc, and copper) were supplemented intravenously and monitored routinely and glutamine ($0.5\,g\,kg^{-1}$) was added to feeds. Persistent diarrhea was problematic with the high feed osmotic and volume load. After 2 weeks the feeds were adjusted to deliver $120\,kcal\,kg^{-1}$ per day and $3.3\,g^{-1}\,kg^{-1}$ per day of protein for persisting hypoalbuminemia $32\,g\,l^{-1}$.

An ophthalmology examination of her eyes was possible after 48 hours, when the swelling had reduced. There was no evidence of corneal burns and routine eye care was continued with the addition of topical antibiotics.

Assessing the interplay between her level of consciousness, pain and sedation were extremely difficult. The only apparent voluntary movement for the first 2 weeks was agitated non-purposeful shaking of her limbs; which appeared to increase with pain or distress. She was initially managed with the combination of morphine (range 60–1000 mcg kg^{-1} per h) and midazolam (range 180–360 mcg kg^{-1} per h). The doses of both drugs escalated as tolerance developed and the morphine was changed to diamorphine (range 360–800 mcg kg^{-1} per h), a more potent opiate, to limit the volume infused. During dressing changes on PICU she had the background infusions increased and additional boluses of diamorphine and midazolam. The infusions were gradually reduced, but she still remained on significant doses (diamorphine 360 mcg kg^{-1} per h and midazolam 180 mcg kg^{-1} per h) at the time of extubation and discharge. In addition to the above regimen, ketamine, clonidine, chlorpheniramine and chloral hydrate were all used at different times, in order to reduce her agitation.

The burn wounds were swabbed during her initial surgery for escharotomy and excision. At the time, the wounds were colonized with *Enterococcus* spp. and *Streptococcus* spp. Her temperature remained elevated at 38 °C and her white blood cell count was initially raised at $55 \times 10^{-9}\,l^{-1}$ but returned to normal range within 5 days. Antibiotics were prescribed for surgical procedures to prevent bacteremia and wounds were regularly swabbed for culture. Blood, modified non-bronchoscopic bronchoalveolar lavage, urine and stool cultures were taken with each suspected episode of sepsis. She had two courses of antibiotics in PICU. Nine days post-burn she was prescribed vancomycin and ciprofloxacin for a sustained fever >40 °C. Cultures were negative so antibiotics were stopped after 48 hours. On the 15th day post-burn she was once again cultured for a sustained fever >40 °C. *Enterococcus faecalis* and *Pseudomonas aeruginosa* were cultured from the central venous line, she was treated with vancomycin and ciprofloxacin for 5 days and new venous and arterial lines were inserted. During the second episode, she developed an inflammatory response for 24 hours requiring volume resuscitation but not inotropic support and, in addition, poor tolerance of enteral feeds necessitated four days of parenteral nutrition.

At the time of discharge from PICU, she was awake, watching her favorite videos and had a sleep–wake cycle.

Discussion

The treatment of children with >80% burns has advanced over the past 30 years with significant improvement in morbidity and mortality. Progress has been made in three areas: burn resuscitation, early excision and closure, and improved general critical care techniques. There are few double-blinded randomized, controlled trials, but a wealth of case series and laboratory evidence.

Initial assessment and management

It is essential, during the initial evaluation, to systematically and thoroughly examine the child in order to identify the degree of injury and to identify or exclude non-burn trauma, allowing the child to be stabilized. A detailed history of the nature of injury, the time it occurred, the duration of exposure, the potential for inhalation injury and any significant previous medical problems, is required.

Primary survey

Airway, Breathing, and *Circulation* remain the primary objective of initial assessment. Early recognition of airway or respiratory compromise, with prompt intubation, can be lifesaving. In circumstances of > 80% TBSA burn, airway, or inhalational burn it is necessary to secure the airway early. Airway and inhalation burns should be suspected with circumoral burns or swelling, singed nasal hair, sooty sputum, stridor, and hoarseness. Intubation should be performed with rapid sequence induction, with cervical spine protection if necessary, using an uncut oral or nasal cuffed endotracheal tube. An uncut ETT allows for the facial and airway swelling that occurs during the first 24–72 hours and a cuff is necessary to avoid perilous re-intubation during the first 72 hours.

Appropriate vascular access, central venous pressure, and arterial blood pressure monitoring should be sited and baseline blood tests sent. Four units of blood should be cross-matched. Fluid resuscitation should start immediately, a nasogastric tube should be passed for gastric decompression and a urinary catheter inserted to monitor urine output as a surrogate for cardiac output and to assess adequacy of volume resuscitation.

Burn-specific secondary survey

It is important to establish the mode of injury, presence or absence of other traumatic injury, carbon monoxide intoxication, and corneal burns. Routine cervical spine, chest, and pelvis X-rays and any further radiological investigations should be examined. Some trauma centers advocate a spiral computer tomography scan, with contrast, from vertex to pelvis rather than X-rays to quickly exclude any other injuries.[5]

An accurate assessment of the extent of the burn is important to inform treatment and transfer decisions. The injuries should be documented on a body map such as the Lund–Browder diagram that compensates for the changes in body proportions with age. A burn is drawn on the cartoon and an age-specific table is used to calculate the body surface area involved (Table 11.3). Alternatively, for areas of irregular or non-confluent burns, the patient's palm, without fingers, represents 0.5% of the body surface area.[6]

Table 11.3. *Adjustment for calculation of total body surface area in children according to age. The relatively large surface area of the head decreases and the surface area of the legs increase from infancy to adulthood*

AREA	Age <1 yr	1 yr	5 yr	10 yr	15 yr	Adult
A: Head	19%	17%	13%	11%	9%	7%
B: Thigh	5.5%	6.5%	8%	9%	9%	9.5%
C: Lower leg	5%	5%	5.5%	6%	6.5%	7%

Both size and depth are frequently underestimated on initial examination. The wound appearance will change over the subsequent few days; accordingly, serial examinations are useful. Partial thickness burns are red, wet, and very painful. They are likely to heal without grafting. Full thickness burns are pale, dry, leathery, and painless and are less likely to heal without grafting. Circumferential or near circumferential burns should be observed closely in close collaboration with the surgical team. Escharotomy of the chest wall should be performed when the burn causes a restriction to chest expansion and high inspiratory pressures are required for ventilation. Abdominal compartment syndrome presents with a tense distended abdomen, <1 ml kg^{-1} per h urine output and raised intra-abdominal pressure >25 mmHg measured transurethrally. Abdominal release can improve threatened organ perfusion until swelling resolves. Peripheral circulation should be monitored closely and fasciotomy performed to ensure peripheral circulation.

Child protection investigations reveal that Non-Accidental Injury (NAI) is associated with approximately a third of children with burns. NAI should always be considered, particularly where the history is not consistent with the clinical picture. The relevant child protection team should be notified and all clinical information and discussions with family members carefully documented.

Intensive care and monitoring

Patients with severe burns should be isolated and barrier nursed in a positive pressure thermoneutral environment. Scrupulous attention must be paid to preventing transmission of infection to these immunologically vulnerable patients. The attachment of external monitoring can be a challenge in children with severe burns. Adequate contact of ECG leads can be achieved by attaching crocodile clips to skin staples. The ETT is best secured with ties that are changed frequently to reduce the risk of infection or accidental dislodgement. Care needs to be taken to avoid pressure from the ties cutting into the angles of the mouth. Small individually made silicon molds can prevent this complication. End-tidal CO_2 measurement provides a useful trend. Invasive blood pressure monitoring with an arterial line enables an accurate blood pressure reading; blood gas analysis and the waveform can provide useful information about the intravascular fluid status.

The goal of burn resuscitation is tissue oxygen delivery. Pulse oximetry is necessary, but may give spurious readings because of reduced perfusion to burnt skin, and unusual sites such as the ears, the tongue, or the penis in boys can sometimes achieve better signals. In addition, falsely high readings can be misleading in association with carbon monoxide poisoning. To avoid unnecessarily high or low levels of oxygenation, the PaO_2 should be measured regularly. The threshold for adequate oxygen delivery has not yet been established.

Studies using subcutaneous fibre-optic oxygenation indices and gastric tonometry have shown that with fluid resuscitation, both oxygen delivery and consumption increase;[7,8] and that there is improved survival with good correlation between delivery and consumption. Burn-specific hemodynamic targets have not been established in children or adults, but expert guidance suggests keeping the hematocrit $\geq 0.30\%$ and central venous pressures $8-12\,cmH_2O$. In adults a study comparing $4\,ml\,kg^{-1}$ per %TBSA resuscitation and goal-directed therapy optimizing cardiac output using the transpulmonary thermodilution technique failed to demonstrate a difference in outcome.[9]

Inhalational burn and ventilation

The management of smoke inhalation is covered in more detail elsewhere in this book.

Children with inhalation burn injuries are more likely to die than those without.[1] The pattern of injury depends on the type of smoke and toxins inhaled. Early problems include airway edema and bronchospasm, and initial chest X-rays are frequently normal. Mucosal edema, leading to sloughing of the endobronchial endothelium, small airway obstruction, and alveolar edema occurs over the next few days and may lead to a clinical and radiological acute respiratory distress syndrome (ARDS) picture. There is no reliable way to stratify severity of injury, but early data using CT in animals seems promising.[10]

Clinical management of inhalational injury relies on protective ventilatory strategies, avoiding large tidal volumes and high inspired oxygen concentrations.[11] High frequency oscillatory ventilation, prone positioning, and inhaled nitric oxide can be of benefit, improving oxygenation in the short term, but have not been shown to improve outcome.[5,12] Despite extensive research in animals, no specific therapies of proven benefit have been identified.

The duration of ventilation following inhalation burn varies. Despite the requirement for long-term ventilation, most children do not require tracheostomy, although this remains contentious.[13–16]

Carbon monoxide binds strongly to hemoglobin to form carboxyhemaglobin, reducing the oxygen-carrying capacity of blood and tissue oxygen delivery. The effect is similar to hypoxic ischemic injury with global effects on the brain, myocardium, liver, kidneys, and bowel. Carboxyhemoglobin levels are normally <0.6%. Levels <7% are seldom associated with the global effects of acute carbon monoxide poisoning, and levels >15% may require further treatment. In most circumstances the levels will reduce with high inspired oxygen alone. The role of hyperbaric oxygen treatment for carbon monoxide poisoning remains questionable.[17] Two randomized control trials in adults have failed to show benefit except in cognitive function at 6 weeks post-injury.[18,19]

Fluid resuscitation and hemodynamics

The mechanisms of capillary leak associated with burns and consequent fluid resuscitation requirements are poorly understood. It is presumed that inflammatory mediators are released from the injured tissue. Fluid redistributes into the soft tissue, and subsequent intracellular and extracellular edema causes significant morbidity with respiratory failure, compartment syndromes of the chest, abdomen, and extremities. Delayed resuscitation is associated with higher fluid requirements and worse inflammatory response.

Fluid requirements include both resuscitation and maintenance volumes. For resuscitation fluid volume, the Parkland or Baxter formula (Table 11.4), described by Charles Baxter from Parkland Hospital in the 1960s, is calculated as $4\,ml\,kg^{-1}$ per %TBSA and is a popular starting point.

Table 11.4. *Fluid prescription for resuscitation and maintenance based on 80% TBSA using the Parkland/Baxter formula compared with prescriptions from the Shriners Hospitals for Children*

Fluid Prescription	Calculation	Fluid per day	Fluid per hour
Resuscitation (Parkland/Baxter)[a] Hartmanns solution (or half Hartmann's solution + half HAS 4.5%)	$4 \times$ weight $\times$ % TBSA $15\,kg \times 80\% \times 4$ $15\,kg \times 30\,ml$	4800 ml 2400 ml 2400 ml	0–8 h 300 ml hr^{-1} 9–24 h 150 ml h^{-1}
Maintenance 5% dextrose, 0.9% saline, 20 mmol KCl l^{-1}	$10\,kg \times 4\,ml\,h^{-1}$ $5\,kg \times 2\,ml\,h^{-1}$	80 ml kg^{-1} per day	50 ml h^{-1}
Total volume 0–8 h Total volume 9–24 h		2800 ml 3200 ml	350 ml h^{-1} 200 ml h^{-1}
Shriners Hospital for Children, Boston 0–8 hr Ringer's lactate + 50 mmol bicarbonate 9–16 hr Ringer's lactate 17–24 hr Ringer's lactate +12.5 g albumin l^{-1}	4 ml kg per %TBSA + 1500 ml m^{-2} BSA	5970 ml	
Shriners Hospital for Children, Galveston Ringer's lactate +12.5 g albumin l^{-1}	5000 ml m^{-2} + 2000 ml m^{-2} BSA[b]	5460 ml	

[a] An extra 30 ml kg^{-1} per day could be added for inhalation burn. [b] Body Surface Area (BSA) is calculated as (87 (height in cm + weight in kg) − 2600) / 10 000. Human Albumin Solution (HAS).

Fluid resuscitation formulae provide a guide but are inaccurate in most individual patients with more than 50% of patients needing resuscitation fluid in excess of the Parkland formula.[20,21] Fluid prescription should be adjusted according to arterial and central venous pressure targets as well as urine output. Half of the fluid deficit is corrected in the first 8 hours and the rest in the following 16 hours. Different centers have preferences for various crystalloid solutions (Table 11.4) and in some centers colloid (human albumin solution or gelofusin) is only used after the first 8 hours because of concerns about osmotic particles leaking into soft tissue and exacerbating tissue edema. Inhalation burns should receive an extra 30 ml kg^{-1} to compensate for additional fluid losses.[22]

The clinical end-points of fluid resuscitation are good peripheral perfusion, stable age-appropriate blood pressure, adequate urine output with sufficient oxygenation and normal lactate. In a child the target output is 1 ml kg^{-1} per h of urine. Oliguria is usually due to hypovolemia and so should be treated by doubling the resuscitation fluids for 1 hour and assessing the need for colloid in the form of blood products. In this case furosemide was given early in the resuscitation for suspected pulmonary edema. Although capillary leak is a problem throughout the early phase, pulmonary edema is seldom a problem. The desaturation was most likely due to atelectasis and inadequate lung recruitment that responded appropriately with increased level of PEEP. Diuretics may give a false impression of urine output and mask hypovolemia. Excessive muscle breakdown causes myoglobinuria visible as pigmented urine and here the fluid intake should be increased to produce $2 \, \mathrm{ml \, kg^{-1}}$ per h urine output. Occasionally in this circumstance mannitol $0.25 \, \mathrm{mg \, kg^{-1}}$ is indicated to enhance urine output and prevent myoglobin from obstructing the renal tubules.

Inflammatory response and burn care

Patients with severe burns can only recover with definitive wound closure. Intensive care can support the patient until coverage is achieved. The burn is the major propagator of the inflammatory response. Early excision promotes healing and reduces the risk of infection thereby reducing the effects of hypermetabolism.

Local tissue damage causes increased capillary permeability and edema with a peak in fluid loss between 1 and 3 hours after the burn. Cytokines orchestrate the systemic inflammatory response, which produces malaise, arthralgia, and resets the hypothalamic temperature control. There is considerable variability but most patients with >25% burns will develop systemic inflammatory response syndrome (SIRS). This is defined as two or more of the following: temperature >38 °C or <36 °C, heart rate $>90 \, \mathrm{min^{-1}}$, respiratory rate $>24 \, \mathrm{min^{-1}}$ or $PaCO_2 < 32 \, \mathrm{mmHg}$, and white cell count >12 or $<4 \times 10^6 \, \mathrm{l^{-1}}$.[23] SIRS is usually evident within 36 hours and the severity correlates with mortality. The capillary leak, increased oxygen demand, and increased carbon dioxide production caused by hypermetabolism often precipitates the need for ventilation.

Surgical expertise is required to correctly differentiate between areas of partial thickness burn that will heal from those areas of full thickness burn that are unlikely to heal and will require excision and grafting. Excision of large surface area can lead to significant blood loss. However, modern surgical techniques have reduced the requirement for blood products by using clysis (adrenaline infiltration into the subcutaneous tissue), euthermia (warm operating theaters), and regional techniques with tourniquets.

The current standard dressings are gauze for temporary cover of partial thickness burns and split skin graft for full thickness burns. To cover extensive excised full thickness burns, the alternatives are allograft (donated human skin), xenograft (porcine skin), cultured keratinocytes, and fibroblasts sprayed onto the wound and a biological membrane Integra. Covering the wound with biological or synthetic skin substitutes appears to reduce hypermetabolism and promote healing.[4,5] All wounds, regardless of dressing, need to be carefully monitored for infection and usually once-daily dressings are required. This time should be utilized to ensure all invasive lines and tubes are clean and well secured as well as using the opportunity to perform range of movement maneuvers and correct positioning to avoid contractures.

Nutrition, energy requirements and hypermetabolism

The stress response to burns is biphasic with an initial phase of shock, profound vasoconstriction and a reduction in the Resting Energy Expenditure (REE); which limits fluid loss and causes hypothermia. Pain, hypovolemia, and starvation switch on catabolic stress hormones that promote metabolism of stored energy. During episodes of starvation fat usually provides energy; in burns, however, skeletal muscle becomes the major source through gluconeogenesis.[24] There is high protein turnover with a net loss, leading to muscle wasting. Extreme loss of lean muscle is associated with a high mortality.

During the second phase of repair, the REE increases, the temperature typically remains at 38.5 °C, circulation becomes hyperdynamic and tissue is repaired. The increased REE is related to the size of the burn and is partly as a result of increased circulating catecholamines, glucocorticoids and glucagon.[25,26] Hyperglycemia is common and is associated with higher mortality.[27] Insulin resistance and suppression increases the catabolic process and, although catabolism cannot be reversed by an insulin infusion, there appears to be a reduction in acute phase proteins with insulin-induced euglycemia.[28,29]

The temperature needs to be maintained at normothermia or mild pyrexia to reduce metabolic demand. The ambient temperature needs to be high, especially when the patient is exposed for surgery or dressing changes. The mild pyrexia is thought to be beneficial but measures should be taken to reduce the temperature below 41 °C. Physical cooling is effective, but peripheral vasoconstriction should be avoided. Antipyretic drugs are not beneficial and may impair healing.

Apart from the obvious risk posed by septicemia in an immunocompromised patient, infection causes increased metabolic demand and should be prevented. Hand washing, regular wound disinfection, and debridement all contribute to wound sterility. The gut is a major source of infection with increased gut permeability and bacterial translocation.[30] However, selective gut decontamination is not recommended.[31]

Early enteral feeding can reduce these risks. Nutrition has emerged as a vital component in the management of critically ill patients supplying vital cell substrate, antioxidants, trace elements, and vitamins. Protein is lost through the surface of the burn and, as amino acids are used for tissue repair and immunological defense, these should be replaced. Catabolism further induces a negative nitrogen balance and an increased protein requirement. Exogenous sources of protein must be supplied to minimize loss of essential amino acids, muscle and bodyweight. The protein target is usually 3 g kg^{-1} per day and the caloric target is usually $1.5 \times$ basal metabolic rate or $1.2 \times$ REE measured by indirect calorimetry.[5] In addition to critical illness and burns, catecholamine infusions and systemic corticosteroids can increase the hypermetabolic state. In contrast, opiates, muscle relaxants, and barbiturates can reduce energy expenditure. This influences the choice of drugs used in the management of children with severe burns.

Monitoring nutrition is important and should be performed regularly using a combination of body weight, muscle mass measurement, urine nitrogen balance, indirect calorimetry (where available), serum protein, and urea measurements under the care of an experienced dietician.

Enteral feeding

There is increasing evidence that starting enteral feeding, as soon as possible, is beneficial. A systematic review in adult patients showed early enteral nutrition was associated with a lower incidence of infection and reduced length of hospital stay.[32,33] In animal studies immediate enteral feeding is associated with a decrease in hypermetabolic rate, lower levels of circulating stress hormones (i.e. glucagons, cortisol, and noradrenaline), increased gastro-intestinal blood flow, a reduction in bacterial translocation from the intestinal tract, and improved outcome There is no clear consensus with regards to how early to start feeds as studies describing "early feeds" range from 2–24 hours after the burn. This would suggest enteral feeding should commence within the first 24 hours.

The long-term addition of glutamine, which acts as an essential amino acid in severe burns, has been successful in reducing intestinal permeability and septicemia, improving wound healing and reducing length of hospitalization.[34,35]

Total Parenteral Nutrition (TPN) is associated with higher mortality in burned patients and the requirement for TPN usually signifies failure of enteral nutrition heralding an infective episode.[36]

Analgesia and sedation

In the emergency situation morphine is the drug of choice and should be titrated to achieve adequate levels of analgesia. Reducing pain associated with burn care has a positive impact on both long-term emotional sequelae for the patient as well as a positive impact on caregivers.[2] A combination of an opiate and a benzodiazepine is most frequently used. Standard pain assessment tools for children are used in the absence of burn specific tools. Tolerance results in increasing requirements and large doses are sometimes required. In a recent report as much morphine as (mean 0.35 ± 0.33, range $0.01–4.38\,\mathrm{mg^{-1}\,kg^{-1}}$ per h) and midazolam (mean 0.14 ± 0.17, range $0.01–1.82\,\mathrm{mg^{-1}\,kg^{-1}}$ per h) were required during long-term ventilation of children with severe burns.[16] Post-traumatic stress disorder is common after severe burns and in some centers early introduction of antidepressants and other drugs as adjunct to analgesia (e.g. gabapentin) have been shown to reduce the prevalence.[5,37]

Neuromuscular blockade is used to assist in effective ventilation. Suxamethonium is avoided after the first 24 hours in burns because of the risk of severe hyperkalemia and arrhythmia. Rocuronium can be used as an alternative for rapid sequence induction and atracurium or cisatracurium can be used in multi-organ failure.

Infection

Constant vigilance is required to detect infection in children with severe burns. In children with >30% TBSA burns, wound infection is the most common source, followed by nosocomial pneumonia, urinary tract infection, septicemia, and Central Venous Catheter infection.[38] Colonization of the burn wound with bacteria is common and surveillance with regular wound swabs usually identifies the likely colonizing organisms. Antibiotics are not necessary for colonization but clinical suspicion of infection should be treated promptly with broad-spectrum antibiotics until cultures can direct specific drug choice. Wound infection can be localized as cellulitis; which presents with redness and swelling of the unaffected skin alongside the burn or invasive, which is caused by rapid proliferation of bacteria in the eschar and progresses to invade the viable tissues below. A low incidence of septicemia is reported with a protocol that requires catheters to be changed over a guide wire every 7 days. The tip of the removed catheter is semi-quantitively cultured and a new catheter is inserted into a new site for cultures growing >15 colony-forming units and inflamed insertion site.[39]

Mortality

Death from burns can occur in the first few days due to shock or associated injuries, in the first few weeks as a result of wound sepsis and later as a result of respiratory insufficiency. In units that routinely care for children with >80% burns the mortality remains high at between 14% and 40%.[1,3]

Learning points

- Early, aggressive fluid resuscitation improves survival.
- Fluid resuscitation should be patient specific using the published formulae as a general guide with the patient's clinical condition and response to fluid.
- Inhalational burn should be suspected with facial burns, a hoarse voice, singed facial hair, and sooty sputum.
- The airway should be secured early with an uncut endotracheal tube following rapid sequence induction. Facial and airway edema will progress for 12–48 hours.

- Unconscious patients, those with >80% TBSA burns and signs of inhalation burn should be intubated and ventilation optimized.

- Carbon monoxide poisoning usually resolves with high-inspired oxygen and effective ventilation. Hyperbaric oxygen should be considered in severe cases (>15% COHb) and where the chamber can easily be accessed.

- Early burn resection and coverage reduces catabolism, pain, and risk of infection.

- Early enteral feeding promotes healing and reduces gut permeability to bacteria.

- High doses of morphine and midazolam are required and should be weaned slowly.

References

1. Sheridan R, Remensnyder J, Schnitzer J et al. Current expectations for survival in pediatric burns. Arch Pediatr Adolesc Med 2000; **154**: 245–9.

2. Sheridan R, Hinson M, Liang M et al. Long-term outcome of children surviving massive burns. J Am Med Assoc 2000; **283**: 69–73.

3. Spies M, Herndon D, Rosenblatt J et al. Prediction of mortality from catastrophic burns in children. Lancet 2003; **361**: 989–94.

4. Sheridan R. Comprehensive treatment of burns. Curr Problems Surg 2001; **38** (9):641–756.

5. Sheridan R, Tompkins R. What's new in burns and metabolism. J Am Coll Surgeons 2004; **198**(2): 243–63.

6. Sheridan R, Petras L, Basha G. Planimetry study of the percent of body surface represented by the hand and palm: sizing irregular burns is more accurately done with the palm. J Burn Care Rehabil 1995; **16**(6): 605–6.

7. Holm C, Melcer B, Horbrand F, von Donnersmarck G, Mulbauer W. The relationship between oxygen delivery and oxygen consumption during fluid resuscitation of burn-related shock. J Burn Care Rehabil 2000; **21**(2): 147–54.

8. Holm C. Resuscitation in shock associated with burns. Tradition or evidence-based medicine? Resuscitation 2000; **44**: 157–64.

9. Holm C, Mayr M, Tegeler J et al. A clinical randomised study on the effects of invasive monitoring on burn shock resuscitation. Burns 2004; **30**(8): 798–807.

10. Park M, Cancio L, Batchinsky A et al. Assessment of severity of ovine smoke inhalation injury by analysis of computed tomography scans. J Trauma 2003; **55**: 417–27.

11. Sheridan R, Kacmarek R, McEttrick M et al. Permissive hypercapnia as a ventilatory strategy in burned children: effect on barotrauma, pneumonia, and mortality. J Trauma 1995; **39**: 854–9.

12. Sheridan R, Zapol W, Ritz R, Tompkins R. Low-dose inhaled nitric oxide in acutely burned children with profound respiratory failure. Surgery 1999; **126**: 856–62.

13. Palmieri T, Jackson W, Greenhalgh D. Benefits of early tracheostomy in severely burned children. Crit Care Med 2002; **30**: 922–4.

14. Saffle J, Morris S, Edelman L. Early tracheostomy does not improve outcome in burn patients. J Burn Care Rehabil 2002; **23**: 431–8.

15. Kadilak P, Sheridan R. Prolonged oral intubation is safe in critically ill children. J Burn Care Rehabil 2001; **22**: S53.

16. Kadilak P, Vanasse S, Sheridan R. Favorable short- and long-term outcomes of prolonged translaryngeal intubation in critically ill children. J Burn Care Rehabil 2004; **25**(3): 262–5.

17. Sheridan R, Shanks E. Hyperbaric oxygen treatment: a brief overview of a controversial topic. J Trauma 1999; **47**: 426–35.

18. Scheinkestel C, Bailey M, Myles P et al. Hyperbaric or normobaric oxygen for acute carbon monoxide poisoning: a randomised controlled trial. Med J Aust 1999; **170**: 203–10.

19. Weaver L, Hopkins R, Chan K et al. Hyperbaric oxygen for acute carbon monoxide poisoning. N Engl J Med 2002; **347**: 1057–67.

20. Friedrich J, Sullivan S, Engrav L et al. Is supra-Baxter resuscitation in burn patients a new phenomenon? Burns 2004; **30**(5): 464–6.

21. Engrav L, Colescott P, Kemalyan N et al. A biopsy of the use of the Baxter formula to resuscitate or do we do it like Charlie did it? *J Burn Care Rehabil* 2000; **21** (2): 91–5.

22. Inoue T, Okabayashi K, Ohtan M et al. Effect of smoke inhalation injury on fluid requirement in burn resuscitation. *J Med Sci* 2002; **51**: 1–5.

23. American College of Chest Physicians/ Society of Critical Care Medicine Consensus Conference: Definitions for sepsis and organ failure and guidelines for the use of innovative therapies in sepsis. *Crit Care Med* 1993; **21**: 476–7.

24. Wilmore DW, Mason AD, Jr, Pruitt BA, Jr, Insulin response to glucose in hypermetabolic burn patients. *Ann Surg* 1976; **183**(3): 314–20.

25. Herndon D, Tompkins R. Support of the metabolic response to burn injury. *Lancet* 2004; **363**(9424): 1895–902.

26. Gore D, Wolf S, Herndon D, Wolfe R. Relative influence of glucose and insulin on peripheral amino acid metabolism in severely burned patients. *J Parenter Enteral Nutr* 2002; **26**: 271–7.

27. Gore D, Chinkes D, Heggers J et al. Association of hyperglycaemia with increased mortality after severe burn injury. *J Trauma* 2001; **51**: 540–4.

28. Jeschke M, Klein D, Herndon D. Insulin treatment improves the systemic inflammatory reaction to severe trauma. *Ann Surg* 2004; **239**(4): 553–60.

29. Wu X, Thomas S, Herndon D, Sanford A, Wolf S. Insulin decreases hepatic acute phase protein levels in severely burnt children. *Surgery* 2004; **135**(2): 196–202.

30. Deitch E. Intestinal permeability is increased in burn patients shortly after burn injury. *Surgery* 1990; **107**: 411–16.

31. Barret J, Jeschke M, Herndon D. Selective gut decontamination of the digestive tract in severely burned pediatric patients. *Burns* 2001; **27**(5): 439–45.

32. Marik P. Early enteral nutrition in acutely ill patients: a systematic review. *Crit Care Med* 2001; **29**: 2264–70.

33. Gianotti L. Role of enteral feeding and acute starvation on postburn bacterial translocation and host defence: prospective, randomised trials. *Crit Care Med* 1994; **22**: 265–72.

34. Garrel D, Patenaude J, Nedelec B et al. Decreased mortality and infectious morbidity in adult burn patients given enteral glutamine supplements: a prospective, controlled, randomised clinical trial. *Crit Care Med* 2003; **31**: 2444–9.

35. Peng X, Yan H, You Z, Wang P, Weber J. Effects of enteral supplementation with glutamine granules on intestinal mucosal barrier function in severe burned patients. *Burns* 2004; **30**(2): 135–9.

36. Wolf S. Enteral feeding intolerance: an indicator of sepsis-associated mortality in burned children. *Arch Surg* 1997; **132**: 1310–13.

37. Sheridan R, Hinson M, Nackel A et al. Development of a pediatric burn pain and anxiety management program. *J Burn Care Rehabil* 1997; **18**(5): 455–9.

38. Sheridan R, Schnitzer J. Management of the high-risk pediatric burn patient. *J Pediatr Surg* 2001; **36**(8): 1308–12.

39. Sheridan R, Weber J, Peterson H, Tompkins R. Central venous catheter sepsis with weekly catheter change in paediatric burn patients. *Burns* 1995; **21**(2): 127–9.

Further reading

1. Henning R. Smoke inhalation. In: Macnab A, Macrae D, Henning R, eds. *Care of the Critically Ill Child*. London, Churchill Livingstone 1999; Chapter 4.2, 348–53.

2. Oliver RI, Spain D. Burns, Resuscitation and Early Management. 12 November 2004. www.emedicine.com/plastic/topic159.htm.

3. Prelack K, Dylewski M, Sheridan RL. Practical guidelines for nutritional management of burn injury and recovery. *Burns* 2007 Feb; **33**(1): 14–24. Epub 2006 Nov 20.

4. Sheridan RL. Comprehensive treatment of burns. *Current Problems in Surgery* 2001; **38** (9): 641–756.

5. Sheridan RL. Burns, Thermal Injuries. 7 November 2003. www.emedicine.com/plastic/topic510.htm.

Coarctation of the aorta in a neonate

Matt Oram and Andrew Wolf

Introduction

Coarctation of the Aorta (CoA) is a vascular abnormality in which the aorta is narrowed, most commonly in the region of the ductus arteriosus and left subclavian artery. This results in an obstruction to blood flow to the lower body. The patient with CoA presenting to the pediatric intensive care unit (PICU) generally falls into one of two groups. They may present in the neonatal period, when closure of the ductus arteriosus precipitates sufficient obstruction to cause symptoms and signs or later in childhood following elective surgery. Those that present in the older child are often discovered as an incidental finding of a murmur or hypertension with or without non-specific symptoms such as fatigue or shortness of breath on exertion.

Case history

A 5-day-old boy was referred from the neonatal intensive care unit (NICU) of a peripheral hospital to the cardiac surgical center for management of a CoA. He had been delivered uneventfully at full term, had initially appeared to be well with no suspected abnormality. On the fifth postnatal day, he was readmitted to hospital having been noted to be feeding poorly, vomiting, and becoming progressively tachypnoic.

Examination and initial management

Examination revealed a tachycardia of 200 beats per minute, a capillary refill time of 5 seconds, impalpable femoral pulses, hepatomegaly, a respiratory rate of 80 breaths per minute and cyanosis, with an oxygen saturation on pulse oximetry of 88% in air. He was found to be hypoglycemic ($2.0 \, \text{mmol} \, l^{-1}$) and acidotic. Capillary blood gases showed a pH of 7.07, $p\text{CO}_2$ 2.0 kPa, bicarbonate $4 \, \text{mmol} \, l^{-1}$ and base excess $-26 \, \text{mmol} \, l^{-1}$. He was placed in headbox oxygen and having secured venous access, given $5 \, \text{ml} \, \text{kg}^{-1}$ of intravenous 10% dextrose and $20 \, \text{ml} \, \text{kg}^{-1}$ of 4.5% human albumin solution then transferred to the NICU. His initial management included intubation, ventilation, and the placement of a nasogastric tube. A right radial arterial catheter was inserted and routine blood tests sent. An ECG revealed a sinus tachycardia and a chest radiograph showed evidence of cardiomegaly with pulmonary congestion. Differential diagnoses of sepsis, a metabolic disorder or a cardiac abnormality were considered. The absence of femoral pulses had alerted the neonatologist to the possible presence of a CoA, and a trans-thoracic echocardiogram was arranged. This demonstrated a discrete narrowing in the descending aorta, at the origin of the left subclavian artery. There was some flow through a patent ductus arteriosus. The child was commenced on an infusion of prostaglandin E_1 (alprostadil) at $10 \, \text{ng} \, \text{kg}^{-1}$ per min and the regional cardiac surgical center contacted.

Case Studies in Pediatric Critical Care, ed. Peter. J. Murphy, Stephen C. Marriage, and Peter J. Davis. Published by Cambridge University Press. © Cambridge University Press 2009.

Progress in the pediatric intensive care unit

Following an uneventful transfer by the retrieval team, the baby was admitted to PICU. A repeat chest radiograph showed the endotracheal and nasogastric tubes to be correctly positioned. Bloods were taken for routine biochemistry, a full blood count, coagulation profile, and blood cross-matching. Arterial blood gases showed some resolution of the acidosis with a base excess of -12 mmol l^{-1} and a serum lactate of 8 mmol l^{-1}. The Prostaglandin E_1 infusion was increased to 30 ng kg^{-1} per min to improve ductal and therefore aortic blood flow. Echocardiography was repeated, confirming the diagnosis and demonstrating a patent ductus arteriosus. Intravenous maintenance fluids were restricted to 80 ml kg^{-1} per day of 10% dextrose/ 0.45% saline. Furosemide 1 mg kg^{-1} 12-hourly was given intravenously. In view of the ongoing lactic acidosis, a right internal jugular central venous catheter was inserted for monitoring of right atrial filling pressure and infusion of vasoactive drugs. Dopamine 5 mcg kg^{-1} per min was commenced.

Over the following 24 hours, the child showed signs of an improved circulation with correction of the metabolic acidosis and maintenance of a good urine output. Having established cardiovascular stability, the decision was made to proceed to surgery. The CoA was repaired via a left thoracotomy incision using a flap from the left subclavian artery (having tied off the subclavian artery distally). The aortic cross-clamp time was 18 minutes and there was no excessive bleeding. During the procedure the baby became progressively hypotensive, requiring an increase in the dopamine infusion to 10 mcg kg^{-1} per min to maintain the mean arterial pressure above 40 mmHg. The prostaglandin infusion was discontinued at the end of the procedure.

Post-operatively, sedation and analgesia was maintained with a morphine infusion at 10–20 mcg kg^{-1} per hour. The femoral pulses and left upper limb perfusion were assessed regularly. The dopamine infusion was weaned off over the following 24 hours with an echocardiogram showing mildly impaired left ventricular function. The intercostal drain was removed on the first post-operative day having drained a minimal amount with no air leak, and the child was extubated 18 hours post-operatively. Fluid restriction was continued at 80 ml kg^{-1} per day. The child was restarted on twice-daily diuretics (furosemide 1 mg kg^{-1} and spironolactone 1 mg kg^{-1}) and regular paracetamol.

Over the following 24 hours, with the slow reintroduction of feeds, increasing abdominal distension was noted along with bilious nasogastric aspirates. An abdominal X-ray was arranged, which showed fluid levels within the bowel as well as gas within the thickened bowel wall. A surgical opinion was sought and a diagnosis of Necrotizing Enterocolitis (NEC) made. As there was no evidence of obstruction or perforation and the baby was relatively systemically well, it was decided to manage the NEC conservatively. The nasogastric tube was left in situ on free drainage and intravenous fluids continued. Enteral nutrition was withheld and total parenteral nutrition commenced. Antibiotics (ampicillin, gentamicin, and metronidazole) were prescribed for the following 7 days. Over that time, the nasogastric aspirates decreased, the abdominal distension resolved and repeated X-rays showed resolution of the intra-mural gas in the bowel. At this point, enteral nutrition with expressed breast milk was cautiously re-introduced, and by 2 weeks the child was on to full enteral feeding and ready for discharge home.

Discussion

CoA is found in around 1 in 2000 live births. CoA accounts for 7% of neonates presenting with cardiac defects. Males are affected more commonly than females. There are two distinct sub-groups of patients, those that present in the neonatal (and indeed antenatal) period and those who present as older children or adults.[1]

The precise etiology of CoA is not known. Proposed mechanisms include: abnormalities of aortic growth, the presence of ductal tissue extending into the vessel wall which contracts after birth and vessel injury occurring before birth.[1] Anatomically, the CoA classically occurs distal to the origin of left subclavian artery and at or distal to the ductus arteriosus (see Fig. 12.1). When viewed from the exterior, the aorta has a localized indentation that corresponds to an internal "shelf," which causes the obstruction to blood flow.

The condition may exist in isolation or be associated with both other cardiac and non-cardiac abnormalities. The most commonly associated cardiac abnormalities include a ventricular septal defect, atrial septal defect, bicuspid aortic valve (or other abnormality of the aortic valve), hypoplastic left heart syndrome, and transposition of the great arteries.[2] Long-term arterial abnormalities may also be associated with the condition including aortic root dilatation and aneurysm formation, both of the aorta and intracranial arteries. Associated non-cardiac conditions include chromosomal abnormalities (Turner's syndrome, Down's syndrome), prematurity, diaphragmatic hernia, and tracheo-esophageal fistula.

Presentation and resuscitation

In the neonatal period, a CoA usually presents within the first 2 to 3 weeks of life when the ductus arteriosus closes. Until this time, a right to left shunt across the duct will maintain lower body perfusion albeit with desaturated blood. Duct closure results in decreased aortic blood flow distal to the origin of the left subclavian artery leading to the key clinical finding of weak or absent femoral pulses. It should be noted that a normal lower limb blood pressure, measured by an automated monitor, does not reliably exclude a CoA. Conversely, a marked

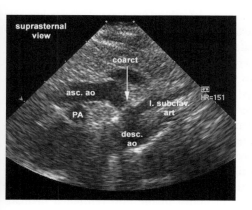

Fig. 12.1. 2-D echocardiogram or the aortic arch showing a CoA at the origin of the left subclavian artery (asc. ao – ascending aorta, coarct – coarctation, desc. ao – descending aorta, l. subclav art – left subclavian artery, PA – pulmonary artery).

Table 12.1. *Initial management of the sick neonate with a suspected CoA*

Airway and breathing	Provide oxygen
	Consider intubation and ventilation
Circulation	Venous access (peripheral, intra-osseous or central venous)
	Check blood glucose
	Check femoral pulses
	Check SpO_2 and BP in all four limbs
Differential diagnosis	Coarctation
	Other cardiac abnormality
	Sepsis
	Metabolic disorder
Having diagnosed a CoA	Prostaglandin E_1 or E_2
	Consider an inotrope, e.g. dopamine
	Echocardiogram if facilities available
	Fluid restrict ± diuretics
	No enteral nutrition initially if unwell/shocked
Make early contact with regional pediatric cardiology center	

difference in blood pressure between limbs is more likely due to random variation than CoA,[3] and the infant will still require echocardiography to confirm or exclude the diagnosis of coarctation.

The decreased blood flow distal to the coarctation leads to regional tissue hypoxia, anaerobic metabolism, and lactic acidosis. The high resistance (or afterload) to left ventricular ejection presented by the infant with CoA results in cardiac failure and, if severe, pulmonary edema. The end-result of this process is a rapid deterioration in the condition of the baby unless the diagnosis is made and resuscitation undertaken.

Resuscitation should follow the standard airway, breathing, and circulation approach (see Table 12.1) with attention to blood glucose as hypoglycemia is a common finding (as with other causes of critical illness in neonates). Early sedation, intubation, and mechanical ventilation of the severely acidotic or hemodynamically unstable neonate may offer some benefit. Airway protection can be provided to the obtunded patient, oxygenation may be improved, left ventricular afterload is reduced, invasive procedures are performed more easily, and a safer inter-hospital transfer can be undertaken.

The key aspect to management is the urgent delivery of intravenous Prostaglandin E_1 or E_2. These prostaglandins usually act by reopening the ductus arteriosus and restoring aortic blood flow distal to the CoA. This allows time for transfer and stabilization of the baby prior to surgery. The starting dose of $10\,ng\,kg^{-1}$ per min may need to be increased to $50\,ng\,kg^{-1}$ per min if there is no improvement in the physiological state of the baby. It must be borne in mind that there is a risk of apnea in the non-ventilated neonate receiving a prostaglandin E_1 or E_2 infusion as well as hypotension, bradycardia, flushing, fever, and coagulopathy. There is also evidence to suggest that prostaglandins may relieve the obstruction of CoA by their effect on ectoptic ductal tissue within the aorta without reopening the duct.[4]

The sick neonate will usually receive fluid boluses during the initial resuscitation efforts whilst diagnostic uncertainty exists. However, these patients are likely to have some degree of left ventricular failure and often also right ventricular failure. Therefore, once the diagnosis of CoA is made, it may be necessary to commence an inotrope, restrict fluids, and give diuretics. Enteral feeding should not be started in the sick neonate (see below). Where a period of relative stability and correction of the acidosis can be achieved, surgery may be deferred for a few days. In the case of the neonate who continues to deteriorate despite intensive care management, surgery is undertaken as an emergency.

Arterial cannulation

If arterial cannulation or sampling is to be undertaken prior to surgery, it should be remembered that only the right radial, brachial, and axillary arteries are available for intra-operative monitoring. The femoral arteries are clearly not useful as they lie distal to the obstruction and the left upper limb arteries are not suitable if the left subclavian artery is ligated during repair. With this limited number of possible sites in mind, arterial cannulation should only be undertaken by experienced practitioners after careful consideration of alternative strategies such as non-invasive blood pressure measurement and the use of capillary blood gases.

Surgery

The most common operations performed are a resection and an "end-to-end" anastamosis or a subclavian flap repair.[5] Another variation on these techniques is the end-to-side aortic anastomosis, which has been reported to be effective and even when performed in the neonatal period to have a low rate of recurrence of coarctation.[6] Operations more rarely performed in neonates are the insertion of an artificial patch into the aorta,[7] although this has a relatively high prevalence of reintervention, for complications such as aneurysm formation, and transcatheter balloon dilatation, which is increasingly used in older children and adults.[8] This technique has been used fairly successfully as a palliative procedure in neonates[9] and has even been reported as a rescue therapy in a 28-week preterm neonate.[10] Endovascular stenting has also been reported as an emergency treatment for neonatal coarctation.[11]

The "end-to-end" anastamosis involves the resection of the narrowed segment and then directly joining the two ends. A subclavian flap repair involves ligation of the left subclavian artery and then rotating a flap of the proximal subclavian artery, which is interposed in the aortic wall to create a wider aorta at the site of the CoA. Both operations require a left thoracotomy incision and cross clamping of the aorta. Neither procedure requires cardiopulmonary bypass. Both procedures are effective for CoA repair in the neonatal period with similar risks for the recurrence of coarctation, the major determinant appearing to be the expertise of the surgeon with the particular technique.[12] Surgery on preterm neonates is possible, with low mortality rates reported, but the rate of re-coarctation is higher in very low-birth weight infants.[13]

During surgery the patient is often cooled to approximately 33 °C in an attempt to protect the spinal cord from ischemic damage as the blood supply to the anterior part of the cord arises from the aorta below the level of the cross clamp. Prior to leaving theater it is essential that the blood flow past the repair is adequate. This is usually assessed by the presence of palpable femoral pulses, a good pulsatile signal from a pulse oximeter on the toe or sometimes a lower limb arterial line.

Post-operative management

Much of the post-operative management of the patient (both neonatal and the older child) following correction of a CoA is common to all cardiac surgery. The patient remains sedated, intubated, and ventilated while they are allowed to warm up, recover from the effects of the general anesthetic and correct any metabolic acidosis. The metabolic acidosis may correct slowly after surgery due to the limited kidney function of the newborn, particularly after a period of renal hypoperfusion.

Intercostal drains should be observed for bleeding and air leakage. Blood loss in excess of $5 \, ml \, kg^{-1}$ per hour should trigger an urgent review by the cardiac surgeon. Blood should be sent for a full blood count, biochemistry, and coagulation profile. Correction of any coagulation abnormality may require the transfusion of fresh frozen plasma or platelets. Regularly checking for the presence of femoral pulses as well as observing for an adequate urine output can monitor blood flow past the surgical repair. Assessment of perfusion of the left arm and hand should be undertaken regularly after a subclavian flap repair, although inadequate blood supply via collaterals is rare. A chest radiograph should be taken to assess the correct positioning of the central venous line, endotracheal tube, nasogastric tube and drains as well as to look for evidence of a hemothorax, pneumothorax, lung collapse, or pulmonary edema. A 12-lead ECG should be performed to look for arrhythmias or ischemia. Analgesia should be provided initially with morphine supplemented with regular paracetamol. Antibiotics to cover skin organisms (e.g. flucloxacillin) are usually continued for a day post-operatively.

Ventricular dysfunction

The left ventricle, which until the operation has been ejecting against a high resistance, may be dilated with impaired systolic function and an abnormally low ejection fraction. As a consequence of back pressure through the pulmonary circulation the right ventricle also commonly fails. As such, the patient may require a period of inotropic support to augment cardiac output. Agents used commonly include dopamine, dobutamine (which has the additional advantage of being able to be given through a peripheral vein if central venous access is not available), adrenaline, or a phosphodiesterase inhibitor such as milrinone. Poor ventricular performance is likely in the presence of cool peripheries, hypotension, oliguria, pulmonary edema, a worsening lactic acidosis, or low central venous oxygen saturation. A trans-thoracic echocardiogram can assess ventricular function and flow through the repair.

Hypertension

Early, short-term hypertension may be present post-operatively. This is much more common in the older child undergoing repair than the neonate. The mechanism of post-operative hypertension may be multifactorial, involving catacholamine and renin release, as well as abnormal baroreceptor mediated autoregulation. The most worrying consequence of uncontrolled hypertension is stress on the aortic suture line risking aortic rupture or aneurysm formation. Blood pressure is therefore kept below the upper limit of normal for the child's age. Having ensured adequate analgesia and sedation, if treatment of hypertension is necessary, a short-acting vasodilator such as sodium nitroprusside may be used. Alternatively, a beta-blocker such as propranolol or combined alpha- and beta-blocker such as labetalol can be used. In infants with poor ventricular function beta-blockers must be used with caution due to their myocardial depressant effects. The successful use of an angiotensin-converting enzyme inhibitor in the immediate post-operative period in older children has also been reported.[14]

The development of late, chronic hypertension is a well-established complication of CoA. It was originally thought that repair in the neonatal period or early childhood would prevent this; however there is evidence to suggest that the elastic properties of the prestenotic aorta of neonates with coarctation are primarily impaired and that they remain abnormal even after successful surgical correction.[15] Follow-up data indicates that neonates undergoing coarctation repair have a significant incidence of hypertension by 10 years of age.[16] Recent research into a polymorphism of the Angiotensin-Converting Enzyme (ACE) gene has suggested that children with a particular ACE genotype may be at greater risk of developing hypertension following coarctation repair in infancy.[17] Patients with CoA therefore require lifelong follow-up and careful management during subsequent surgery and anesthesia.[18]

Respiratory failure

Causes of post-operative respiratory failure include:

- Cardiac failure
- Pleural effusions
- Pneumothorax
- Lobar/segmental lung collapse
- Pneumonia
- Upper airway obstruction.

A chest X-ray is essential to aid the management of a child who either fails to wean from ventilation or develops respiratory failure after extubation. Pleural effusions may be due to the presence of blood, reactive exudates, left ventricular failure, or a chylothorax. A chylothorax is the presence of lymph in the pleural space following damage to the thoracic duct or back pressure from right ventricular failure. Both pleural effusions and pneumothoraces may require repositioning or replacement of intercostal drains. Chylothorax may necessitate the institution of a medium chain triglyceride diet, or in more intractable cases, the stopping of all enteral feeds and the use of parenteral nutrition. The use of octreotide, a somatostatin analog, for post-operative chylothorax remains uncertain, and in one neonate who underwent coarctation repair, its use was associated with the development of necrotising enterocolitis, possibly secondary to its effects on splanchnic perfusion.[19]

Lung collapse is managed with good analgesia, chest physiotherapy, and sometimes, continuous positive airways pressure (CPAP). An unresolving left lower lobe collapse after a CoA repair should raise the concern of phrenic nerve damage causing diaphragmatic paralysis. Pneumonia is managed in a similar fashion to lung collapse with the addition of appropriate antibiotics after cultures have been sent. Upper airway obstruction may develop immediately after extubation due to vocal cord edema following intubation. Alternatively, damage to the left recurrent laryngeal nerve where it loops around the aortic arch can cause vocal cord paralysis, although this appears to be a greater risk in older children and adults undergoing coarctation repair.

Necrotizing enterocolitis

In this case, one of the presenting features was vomiting. Later, the infant developed abdominal distension and features of an ileus. This should raise the suspicion of necrotizing enterocolitis (NEC). NEC is often associated with prematurity and low birthweight infants, although the etiology is not always clear. In the case of a baby with CoA, it is likely that there is a hypoxic injury to the bowel secondary to low cardiac output. This is brought about by mucosal hypoperfusion as the arterial supply to the bowel arises from the aorta in the abdomen, below the area of aortic narrowing. Enteral feeding causes an increase in oxygen demand in the gut mucosa. If this increased demand cannot be met because of a poor blood supply, bowel ischemia may result. A case-control study of necrotizing enterocolitis in neonates with congenital heart disease[20] found that diagnoses of hypoplastic left heart syndrome and truncus arteriosus were independently associated with the development of NEC by multivariate analysis, along with earlier gestational age of the infant and episodes of low cardiac output. For this reason, babies are commonly not enterally fed after CoA repair, especially those who had a degree of shock at presentation. In the absence of evidence of NEC, feeding is usually reintroduced around day 2 to 5 post-operatively. Where enteral feeding is to be withheld for more than a few days, parenteral nutrition will be necessary.

Other complications
Other uncommon complications related to cross-clamping the aorta include ischemia of the spinal cord causing paraplegia and renal failure due to acute tubular necrosis.

Learning points
- Early diagnosis and prompt treatment are essential.
- Examination of the femoral pulses is mandatory in all sick neonates.
- Where a CoA is suspected in an unwell neonate, prostaglandin E_1 or E_2 10 ng kg^{-1} per min must be started immediately in a closely monitored environment.
- Contact regional cardiothoracic unit immediately for advice and referral
- Consider: intubation, ventilation, inotropic support, fluid restriction, and diuresis.
- Stop enteral feeding until formally assessed.
- Following repair, femoral pulses should be regularly assessed.
- Enteral nutrition should be reintroduced with caution especially when the neonate is or has been cardiovascularly unstable.
- Hypertension should be carefully controlled post-operatively.

Acknowledgments
The authors are grateful to Dr. Graham Stuart for allowing us to use the echocardiogram in Fig. 12.1.

References
1. Benson LN, McLaughlin PR. Coarctation of the aorta. In: Freedom RM, Yoo S-J, Mikailian MRT, Williams W, eds. *The Natural and Modified History of Congenital Heart Disease.* New York, Blackwell Publishing, 2004.
2. Schwengel DA, Nichols DG, Cameron DE. Coarctation of the aorta and interrupted aortic arch. In: Nichols DG, Cameron DE, Greeley WJ, Lappe DG, Ungerleider RM, Wetzel RC, eds. *Critical Heart Disease in Infants and Children.* Missouri, Mosby, 1995.
3. Crossland DS, Furness JC, Abu-Harb M *et al.* Variability of four limb blood pressure in normal neonates. *Arch Dis Child* 2004; **89:** F325-7.
4. Liberman L, Gersony WM, Flynn PA *et al.* Effectiveness of prostaglandin E1 in relieving obstruction in coarctation of the oarta without opening the ductus arteriosus. *Pediatr Cardiol* 2004; **25:** 49–52.
5. Gibbs JL. Treatment options for coarctation of the aorta. *Heart* 2000; **84:** 11–13.

6. Younoszai AK, Reddy VM, Hanley FL, Brook MM. Intermediate term follow-up of the end-to-side aortic anastomosis for coarctation of the aorta. *Ann Thoracic Surg* 2002; **74**: 1631–4.

7. Quaegebeur JM, Jonas RA, Weinberg AD *et al.* Outcomes in seriously ill neonates with coarctation of the aorta. A multiinstitutional study. *J Thorac Cardiovasc Surg* 1994; **108**: 841–51.

8. McCrindle BW. Coarctation of the aorta. *Curr Opin Cardiol* 1999; **14**: 448–52.

9. Rao PS, Jureidini SB, Balfour IC *et al.* Severe aortic coarctation in infants less than 3 months: successful palliation by balloon angioplasty. *J Invas Cardiol* 2003; **15**: 202–8.

10. McMahon CJ, Alromani A, Nihill MR. Balloon angioplasty of critical coarctation in a 970-gram premature neonate. *Cardiol Young* 2001; **11**: 468–71.

11. Fink C, Peuster M, Hausdorf G. Endovascular stenting as an emergency treatment for neonatal coarctation. *Cardiol Young* 2000; **10**: 644–6.

12. Cobanoglu A, Thyagarajan GK, Dobbs JL. Surgery for coarctation of the aorta in infants younger than 3 months: end-to-end repair versus subclavian flap angioplasty: is either operation better? *Eur J Cardiol Thorac Surg* 1998; **14**: 19–25.

13. Bacha EA, Almodovar M, Wessel DL *et al.* Surgery for coarctation of aorta in infants weighing less than 2 kg. *Ann Thorac Surg* 2001; **71**: 1260–4.

14. Rouine-Rapp K, Mello DM, Hanley FL *et al.* Effect of enalaprilat on postoperative hypertension after surgical repair of coarctation of the aorta. *Pediatr Crit Care Med* 2003; **4**: 327–32.

15. Vogt M, Kuhn A, Baumgartner D *et al.* Impaired elastic properties of the ascending aorta in newborns before and early after successful coarctation repair: proof of a systemic vascular disease of the prestenotic arteries? *Circulation* 2005; **111**: 3269–73.

16. O'Sullivan JJ, Derrick G, Darnell R. Prevalence of hypertension in children after early repair of coarctation of the aorta: a cohort study using casual and 24-hour blood pressure measurement. *Heart* 2002; **88**: 163–6.

17. Zadinello M, Greve G, Liu XQ *et al.* Angiotensin I converting enzyme genotype affects ventricular remodelling in children with aortic coarctation. *Heart* 2005; **91**: 367–8.

18. Celermajer DS, Greaves K. Survivors of coarctation repair: fixed but not cured. *Heart* 2002; **88**: 113–14.

19. Mohseni-Bod H, Macrae D, Slavik Z. Somatostatin analog (octreotide) in management of postoperative chylothorax: Is it safe? *Pediatr Crit Care Med* 2004; **5**: 356–7.

20. McElhinney DB, Hedrick HL, Bush DM *et al.* Necrotizing enterocolitis in neonates with congenital heart disease: risk factors and outcomes. *Pediatrics* 2000; **106**: 1080–7.

Chapter 13

The 2-month-old with severe pertussis (whooping cough)

Emma J. Bould and Mark J. Peters

Introduction

Whooping cough is a highly contagious illness of the respiratory tract caused by *Bordetella pertussis*. It is prevalent worldwide (20–40 million cases per year) and is responsible for an estimated 200 000–300 000 deaths per year (WHO). Since the introduction of vaccines, the total number of cases per year has fallen dramatically, but more than 1000 cases are still reported each year in England and Wales. Most vulnerable are unvaccinated or inadequately vaccinated small infants and children.

Case history

A 2-month-old girl was brought to her general practitioner (GP) with a 5-day history of worsening cough, difficulty in breathing, and poor feeding. She had been born in good condition at 30 weeks' gestation, and discharged home, well, from the Special Care Baby Unit (SCBU) 2 weeks previously. She had not yet received any immunizations. The GP referred her urgently via ambulance to her to the local hospital emergency department.

Examination

On arrival at hospital she was breathing spontaneously but was tachypnoic (80 breaths min^{-1}) and grunting with notable intercostal and subcostal recession. Her oxygen saturation was 88% in air and improved to 92% with supplemental oxygen at $5 \, l \, min^{-1}$ via reservoir face mask. Her temperature was 37 °C. She was pale, tachycardic (180 beats min^{-1}), and peripherally shut down with a capillary refill time of 4–5 seconds. Her mean blood pressure was 45 mmHg. On auscultation bilateral crackles and transmitted upper airway noise was heard. She became agitated on handling and was seen to have a number of apneic episodes in quick succession that responded to stimulation, and therefore a senior pediatrician and an anesthetist were called urgently.

Intravenous (IV) access was obtained and 32 ml ($10 \, ml \, kg^{-1}$) of normal saline given intravenously with a marked improvement in her peripheral perfusion and heart rate. Further IV access was then obtained via another cannula and blood samples were obtained (see Table 13.1).

A decision was made to institute artificial ventilation because of the frequency of the episodes of apnea. Anesthesia and paralysis was induced with thiopental ($3 \, mg \, kg^{-1}$) and suxamethonium ($2 \, mg \, kg^{-1}$), respectively, and cricoid pressure applied during intubation. A size 3.5 endotracheal tube (ETT) was secured at 8 cm at the lips. There was no significant desaturation during intubation and a mild bradycardia resolved spontaneously without medication.

ETT placement was confirmed with end-tidal CO_2 monitoring and symmetrical chest movement with bilaterally air entry were observed. Oxygen saturation improved to 95% in 40%

Case Studies in Pediatric Critical Care, ed. Peter. J. Murphy, Stephen C. Marriage, and Peter J. Davis. Published by Cambridge University Press. © Cambridge University Press 2009.

Table 13.1. *Investigations sent during resuscitation and results*

Tests sent	Results on arrival
Blood gas	Venous pH 7.21, pCO_2 9.8 kPa, pO_2 6.4 kPa, Bicarbonate 29 mmol l^{-1}, BE −9, HB 7.8 g dl^{-1}, Na^+ 131 mmol l^{-1}, K 4.0 mmol l^{-1} (post-intubation capillary gas: pH 7.33 pCO_2 6.0 kPa, pO_2 13.0 kPa, BE −5 mmol l^{-1})
Blood culture	Negative at 48 hours
Urea and electrolytes	Na+ 131 mmol l^{-1}, K 3.9 mmol l^{-1}, Urea 4.0 mmol l^{-1}, Creatinine 70 µmol l^{-1}
Blood glucose	4.2 mmol l^{-1}
Full blood count	Hemoglobin 8.0 g dl^{-1}, white cell count $24 \times 10^9 \ l^{-1}$, (differential 71% lymphocytes), Platelets $545 \times 10^9 \ l^{-1}$
Group and save	O +ve, no atypical antibodies Maternal serum was still available for future cross-match from her time in SCBU
Coagulation	International normalized ratio 1.4
Liver function tests	Total Bilirubin 14 µmol l^{-1}, Alkaline phosphatase 430 IU l^{-1}, Aspartate transaminase 74 IU l^{-1}, Albumin 30 g l^{-1}
C-reactive protein	40 mg l^{-1}
Respiratory serology	Rising anti-*Bordetella pertussis* IgA and IgM titers
Nasopharyngeal aspirate (NPA)	Pertussis culture and PCR positive. MC&S negative. Respiratory viral immunofluorescence negative

inspired oxygen. Ventilation was continued with synchronized intermittent mandatory ventilation (SIMV) at 40 breaths per minute with a peak inspiratory pressure (PIP) of 22 cm H_2O and a positive end-expiratory pressure of 4 cmH_2O. A nasogastric tube (NGT) was then placed and stomach contents aspirated. A urinary catheter was then inserted. Sedation and analgesia was achieved with a morphine infusion at 20 mcg kg^{-1} per min. A chest X-ray confirmed satisfactory positioning of both ET and NG tubes and revealed diffuse bilateral shadowing.

10% dextrose/saline 0.45% maintenance fluids with potassium were then started at a restricted volume of 80 ml kg^{-1} per day and a dose of IV clarithromycin was given. A capillary blood gas confirmed that minute ventilation was adequate (Table 13.1) and she was transferred to the pediatric intensive care unit (PICU) where she was isolated.

Progress on pediatric intensive care

On admission to intensive care she presented a picture of isolated respiratory failure of moderate severity. The ratio of measured partial pressure of oxygen to the inspired oxygen fraction (PF ratio) was 162, and the alveolar-arterial oxygen tension gradient (AaDo$_2$) was 146. The estimated risk of mortality was 17% using the paediatric index of mortality (PIM) tool.

She was conventionally ventilated for 24 hours and she remained cardiovascularly stable. Ventilation was aimed at tidal volumes of 5–7 ml kg^{-1} together with a permissive hyper-capnia strategy to maintain the arterial pH >7.25. Sedation and analgesia was continued. A heparinized double-lumen femoral venous line was inserted under sterile conditions using the Seldinger technique. Radial arterial access was also obtained.

Further blood cultures and a bronchoalveolar lavage for immunofluorescence for respiratory viruses and microscopy and culture were negative.

Clarithromycin was continued and milk NGT feeds were started, which were well tolerated.

On day 2, her condition deteriorated with episodes of desaturation. Fraction of inspired oxygen (FiO_2) was increased gradually to 0.8 to maintain oxygen saturations between 88% and 92%. Thicker ETT secretions were noted by the physiotherapists, but the ETT itself remained patent, easy to suction and in a good position. Lingular and left upper lobe collapse were noted on chest X-ray. In response to poor gas exchange (arterial gas pH 7.10, pCO_2 9.5 kPa, pO_2 7.0 kPa, bicarbonate 20 mmol l^{-1}, base excess −7 mmol l^{-1}), morphine sedation was increased (30 mcg kg^{-1} per min), neuromuscular blockade was started with IV vecuronium (20 mcg kg^{-1} per min) and ventilatory pressures were increased to 28/10. She remained cardiovascularly stable but became febrile (38.5 °C). Repeat bloods showed an increasing white cell count ($35 \times 10^9 l^{-1}$). Blood and urine cultures were repeated and cefotaxime given. Nasogastric feeds were stopped and maintenance fluids started. A per-nasal swab culture confirmed the presence of Bordetella pertussis.

High frequency oscillatory ventilation (HFOV) with a mean airway pressure (MAP) of 26 and ΔP of 38 in 60% oxygen was commenced because of persistent hypoxia. She showed some improvement after this, and a repeat chest X-ray confirmed re-expansion but no hyperinflation of the lungs.

She remained unstable over the next 12 hours and required an FiO_2 of 1.0 and MAP 34 (ΔP 50) to maintain oxygen saturation >85% and PaO_2 >6.0 kPa, despite being turned prone. She developed profound desaturation and variability in blood pressures. An echocardiogram demonstrated a dilated right heart and pulmonary pressures estimated to be approaching systemic values. Inhaled nitric oxide (iNO) was started at 20 ppm resulting in a brief initial improvement in PaO_2 to 7.6. Methemoglobin concentration remained less than 3% during NO treatment.

All calculated parameters that are used to quantify the severity of abnormalities of gas exchange were severely abnormal: the oxygenation index (MAP × FiO_2/ PaO_2 (mmHg) × 100) was 67; PaO_2/ FiO_2 ratio 57; and the alveolar–arterial O_2 tension gradient (AaDo2) 584. The treating team felt that she had potentially reversible lung disease and was therefore a candidate for extracorporeal life support. An extra-corporeal membrane oxygenation (ECMO) center was then contacted and transfer arranged.

Transfer to cardiac intensive care unit with Extra-Corporeal Mandatory Oxygenation (ECMO) facilities

For transfer, HFOV was changed to conventional ventilation. Fluids and infusions, including paralysis, were continued. Monitoring, resuscitation drugs, and equipment were available and checked before transfer. Maternal blood for future cross-match was taken for the receiving hospital.

The transfer was uneventful until shortly after arrival at the ECMO center, when she became profoundly desaturated (<40%). She was manually ventilated until there was improvement in saturations to 70%. A decision was made to institute veno-venous ECMO support urgently. A dual lumen, 12 French, right internal jugular cannula was inserted by the cardiothoracic surgeon. After a brief period of bradycardia going on to ECMO, there was a rapid improvement in oxygen saturation to 98%.

Progress on ECMO

Despite ECMO she deteriorated over the next few days. Ventilation was continued with rest mechanical ventilator settings of peak inspiratory pressure (PIP) 20 cmH$_2$O, peak end expiratory pressure (PEEP) 10, FiO$_2$ 0.21, ventilator rate of 10 breaths min^{-1}, and inspiratory time of 1 second. Rigid bronchoscopy, surfactant, steroid, and DNAse therapy were initiated but repeated CXRs showed a "white-out", no chest movement was seen, and there was no evidence of recovery of respiratory function (Fig. 13.1)

Antibiotics, morphine, and vecuronium infusions were continued. Regular blood products were given to optimize the hematocrit (HCT >0.4), and maintain hemoglobin above 12, fibrinogen above 1.5 and platelets above 100. A heparin infusion was started and the activated clotting time maintained between 180 and 220 seconds.

Lactate and blood gases showed a worsening metabolic acidosis and inadequacy of oxygen delivery. Her perfusion remained very poor and in view of significant hemodynamic compromise she was converted to veno-arterial ECMO with some effect, although this was not maintained. An infusion of noradrenaline (0.01–0.5 mcg kg^{-1} per min) was given to maintain blood pressure. She also developed pleural and pericardial effusions, which were drained.

She showed evidence of worsening multi-organ failure. Cranial ultrasound showed periventricular high reflectivity but no intracranial bleeding. Epileptiform discharges were seen on electroencephalogram (EEG), thought to reflect pertussis encephalopathy. The anticonvulsant phenytoin was started. No visual evoked potentials could be identified, and there was an inconclusive result for auditory evoked potentials. Echocardiography showed left ventricular hypertrophy and right ventricular pressures approaching systemic values. A conjugated hyperbilirubinemia was noted with normal liver ultrasound scan. Renal failure with poor urine output and rising urea and creatinine developed, which necessitated hemofiltration which was undertaken from the ECMO circuit.

By day 7 there was no evidence of recovery. After taking a second opinion from an independent consultant, a multidisciplinary decision was made with the agreement of the parents to withdraw care. The child was decannulated and died a short time later.

After discussion with the Coroner, a death certificate was issued which gave the cause of death as:

Multiple Organ failure secondary to *Bordetella pertussis* infection.

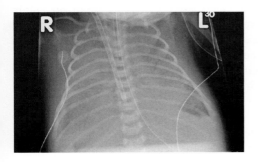

Fig. 13.1. Chest X-ray on ECMO: the tip of the endotracheal tube lies approximately 1 cm above the carina and the tip of the NG tube lies beneath the diaphragm. The ECMO catheter lies in the right internal jugular vein. There is white-out of both lungs, with air bronchograms present. These appearances are consistent with ECMO.

Discussion

Epidemiology, presentation, and complications

Bordetella pertussis is a Gram-negative bacillus transmitted by droplet spread. Typically, catarrhal symptoms and cough develop after an incubation period of 7–10 days. Later, the classical whooping or paroxysmal coughing starts that can last for some weeks.

Before vaccination against *Pertussis* was first introduced in the 1950s, the average annual number of notifications in England and Wales exceeded 100 000. By 1972, when vaccine take-up was >80%, there were only 2069 notifications of *Pertussis* (WHO). Currently, the inactivated whole cell *Pertussis* vaccine is given as part of a combined DTP-Hib vaccine at 2, 3, and 4 months of age. A full course of whooping cough vaccination has at least 90% efficacy. Vaccination scares in the 1970s and 1980s led to decreased vaccine uptake with *Pertussis* epidemics and deaths as a result.

In the late 1990s there was good DTP vaccination uptake; however, an increasing proportion of *Pertussis* cases in unvaccinated infants under 6 months of age was seen. Studies showed that adults and adolescents from the same household acted as a reservoir for *Pertussis* infection in these very young infants. This led to the introduction of a booster vaccine dose in 2001.

High levels of herd immunity from *Pertussis* remain important as untreated patients frequently remain contagious for 3–5 weeks. Erythromycin may be effective in reducing infectivity.

Most serious complications from *Pertussis* occur in the very young and the vast majority of deaths from *Pertussis* worldwide are young infants. As in our case, those who are ex-premature, unvaccinated, and still neonates are at particular risk of severe *Pertussis* infection. Such children have not completed the full vaccination course and are not always protected by maternal antibodies. Infants may present with non-specific features including feeding difficulties, fever, vomiting, tachypnea, cough, gagging, cyanosis, bradycardia, and apneas. Blood results may lack the characteristically high white cell count initially.[1]

Complications include vomiting, weight loss, subconjunctival hemorrhages, pneumonia, pneumothorax, pneumomediastinum, seizures, subarachnoid hemorrhage, encephalopathy, cortical atrophy, cardiac arrest, delayed motor and cognitive development, and death. Co-infection with respiratory syncytial virus and other respiratory infections occurs often and screening for these should also be done.

Laboratory diagnosis

Bordetella pertussis is difficult to grow in the laboratory but diagnosis of *Pertussis* infection can be undertaken by culture on special artificial media from per nasal swab or preferably from nasopharyngeal aspirates. Culture and direct fluorescent antibody testing is positive in 80% cases collected in first 2 weeks provided antibiotics had not been given. Polymerase Chain Reaction (PCR) is more sensitive than culture, but yields high false positives. In one study PCR had a sensitivity of 61% and specificity 80%. Diagnosis can also be made by demonstrating presence of specific antibodies in the serum.

Pathogenesis

It is thought that *Bordetella pertussis* first attaches to the cilia of ciliated epithelial cells of the respiratory tract. This is facilitated by the adhesins Filamentous Hemagglutinin (FHA), Pertussis

Toxin (PT), fimbriae (FIM), lipopolysaccharide (LPS), and Tracheal Colonization Factor (TCF). Then, paralysis of cilia and death of ciliated cells leads to defective mucociliary clearance.

Release of *Pertussis* toxin causes further damage to respiratory tract and interferes with the immune response by preventing migration of lymphocytes and macrophages to areas of infection, and adversely effecting phagocytosis and intracellular killing. This leads to the symptoms of whooping cough and, if the bacteria reach the alveoli, pneumonia develops, which has a high morbidity. At autopsy, inflammation of the mucosal lining of the respiratory tract ciliary epithelium is seen with congestion and infiltration of the mucosa by lymphocytes and polymononuclear leukocytes and inflammatory debris in the bronchi.

Ventilation of infants with *Pertussis*

Evidence has suggested that the disease process in infants with *Pertussis* may be attenuated by early intervention for apneic episodes and respiratory distress by instituting ventilatory support. Ideally, this should be done electively and in controlled conditions.

In the emergency situation with evidence of cardiovascular compromise, care should be taken with the choice of induction agent as drugs with myocardial depressant activity (thiopental, propofol, and midazolam) may worsen the situation. Consideration should be given to using ketamine, fentanyl, or simply reducing the dose of induction agent if these are not readily available. Appropriate levels of sedation, analgesia, and paralysis should be maintained while ventilation is stabilized.

Ventilation should be aimed at preservation of adequate gas exchange, while protecting the lung from further ventilator-induced lung injury. Suggested lung protective ventilation strategies include limitation of tidal volumes to 4–7 ml/kg, limiting plateau pressures to $\leq 30 \, cmH_2O$, while allowing permissive hypercapnia with $pH_{arterial} > 7.2$ and tolerance of oxygen saturation of >85%.[2] Attempting to optimize lung volumes with PEEP and prone positioning, use of HFOV especially when a mean airway pressure $>16 \, cmH_2O$ may be helpful. There is some evidence to suggest that administration of surfactant may improve outcomes.[3]

Pulmonary hypertension in *Pertussis*

Pulmonary hypertension is a devastating complication of severe *Pertussis* infection in young infants. It is particularly difficult to treat and only rarely responds to conventional therapies such as alkalization and inhaled nitric oxide. Mechanisms underlying this intractable form of pulmonary hypertension that differ from those in other forms of infant respiratory failure have been suggested. One is that extreme leukocytosis predisposes to the formation of lymphocyte aggregates in the pulmonary vasculature, resulting in increased pulmonary vascular resistance via obstruction rather than vasoconstriction.[4] Several lines of evidence support this theory, including the striking association between hyperleukocytosis (WCC $>100 \times 10^9 \, l^{-1}$) and risk of death with pulmonary hypertension and post-mortem leukocyte thrombi found in pulmonary arterioles. Attempts to reduce lymphocyte numbers and adhesiveness in the acute stage of *Pertussis* with hyperleukocytosis may be appropriate. Strategies include high dose corticosteroids and administration of HMG-CoA reductase inhibitors (statins). Rapid lympho-depletion with exchange transfusions and/or leukofiltration have been associated with improved outcomes in short case studies.[5]

ECMO and *Pertussis*

Any child with *Pertussis* who is failing to stabilize with standard pediatric intensive care support should be discussed with the local ECMO center.

While the value of ECMO in these cases of intractable pulmonary hypertension has been questioned, there are undoubtedly a significant proportion of cases of *Pertussis* referred for ECMO who do survive.[6] These may represent more of a bronchopneumonia/acute respiratory distress syndrome pathophysiology than the severe and resistant pulmonary hypertension described above.

ECMO should be considered in those infants and children thought to have potentially reversible lung disease who have been ventilated for less than 7 days, and hence avoided irreversible ventilator induced lung damage.

Oxygenation indices are derived variables intended to aid the interpretation of arterial blood gas measurements and to assess the efficiency of pulmonary uptake of oxygen. They may be used to decide when ECMO may be appropriate for a patient. Some authors suggest that the following thresholds should prompt referral for ECMO: Oxygenation Index >35, A-a gradient >500 mmHg and Oxygen (PF) ratio <100.

Perhaps a more logical view is not to focus on a particular threshold of gas exchange abnormality but to refer for ECMO at a stage when there is evidence that conventional management is not achieving stability – an example might be recurrent air-leak with a continued requirement for high pressure ventilation.

Learning/practice points

- The importance of the pertussis vaccine programme in reducing *Pertussis* deaths worldwide.
- Consideration of diagnosis and treatment of pertussis in adults to prevent reservoirs of infection.
- Treatment of contacts with erythromycin and informing public health.
- Atypical presentation of *Pertussis* in infants.
- Young infants are those at highest risk of morbidity and mortality.
- Consideration of co-infection and screening for them on admission.
- Early intervention and ventilatory support may attenuate the disease.
- Ventilation strategies should be employed that minimize ventilator induced injury.
- Early echocardiography and consideration of PHT in sick infants.
- Early consideration of need for ECMO.
- WCC is an independent predictor of mortality.
- Additional therapies such as steroids should be considered in the most severe cases with hyperleukocytosis and resistant pulmonary hypertension.

References

1. Crowcroft NS, Booy R, Harrison T *et al.* Severe and unrecognised: pertussis in UK infants. *Arch Dis Child* 2003; **88** (9): 802–6.
2. The Acute Respiratory Distress Syndrome Network. Ventilation with lower tidal volumes as compared with traditional tidal volumes for acute lung injury and the acute respiratory distress syndrome. *N Engl J Med* 2000; **342**(18): 1301–8.
3. Willson DF, Thomas NJ, Markovitz BP *et al.* Pediatric acute lung injury and sepsis investigators effect of exogenous surfactant (calfactant) in pediatric acute lung injury: a randomized controlled trial. *J Am Med Assoc.* 2005; **293**(4): 470–6.

4. Pierce C, Klein N, Peters M. Is leukocytosis a predictor of mortality in severe pertussis infection? *Intens Care Med* 2000; **26** (10): 1512–14.
5. Romano MJ, Weber MD, Wiesse ME, Sin BL. Pertussis pneumonia, hypoxaemia, hyperleukocytosis, and pulmonary hypertension: improvement in oxygenation after a double volume exchange transfusion. *Pediatrics* 2004; **114**(2): e264–6.
6. Williams GD, Numa A, Sokol J, Tobias V, Duffy BJ. ECLS in pertussis: does it have a role? *Intens Care Med* 1998; **24** (10): 1089–92.

Further reading

Health Protection Agency Website
http://www.hpa.org.uk/infections/topics_az/
    whoopingcough/menu.htm.

Pericardial effusion in a child

Patricia M. Weir

Introduction

Pericardial effusion can be thought of, simply, as excess fluid within the pericardial sac. Cardiac tamponade can be defined as compression of the heart due to accumulation of fluid in the pericardium. Pericardial effusions are not uncommon in pediatric critical care. Cardiac tamponade, although much less common than simple pericardial effusions, is an emergency situation, which must be recognized and dealt with immediately. Pericardial effusion has multiple potential causes and a variable presentation. A high index of suspicion of pericardial effusion is therefore very important to prevent missing the diagnosis. Failure to recognize the problem, and deal with it appropriately, may result in the death of the child. Presentation to an emergency department of a child with a pericardial effusion is a rare but potentially life-threatening event.

Case history

A 6-month-old, 5 kg boy underwent a patch repair of a large Ventricular Septal Defect (VSD). He had been born at 34 weeks' gestation with a degree of intra-uterine growth retardation. He had spent much of his first 6 months of life in hospital and satisfactory enteral feeding, and growth, had never been established prior to repair of the VSD. Pre-operatively he had been managed on furosemide and captopril, for cardiac failure, and was noted, on Echocardiography (ECHO), to be pulmonary hypertensive.

Following surgery, his post-operative course in the Pediatric Intensive Care Unit (PICU) had been somewhat slow and, in the immediate post-operative period, was complicated by a moderate degree of pulmonary hypertension. He was managed using diuretics and sildenafil and was discharged to the cardiac ward 5 days after his operation. ECHO at that time showed a tiny patch leak across the VSD, good ventricular function, and a tricuspid regurgitant jet, suggestive of improved, but still raised, pulmonary artery pressures. He made steady progress on the ward and on day 11 post-operatively he was deemed well enough to be transferred back to his local District General Hospital (DGH) for further monitoring of his feeding and growth prior to discharge home.

After transfer he was well for 3 days then, on Day 15 post-operatively, he was noted to be "off feeds," to have an increased oxygen requirement, and to have developed a low grade fever (38–38.5 °C). A chest infection was suspected and he was commenced on co-amoxiclav (Augmentin). Over the next 24 hours he had two episodes of becoming pale and mottled and he was discussed with the cardiologists in the lead center. These episodes were thought to be pulmonary hypertensive events, precipitated by infection. The following day there was concern that he was not improving with the antibiotics, and he was again discussed with the cardiologists, who felt he should be transferred back to the cardiac unit for review. The arrangements for transfer were discussed with PICU and it was decided that he should be

Case Studies in Pediatric Critical Care, ed. Peter. J. Murphy, Stephen C. Marriage, and Peter J. Davis. Published by Cambridge University Press. © Cambridge University Press 2009.

transferred by the Pediatric Intensive Care Unit Retrieval Team. On arrival at the referring hospital, the Retrieval Team found him to have a heart rate of 160 b min^{-1}, mild respiratory distress with oxygen saturations of 95% or greater in high flow oxygen. His capillary refill time was 2 seconds and his blood pressure was 100/65. It was felt that no further intervention was required prior to transfer and he was brought back to PICU spontaneously ventilating in face mask oxygen. He remained stable throughout the transfer.

On arrival on PICU an echocardiogram was performed, which showed a 10–12 mm pericardial effusion around the lateral wall of the left ventricle and inferior to the right atrium. The cardiologists felt the effusion was hemodynamically significant and a plan was made to perform a needle pericardiocentesis and placement of a pigtail drain, using the Seldinger technique, as a semi-urgent procedure. He was subsequently anesthetised for this procedure in PICU using ketamine, midazolam and suxamethonium initially, supplemented by fentanyl and vecuronium subsequently. Following pre-oxygenation and induction of anesthesia, he was intubated and ventilated and remained cardio-respiratorily stable throughout. Needle pericardiocentesis was attempted twice under ECHO guidance using the subxiphoid approach. However, on both occasions, blood was aspirated and the needle could be seen entering the right atrium on ECHO. The cardiac surgeons were therefore called and they proceeded to drain the effusion by re-opening the bottom end of the sternotomy wound. There was an immediate hemodynamic improvement noted on drainage of the effusion with a rise in blood pressure and drop in heart rate. The fluid drained initially was blood tinged then cleared to a straw-coloured fluid. In total, approximately 40 ml of fluid was drained. A drain was left *in situ* for 2 days without any further drainage and there was no re-accumulation of fluid evident on follow up ECHOs after drain removal.

The child remained intubated for 3 days, since he again became pulmonary hypertensive on attempts to wean ventilation. Eventually, 2 days later, he was uneventfully extubated and has made good progress since, with no further complications. A 5-day course of antibiotics was completed; however, there was no evidence of infection in sputum, blood, or pericardial fluid cultures and his infective markers in blood remained low.

When seen for follow-up, 6 months later, he remained well, was gaining weight and showed no evidence of recurrence of a pericardial effusion.

Discussion

This case has been chosen as it illustrates many of the features commonly associated with pericardial effusion. Namely, that pericardial effusions are relatively common after cardiac surgery, that presentation and diagnosis are not always clear cut, and that treatment is not always straightforward.

Causes of pericardial effusion

Pericardial effusion is simply excess fluid in the pericardial space and therefore there are multiple potential etiologies. In our patient the cause of the effusion was post-surgical inflammation. There are, however, many potential causes. Table 14.1 lists the more common causes and gives a flavor of how variable the etiology can be. In institutions, where there is a cardiac surgical program, previous cardiac surgery will be the most frequent cause of pericardial effusions. In non-cardiac surgical patients, the effusion is often part of a spectrum of acute pericarditis, caused by an inflammatory process in the pericardium, which again may have multiple potential etiologies.

Table 14.1. *Causes of pericardial effusions*

Post-cardiac surgery
- Early (blood)
- Late (serous/inflammatory exudates)

Traumatic
- Chest trauma
- Secondary to cardiac catheterization
- Central venous catheter related
- Foreign body ingestion

Infection
- Bacterial
- Viral
- Rheumatic fever

Inflammatory
- Nephrotic type syndromes
- Auto-immune disorders

Renal failure
- Fluid overload
- Uremia
- Peritoneal dialysis

Others
- Secondary to neoplasia (esp. leukemia)
- Down's syndrome
- Anorexia nervosa
- Hypothyroidism
- HIV
- Recurrent pericarditis

Idiopathic
- Cause unknown in up to 50% of non-post-cardiac surgical pericardial effusions

Trauma is an uncommon but important cause of cardiac tamponade, since it may present very acutely, requiring urgent decompression. A high index of suspicion is necessary and it must be remembered that tamponade is frequently described secondary to central venous lines and cardiac catheterization as well as direct chest trauma.

In some areas of the world, infection and acute rheumatic fever will be the commonest causes. Up to 50% of pericarditis will have no definitive etiology identified and will be labelled as "idiopathic" or "presumed viral."

The pathophysiology of pericardial effusion remains poorly understood. With the exception of traumatic effusions or bleeding post-surgery, the mechanism is immunologically mediated. Engle in 1980 demonstrated the presence of high levels of anti-heart antibodies in 100% of cases of Post-Pericardiotomy Syndrome (PPS). These antibodies are also found in other causes of myocardial injury but rarely in such high titers. She also found high levels of antiviral antibodies and theorized that either fresh viral infection or reactivation of a virus may play a part in the development of PPS.[1]

Post-cardiac surgery

The percentage of children found to have pericardial effusion after cardiac surgery is reported as being between 13.6% and 53%. This large range is, in part, due to differences in definition of pericardial effusion and how carefully effusions have been looked for. After cardiac surgery, early pericardial collections are usually due to post-operative bleeding and become evident in the first few hours post-operatively in PICU. Alternatively, they may present days to weeks later as part of an inflammatory response known as PPS. This consists of fever and signs of pericardial inflammation usually occurring more than a week post-operatively. A recent study of 336 children after open heart surgery found that 77 (23%) of the patients had pericardial effusions.[2] Of these 43 were classified as moderate or large and 18 (5%) were symptomatic; 12 children (4%) required drainage; and 97% of effusions occurred within the first 28 days post-operatively with a mean onset time of 11 days. Effusions were significantly more common in children undergoing Fontan-type procedures, in children with post-pericardiotomy syndrome, in female children and in those on warfarin. Effusions can occur after what is often considered "minor" surgery and one retrospective review of 87 patients reported that one in nine patients following repair of secundum ASD closures required drainage of pericardial effusions.[3] Chylopericardium following cardiac surgery has also been described.[4]

In our patient the deterioration occurred between the second and third week post-operatively. Fever and tachycardia were present, with two acute episodes of low cardiac output state. This was interpreted as a chest infection, triggering an exacerbation of his pulmonary hypertension. This illustrates the need to keep a high index of suspicion for pericardial effusion in post-cardiac surgical cases.

Traumatic effusions

Effusions may occur secondary to blunt or penetrating chest trauma, although this is rare in children in the UK. It is a well-recognized complication of cardiac catheterization, both seen at the time of catheter and as a post-procedure problem. Traumatic pericardial effusion is also well documented as a complication of indwelling Central Venous Catheters (CVC). This can occur due to misplacement of the catheter in the pericardium at the time of insertion or as a subsequent catheter migration. In the latter scenario it has been shown, in infants, that the pericardial fluid is frequently consistent with the infusate, even when original catheter placement was definitely intravascular.[5] It is theorized, in this group, that there is either frank migration of the catheter through the myocardial wall or adherence to the wall and diffusion of infusate through the wall of the atrium. It is therefore recommended that a CVC is not left long term in the right atrium, but should ideally be positioned at the SVC or IVC/atrial junction or 1–2 cm back from this point. In small infants with an internal jugular line the problem of pulling back a short (e.g. 6 cm) line with the subsequent risk of leakage of the proximal port or poor line fixation and subsequent loss of a vital line has to be weighed against the risk of leaving the tip in the atrium. Pericardial effusion secondary to CVC placement carries a significant morbidity and mortality since it is often not recognized and the effusion is often compounded by use of the misplaced catheter for resuscitation. Effusions are also described following repair of pectus excavatum and pacemaker insertion.

Infective
In less-developed parts of the world infective pericardial effusions are not uncommon. These are predominantly Staphylococcal infections, but effusions have also been described secondary to other bacterial infections, including mycoplasma, tuberculosis, parasites, Familial Mediterranean fever and viruses (Influenza, CMV, Adenovirus, Coxsackie). They are also found as a feature of acute rheumatic fever. Cardiovascular involvement in HIV is well described especially in developing countries and a study from Thailand of 27 children with CVS symptoms, principally dyspnea, found that 44% had pericardial effusions on ECHO.[6]

Other inflammatory causes
Pericardial effusions occasionally occur as part of a systemic inflammatory response to sepsis. They also occur with a multitude of inflammatory and auto-immune type syndromes, such as nephrotic syndrome, granulomatous disease, Kawasakis, collagen vascular disorders, and certain forms of metabolic disease. Pericardial effusions are also seen secondary to neoplastic disease, especially leukemia.

Renal
Pericardial effusions are relatively common in children with chronic renal failure and can occur secondary to fluid overload, uremia, peritoneal dialysis, or as part of the underlying etiology.

Idiopathic
A 21-year review from Melbourne Children's Hospital found 31 patients with pericardial effusions of an inflammatory origin not related to either cardiac surgery or malignancy. Of these, 15 (48%) patients had no specific identifiable etiology despite extensive investigation.[7]

Others
There is an increased incidence of pericardial effusions in children with Down's Syndrome. They are also found in patients with anorexia nervosa.

Recurrent pericarditis
A small number of children develop recurrent pericarditis and pericardial effusions. These often occur in cases of uncertain initial etiology but can occur following cardiac surgery and in association with chronic inflammatory conditions.[8] They can prove very resistant to treatment. Colchicine has been used with good results however this may depend on the underlying etiology and may be more successful in areas with a high incidence of familial Mediterranean fever.

Presentation and diagnosis
The presentation of pericardial effusion is classically very non-specific (see Table 14.2). Therefore, a good history, which identifies any risk factors, and a high index of clinical suspicion, are very important. This case provides a good example of how signs and symptoms can be attributed to other causes such as infection and pulmonary hypertension. Generally, as the effusion increases in size, then the symptoms will become those of a low cardiac output state. The rate of development of the effusion affects the clinical signs and symptoms. A slowly accumulating effusion can remain asymptomatic until very large, whereas acutely a small amount of fluid, especially in an infant, may cause cardiac compromise.

Table 14.2. *Diagnosis of pericardial effusion*

Symptoms
- Non-specific malaise, vomiting, fatigue
- Pain: chest or abdominal
- Fever
- Hoarseness

Signs
- If large: Low cardiac output state – poor perfusion, prolonged capillary refill time, "shock," acidosis
- Muffled heart sounds
- Tachycardia
- Hepatomegaly
- Pericardial rub
- Pulsus paradoxus
- Jugular venous distension

Investigations
- Low-voltage ECG
- ECG: ST elevation, PR depression
- Chest X-ray – large globular heart
- Echocardiography – excess fluid seen in pericardial space

Common symptoms of pericardial effusion are non-specific malaise, tiredness, dyspnea, and vomiting. The child may complain of chest pain or abdominal pain and fever. Hoarseness can occur as a result of stretch on the recurrent laryngeal nerve and, occasionally, the patient will present with hiccoughs. In large, or rapidly expanding, effusions the child may present with altered mental state and symptoms of shock.

On examination, the majority of these children will be tachycardic and, in severe cases, will have low blood pressure. Tachycardia is an important sign and should not be dismissed as agitation, especially if persistent. Hypotension occurs late and is an indication for immediate drainage of the effusion. The child may be pale, clammy with poor volume pulses and a delayed capillary refill time. Hepatomegaly is often detectable. Pulsus paradoxus (an exaggerated fall of systolic BP in inspiration) is commonly present, but is difficult to elicit clinically in children. It can often be seen as a large fall in inspiration in the peak of the trace on an oxygen saturation monitor.[9] Tachypnea may be present and the classical signs of engorged neck veins and muffled heart sounds may be elicited. Pericardial friction rubs are commonly heard in early PPS but may disappear as fluid accumulates in the pericardium. These classical signs are often not present or difficult to elicit.

In a patient presenting in a low cardiac output state, with a large heart and raised central venous pressure, it is important to differentiate pericardial effusion from poor ventricular function. Cardiac tamponade from pericardial fluid must be considered until proven otherwise. This can be rapidly assessed at the bedside with the use of a portable ultrasound or ECHO probe, even by those with minimal cardiological expertise.

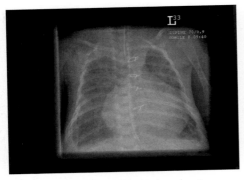

Fig 14.1. AP chest X-ray showing large heart secondary to pericardial effusion and a right-sided pleural effusion.

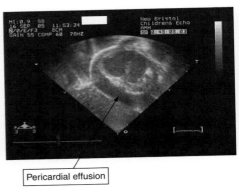

Pericardial effusion

Fig. 14.2. Echocardiograph showing a pericardial effusion.

In this case early echocardiography would have demonstrated the presence of an effusion, allowing a timely assessment and drainage.

Investigations

An electrocardiograph (ECG) will classically show low voltage complexes. ST segment elevation in all leads other than V1 and aVR are a specific sign of pericardial inflammation. PR depression in both limb and precordial leads of greater than 0.5 mm has been described in adults as being present in 23% of patients with asymptomatic pericardial effusion.[10]

Chest X-ray (Fig. 14.1) may show an enlarged or globular heart. Change in heart size may be a clue to development of effusion, but can be difficult to assess in children if the film is not taken at the same point in respiration.

The definitive diagnosis is made by ECHO (Fig. 14.2). This will allow estimation of the size and position of the effusion and an assessment of the presence or absence of cardiac compromise. In cardiac tamponade, fluid interferes with the diastolic filling of the chambers and therefore diastolic collapse on ECHO indicates cardiac compromise.

Portable ultrasound devices allow a rapid check for large effusions to be performed in emergency situations by non-cardiologically trained practitioners.

Only around half of cases will have the classical changes to heart sounds, low-voltage ECG, or hepatomegaly.

CT and MRI can both be useful for evaluating loculated or hemorrhagic effusions, pericardial masses, and constrictive pericarditis but are not suitable in the acute situation with a hemodynamically unstable child.

Percutaneous pericardial biopsy has been described as a safe and efficacious method of establishing an underlying diagnosis in children and adolescents.

Management

This must take into account both the size of effusion and likely underlying etiology. If the effusion is small, then the treatment can be expectant with diuretics and the addition of aspirin, if an inflammatory cause is likely. Debate exists around the efficacy and dose of aspirin in post-pericardiotomy syndrome (PPS). Frequent clinical assessments and repeated ECHO examinations will be required to monitor size of effusion.

If the effusion is large or causing cardiac compromise, then drainage will be required. Drainage may also occasionally be required for diagnostic purposes. In most instances, drainage will be an elective or semi-urgent procedure, as in this case. This would, usually, be performed by cardiologists or cardiac surgeons. Very occasionally emergency pericardiocentesis will need to be performed. If no echocardiography is available, this should only be done as a blind procedure in a dire emergency, for example, a cardiac arrest or near arrest setting.

The presentation of a sick child with a pericardial effusion and a degree of cardiac compromise to a non-cardiac center can present difficult issues. The problems include the potential difficulty in making a definitive diagnosis without echocardiography, and issues relating to potential transfer. These problems are best dealt with by discussion between the presenting hospital and the cardiologists and pediatric intensivists at the lead cardiac center. Usually, the child can be safely transferred prior to definitive treatment. However, on occasions, it may be necessary to drain the effusion before transfer. The development of telemedicine links will potentially assist the transfer of ECHO data and assessment in these patients.

Initial resuscitation of a sick child will follow the principles of Advanced Pediatric Life Support management.[11] After assessment of airway, breathing, and circulation an initial fluid bolus may well be beneficial in improving cardiac filling and therefore increasing cardiac output despite signs of high central venous pressure (distended neck veins and hepatomegaly). Fluid should be given in small increments (5 ml kg^{-1}) and the effect assessed. As in all resuscitation situations the fluid used should be either a near isotonic crystalloid such as normal saline or Hartmann's solution or a colloid.

Emergency pericardiocentesis

Pericardiocentesis without ECHO imaging should only be carried out in the event of very severe cardiac compromise where waiting for an ECHO or presence of a cardiologist would clearly result in death or serious morbidity. It often occurs in the situation of a cardiac arrest where cardiac tamponade is a potential or suspected etiology or as a last resort if resuscitation has not been successful and it cannot be ruled out. In this scenario it is most likely that some electrical activity will have been present but no palpable cardiac output (pulseless electrical activity– PEA arrest).

There are specific kits available for emergency pericardiocentesis, which consist of an insertion pack, containing a needle through a catheter, and a lead with an alligator clip for attachment between the needle and an ECG. This can be used to detect ECG changes on contact with myocardium. In the absence of a specific set any cannula of sufficient length can be used. This generally means using cannulas that are longer than those traditionally used for IV access in this patient's age group. In younger children this can be got round by using a larger diameter catheter, which is usually longer, e.g. 18G (gauge) or 20G 51 mm. For older children longer catheters, such as a 16 or 18G, 10–15 cm catheters, should be available in emergency areas. In a true emergency, if no appropriate cannula is available, a spinal needle of appropriate length may be available in clinical areas.

Technique

If at all possible this should be performed aseptically. Ideally this should be done under ultrasound or ECHO guidance if available.

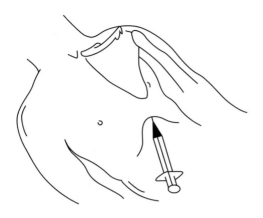

Fig. 14.3. Needle position for emergency pericardiocentesis.

1. First identify the xiphisternum.
2. Ensure an ECG is attached.
3. Take an appropriate cannula (see above) with a syringe attached.
4. Insert 1–2 cm below xiphisternum at an angle of 45 degrees to the skin aiming cephaladly and slightly to the left, imagining you are aiming at the tip of the scapula. Aspirate as you insert the cannula.
5. As soon as you aspirate fluid, advance the cannula and remove the needle.
6. If the fluid is blood or heavily blood stained, the question is whether it is from the pericardium or accidental penetration of the right ventricle. Empty the "blood" into a pot and look for clotting. Fluid from the pericardium should not clot due to the presence of endogenous fibrinolytic compounds, whereas blood aspirated from the heart will clot unless there is a systemic coagulopathy. Drainage of even small amounts of fluid from the pericardium usually results in a significant improvement in hemodynamics, which also indicates correct placement of the cannula (see Fig. 14.3).

ECG monitoring can be helpful in indicating that the needle is touching or entering ventricular muscle. You may see the onset of ectopic beats or a change in the QRS complex morphology.

Complications largely involve damage caused by the needle and include aspiration of ventricular blood, laceration of epicardial or coronary arteries or veins, pneumothorax, and dysrthythmias. Thus, blind pericardiocentesis should be reserved for immediately life threatening situations.

Semi-urgent drainage

In this case semi-urgent drainage was required and this was performed on PICU with a consultant cardiologist and consultant intensivist. These children are seriously compromised and should be anesthetized and operated on by experienced staff at a senior level. The decision as to whether to drain the effusion percutaneously or as an open procedure will be taken depending on the size and position of the effusion. Posterior effusions can be quite sizeable but not amenable to percutaneous access. It was thought that it would be possible to drain this effusion percutaneously by a cardiologist, but as it was performed out of hours the consultant pediatric cardiac surgeon on call was advised that the procedure was taking place. Percutaneous drainage by cardiologists has a good safety record, although as seen in this case it will not always be successful and therefore, except in emergency situations, this should be performed in a centre with a surgeon, capable of performing a sternotomy and drainage, if required.

Anesthetic technique

These children will usually have a high intrinsic sympathetic drive, which will be lost on induction of anesthesia. They may well also be intravascularly depleted, despite having signs of raised central venous pressure. Therefore, a cardiostable induction regime should be used. There are many different options available, but ketamine 2 mg kg^{-1}, midazolam 0.5–1 mg kg^{-1} and a muscle relaxant (suxamethonium, followed by pancuronium or vecuronium) would be a good choice in a sick child. Be prepared to give volume intravenously (have 10 ml kg^{-1} drawn up and ready to deliver before induction).

A useful addition is to prepare a dilute solution of adrenaline, 1 in 100 000 solutions can be made by putting 1 mg (1 ml of 1 in 1000) into a 100 ml bag of saline. This allows you to give small doses of adrenaline (from 1 mcg upwards) in the event of cardiovascular collapse during or shortly after induction of anesthesia. It is better to give a small dose (often as little as 1–5 mcg total dose is effective) if the blood pressure is sagging and coronary perfusion is compromised (seen as any change in ECG complexes) rather than wait for full-blown cardiac compromise.

Percutaneous drainage

This is performed under ECHO guidance and aseptic conditions. This may be performed in theater, a cardiac catheterization laboratory, or an intensive care unit. The patient should be monitored with an ECG, saturation monitor, and blood pressure measurement. This procedure is not free from complication such as entering the heart, damage to the myocardium or coronary arteries. Therefore, it is our practice to inform the cardiac surgeons when undertaking a percutaneous drainage.

The pericardium is entered with a seeking needle under ECHO control usually from the subxiphisternal area (similar to emergency pericardiocentesis). Following aspiration of fluid, a guide wire is inserted and a pigtail-type catheter is usually left *in situ* in the pericardium. Fluid should be sent for microscopy and culture. Cytology should be performed if neoplasia is suspected.

Surgical drainage

This is usually performed by opening the pericardium immediately below the xiphisternum. In the case of post-operative patients this will involve opening the bottom end of the sternotomy wound, although occasionally the full sternotomy will require to be re-opened. This is usually a semi-elective or urgent procedure. However, in cases of cardiac tamponade, in the post-operative cardiac surgical patients, re-opening of a sternotomy wound may be a life saving procedure which will have to be performed as an emergency procedure. This should ideally be performed by cardiac surgeons but may occasionally have to be performed, or at least started, by intensive care staff, while awaiting the arrival of the surgeon. This should be undertaken in as aseptic a method as possible. In cardiac surgical centers a chest opening trolley with the necessary equipment, including sternal wire cutters, should be readily available.

In cases of recurrent effusion a pericardial window can be made to allow continued drainage. This would usually be performed in theater as a semi-elective or urgent procedure. Percutaneous balloon pericardiotomy has been described as an alterative to a surgical pericardial window.

Post-drainage care

The patient should be closely monitored hemodynamically, and, indeed, require a period of observation and ventilation in an intensive care or high-dependency unit depending on their clinical condition. Repeat ECHO examination will be required to monitor potential recurrence of the effusion.

In our patient the post-operative period was complicated by the development of pulmonary hypertensive events when we attempted to wean the child from ventilation. This was related to the pre-existing pulmonary hypertension, secondary to a large VSD. It does demonstrate, however, that pericardial effusions and cardiac tamponade will most commonly exist alongside other pathophysiology.

Purulent pericarditis

Installation of streptokinase, into the pericardium, has been described in purulent pericarditis. This helps to breakdown fibrin and prevent the development of constrictive pericarditis.[12]

Outcome

With appropriately timed recognition and intervention, the mortality from pericardial effusion should be extremely low and related to the underlying cause.

In our patient the effusion did not recur and the pulmonary hypertension slowly resolved. Feeding was gradually established and at a 6-month review he was thriving and gaining weight.

Recurrent pericardial effusion is rare and difficult to manage when it occurs. Development of constrictive pericarditis post-pericardial effusions is a rare but serious sequelae, usually occurring in the first year after initial presentation.

Learning points

- Signs and symptoms of pericardial effusion are often non-specific and therefore a clinical index of suspicion is necessary to make the diagnosis.
- A good history will identify risk factors for pericardial effusion.
- Recent cardiac surgery places patients at a high risk in the first month after surgery of pericardial effusion and potential cardiac compromise.
- Pericardial tamponade can occur early or late after any cardiac surgical procedure even those that are considered "straight-forward" such as secundum ASD repair. Ninety-seven percent will present within 28 days of surgery.
- In a patient with a low cardiac output state and signs of a raised central venous pressure a diagnosis of pericardial effusion with cardiac tamponade must be considered until it can be eliminated.
- Echocardiography is the definitive diagnostic test for pericardial effusions.

- The availability of portable ultrasound devises allows a quick check for large effusions to be performed by non-experts in an emergency situation and allows rapid differentiation from severe ventricular dysfunction.
- Co-existing pathophysiology is commonly present.

Problems in practice

- Drainage of pericardial effusion even under ultrasound guidance is not a risk-free procedure and should be undertaken if at all possible by trained personnel in a setting with cardiac surgical back-up available.
- In the emergency situation with cardiac arrest or near arrest it can be difficult to tell whether blood aspirated during a needle pericardiocentesis is from the pericardium or the ventricle. Clotting of the blood and worsening or failing to improve hemodynamics would suggest intraventricular placement of the needle or catheter.
- The transfer of a sick patient with a large pericardial effusion causing cardiac compromise presents a difficult management problem and needs to be discussed with the lead pediatric cardiac center. In rare cases it may be necessary to drain the effusion prior to transfer.

References

1. Engle M, Zabriskie J, Senterfit L, Gay W, O'Loughlin J, Ehlers K. Viral illness and the postpericardiotomy syndrome. *Circulation* 1980; **62** (6): 1151–8.
2. Cheung E, Ho S, Tang K, Chau A. Pericardial effusion after open heart surgery for congenital heart disease. *Heart* 2003; **89** (7): 780–3.
3. Jones DA, Radford DJ, Pohlner PG. Outcome following surgical closure of secundum ASD. *J Paediatr Child Health* 2001; **37** (3); 274–7.
4. Campbell RM, Benson LN, Williams WW, Adatia I. Chylopericardium after cardiac operations in children. *Ann Thorac Surg* 2001; **72**(1): 193–6.
5. Nowlen T, Rosenthal G, Johnson G, Tom D, Vargo T. Pericardial effusion and tamponade in infants with central catheters. *Pediatrics* 2002; **110** (1): 137–42.
6. Pongprot Y, Sittiwangkul R, Silvilair S, Sirisanthana V. Cardiac manifestation of HIV-infected Thai children. *Ann Trop Paediatr* 2004; **24** (2): 153–9.
7. Mok G, Menahem S. Large pericardial effusions of inflammatory origin in childhood. *Cardiol Young* 2003; **13**: 131–6.
8. Raatikka M, Pelkonen PM, Karjalainen J, Jokinen EV. Recurrent pericarditis in children and adolescents. *J Am Coll Cardiol* 2003; **42** (4) 759–64.
9. Tamburro R, Ring J, Womback K. Detection of pulsus paradoxicus associated with large pericardial effusions in pediatric patients by analysis of the pulse-oximetry waveform. *Pediatrics* 2002; **109** (4): 673–7.
10. Kudo Y, Yamasaki F, Doi Y, Sugiura T. Clinical correlates of PR-Segment depression in asymptomatic patients with pericardial effusion. *J Am Coll Cardiol* 2002; **39**(12): 2000–4.
11. Advanced Life Support Group *Advanced Paediatric Life Support The Practical Approach*. 4th edn. Oxford, Wiley-Blackwell, 2005.
12. Ekim H, Demirbag R. Intrapericardial streptokinase for purulent pericarditis. *Surg Today* 2004; **34** (7): 569–72.

Chapter 5

Management of non-accidental injury on the Pediatric Intensive Care Unit

Robert Ross Russell and Duncan McAuley

Introduction

In the UK 2–3% of children are abused each year, with serious injury occurring in 1 in a 1000.[1] Doctors and allied professionals having contact with children should be aware of the possibility of abuse. In 2003, Lord Laming stated that the *"rigorous investigation and management of actual or possible abuse in children requires the systematic, comprehensive and timely documentation of concerns, and evidence that they have been properly addressed."*[2] Awareness of the commonness of abuse and the variety of presentations are important steps towards its recognition.

Case history

A 21-month-old boy presented to his local emergency department having reportedly fallen down the stairs. His mother and younger sister, aged 6 months, were in attendance. The mother said she left the stairguard open and the boy tripped on the top step, falling the whole flight of 16 stairs, landing on a carpeted floor, but striking his head on the wall. He was brought to hospital 3 hours after the fall, complaining of pain in his left upper arm and a wound on his head. The boy was one of two siblings living with their mother and her partner. He did not have any significant birth history or previous medical history.

Examination

The boy appeared small for his age with a grossly normal developmental state. There was bruising and tenderness over the left humerus, bruising over the left buttock and a 3 cm laceration over his occiput. The boy had vomited once and complained of a sore head. He appeared slow to answer questions but was fully alert and orientated. He did not have any tenderness over his chest or abdomen and vital signs were normal.

An X-ray of his arm revealed an oblique fracture of the lower shaft of the humerus. His head wound was cleaned and glued using tissue adhesive. The boy vomited a further two times and was therefore referred to the inpatient pediatric ward for continued neurological assessment. His arm was placed in an above-elbow Plaster of Paris back slab. Over the next 4 hours his conscious level dropped to a Glasgow Coma Score (GCS) of 11/15; he opened his eyes to pain (E2), was persistently irritable (V3) and was able to localize a painful stimulus (M5). A 22G cannula was inserted and blood sent for full blood count (FBC), urea and electrolytes (U and E), glucose and clotting screen. A CT brain scan was undertaken, which was grossly abnormal (Fig. 15.1).

The pediatric consultant on-call discussed the case with the regional pediatric intensive care unit and it was decided he should be intubated and ventilated prior to transfer for

Case Studies in Pediatric Critical Care, ed. Peter. J. Murphy, Stephen C. Marriage, and Peter J. Davis. Published by Cambridge University Press. © Cambridge University Press 2009.

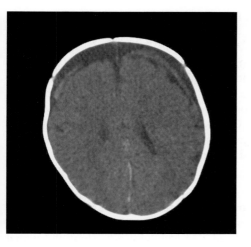

Fig. 15.1. CT scan showing mixed density subdural collections.

neurosurgical evaluation. A rapid sequence induction was performed, using thiopental 4 mg kg^{-1} and suxamethonium 1.5 mg kg^{-1}, and a size 5 uncuffed endotracheal tube inserted. Whilst in the local hospital adult ITU, he was monitored with ECG, oxygen saturation, non-invasive blood pressure, and end-tidal CO_2. Having been stabilized, the child was transported to the regional pediatric intensive care unit by ambulance with an 80-minute journey time.

Progress on PICU

On arrival at the regional centre the child and his CT scan were reviewed by the neurosurgeons. The CT was interpreted as showing acute on chronic subdural collections, but with minimal mass effect and no decompression was attempted. An intracranial pressure (ICP) bolt was inserted, which showed an opening pressure of 20 cmH$_2$O, and subsequently read between 10 and 15 cmH$_2$O. He was sedated with midazolam (200 mcg kg^{-1} per h) and morphine (20 mcg kg^{-1} per h). His ET tube was converted to a nasal tube and ventilation was adjusted to a rate of 30 breaths per minute at pressures of 24/4 and in 30% oxygen. Fluids were restricted to 70 ml kg^{-1} per day (70% maintenance). Ranitidine was started, as were enteral feeds, but no antibiotics were prescribed.

Further history was taken from the child's carers. The boy's father had left home 3 months previously, and the mother had a new partner. The history of the injury changed somewhat in that the mother now said that the boy had been in her partner's arms and he had slipped on the stairs, subsequently dropping him. She denied any previous significant injuries to the child, but the family did have a designated social worker.

On contacting social services to discuss the family, it transpired that the family had had several previous visits to their local emergency department in the previous 2 months. There was also a history of domestic violence between the two carers, and mother's new partner had a police record of violence.

Full examination of the infant was undertaken. A variety of bruises of different ages were found on the arms and legs, and these were marked on a body diagram in the notes and also photographed. A consultant ophthalmologist review was requested, identifying widespread retinal hemorrhages in both eyes, suggestive of a shaking injury. Detailed clotting studies were taken, which were all normal.

In view of the concerns over the possibility of non-accidental injury (NAI), the social services (both local to the PICU as well as to the family) were formally informed of the child's admission on the first day and a strategy meeting organized. The 6-month-old sister was removed from the family's care pending further reviews. The local police were also notified. A pediatrician was assigned as lead consultant for the child. A case meeting was held on day 3, and a formal case conference followed later. Over several days the child woke and was eventually extubated successfully, at which stage a complete skeletal survey was undertaken. An MRI scan was also obtained whilst the child was anesthetized.

Discussion

This case demonstrates many of the difficulties in caring for children where NAI is suspected. This child has many features found in such cases, including a history that changes with time, some delay in presentation, two cardinal features of NAI (subdural collections and retinal hemorrhages) and a family with a history of violence. Nevertheless, the history given is of a serious accident that could also cause substantial injury.

It is not the role of the PICU team to make an early judgment on the cause of injuries in these children, but it is crucial that the possibility of NAI is considered, and that appropriate investigations (including careful examination) are undertaken and clearly documented. The Laming report[2] has also recently emphasized the importance of communicating with all agencies that might have additional information (primary care physician, social services, Police, etc.) to ensure that all parties have a full picture of the concerns. Serious non-accidental injury is more likely in those under 2 years of age, although death is unusual after 1 year.[3] Serious head injury is the commonest cause of death in abused children but is rare in accidental falls.[4] Approximately 1% of accidental falls of less than 3 feet result in skull fractures, and, although serious intracranial injury can occur in such falls, it is extremely rare. Most abuse is perpetrated by the child's parents, with men more likely to fatally injure a child. Child abuse is associated with poor parenting skills, domestic violence, and animal maltreatment. It can occur, however, irrespective of race, religion, social class, or cultural background.

Assessment

A meticulous history and examination are important in assessing non-accidental injury. Where possible, a full history should be taken from the child, if necessary in the absence of the parents. This may be difficult in the PICU setting due to use of sedation or the age of the child. History should include development and social history and family details. It is important not to rely on previous histories taken by other healthcare workers. Weight, height, and head circumference should be measured and plotted on a centile chart. A thorough physical examination should include hair, mouth, nose and nails. Any injuries should be carefully recorded as to their site, size, shape, colour and stage of healing. There is a correlation between site and size of bruising and probability of abuse.[5] Where appropriate, medical photographs are extremely valuable.

The presence of the following indicates possible abuse, although none are diagnostic:

1. Delay or failure to seek medical attention
2. Vague or inconsistent histories
3. History incompatible with the child's injuries

4. Abnormal parental affect, such as lack of concern, hostility, or preoccupation with their own problems

5. Abnormal appearance of child or abnormal interaction with parents

6. Direct history from child

7. Injuries of different ages.

Some forms of injury are highly associated with non-accidental injury. These include finger-tip bruising, adult human bite marks, cigarette burns, lash marks, and a torn frenulum. Imprints of bites can yield useful forensic information. Unexplained subdural hematomata and retinal hemorrhages are highly suggestive of abuse. Bruises of different ages are a common feature of abuse and it is useful to be able to estimate the age of a bruise, although the accuracy of the timings is poor. Although accurate aging is impossible, the following is a rough guide for superficial bruises:

- <24 hours   red/purple
- 12–48 hours   purplish blue
- 48–72 hours   brown
- >72 hours   yellow

Red coloration may persist for a week and bruising in pigmented skin can be better demonstrated using ultraviolet light.[6]

Good note-keeping is important. Medical notes may be scrutinized at a later date and constitute a legal document. Any discrepancies between initial history and that given on PICU may be significant. All conversations with parents should, ideally, be recorded and it is advisable to have a witness present as a precaution against subsequent complaints by the parents. As well as recording examination findings, photographs can be very useful evidence and do not require consent if there is genuine suspicion of NAI. It remains good practice, however, to inform families of all procedures and of the reasons for those tests. All written notes must be dated and timed, signed and have the name of the signatory clearly stated on every page.

Investigations

The types of investigations appropriate for cases of suspected non-accidental injury depend on the presenting features. As in this case, when non-accidental bruising is suspected, investigations should be aimed at excluding medical causes of excessive bruising. There is wide individual variation in the degree to which a child will bruise following a defined episode of trauma. Toddlers often develop bruises from mild head trauma, while older children commonly develop lower limb bruises. The infant who is not walking, however, will rarely fall far enough to bruise themselves, and bruising in the under-1-year-old is very concerning. Unusual patterns of bruising or the presence of petechiae or significant mucosal bleeding lead to the suspicion of abuse or an underlying bleeding disorder. A drug history can be significant; even one dose of a non-steroidal anti-inflammatory drug can predispose to easy bruising, which may persist for weeks or months.[7]

Initial laboratory investigation of suspicious bruising should include a full blood count and film, coagulation screen, renal, and hepatic function tests. Cases of suspected non-accidental bruising should be discussed with a pediatric hematologist (Table 15.1).

The incidence of non-accidental fractures is highest in the first year of life; 4 in 10 000 children under 18 months and 0.4 in 10 000 children aged 19–60 months.[8] Unexplained fractures in pre-ambulant infants are highly suspicious.[9] The humerus is the most commonly fractured long bone

Table 15.1. *Important medical causes of bruising*

Hemophilia A or B
von Willebrand's disease
Glanzmann's thromboasthenia
Factor XIII deficiency
Ehlers–Danlos and Marfan's syndromes
Malignancy

in non-accidental injury with spiral or oblique fractures being typical. Long bone fractures from abuse are often at the distal end (involving the corners of the epiphyses). Metaphyseal-epiphyseal fractures are classic signs of abuse in infants. These injuries occur from acceleration and deceleration as the infant is shaken and usually occur at the knee, wrist, elbow, or ankle.

Rib fractures occur in 5%–26% of abused children.[9] Such fractures in children under 2 years of age, especially if multiple, are very suspicious for abuse. There are particularly associated with the shaken infant syndrome, caused by thoracic compression. Cardiopulmonary resuscitation is unlikely to be responsible for rib fractures in young children.

A skeletal survey should be performed in all children less than 24 months with a suspicious fracture or with severe bruising. A radiological survey will detect occult lesions and has a high level of specificity. Radionucleotide bone scanning is more sensitive and can be used if conventional radiography is normal.[10] However, bone scanning can miss metaphyseal lesions around normally active joints or healed injuries. Fractures may occur after minimal trauma in conditions with increased bone fragility such as osteogenesis imperfecta or metabolic bone disease. These are much rarer than child abuse and can usually be diagnosed on a clinical and radiological basis. Expert radiological, pediatric and biochemical help may be required in some cases. Temporary brittle bones have been postulated as an explanation for some infant fractures, although there is a paucity of evidence to support this. Imaging of the brain with CT or MRI is required to investigate suspected non-accidental head injury. CT scans are more readily available and can demonstrate scalp, bone, extra axial hematomas, and parenchymal injury although MRI is better at excluding diffuse axonal injury and may also be better able to assess the timing of the injury[10A]. Given the reports of cervical cord damage in cases of severe non-accidental head injury, some authors have suggested that neuroimaging should include the spinal column.[17] Ultrasound imaging has no place in the initial assessment of suspected NAI head injury.

A formal ophthalmic opinion from an experienced and senior ophthalmologist is important. Although there remains some controversy[11] about the precise interpretation of eye findings in such infants, a detailed report is essential.

Non-accidental head injury

Head injury is the commonest reason for abused children to require admission to a PICU. Most subdural hemorrhages (SDH) in infancy result from non-accidental injury when the infant has been shaken.[4] The morbidity and mortality of these patients is very high.[12] Two major patterns of head injury can occur: focal injury from impacts, e.g. punching or hitting head after throwing or swinging, and diffuse injury from acceleration–deceleration phenomena (shaking). There is debate about the forces involved and whether diffuse axonal injury or hypoxic–ischemic injury is more important[13,14] but it is now generally agreed that shaking alone can cause SDH. The term "shaken baby syndrome" has been used to describe cases of subdural and subarachnoid hemorrhages, retinal hemorrhage, and associated long bone changes.

SDHs arise from tearing of the bridging subdural veins; those seen in non-accidental head injury are usually small and exert little mass effect. The SDH is rarely responsible for the severe long-term outcomes seen, which are probably related to the degree of hypoxic–ischemic damage[15] as well as associated impact injury, secondary cerebral hypoperfusion, and refractory seizures. Data on long-term outcomes from non-accidental head injury are scarce, although it is known that morbidity is profoundly worse than for accidentally head injured children.[16]

Geddes *et al.* reported a high incidence of diffuse microscopic neuronal hypoxic brain damage in children with non-accidental head injury.[15] It has been suggested that, in children presenting with a history of apnea and hypoxic brain damage, cervical hyperextension/flexion during shaking causes damage to brain stem respiratory centres.[15,17] This is supported by earlier work that described damage to the cranio-cervical junction in babies where there was no evidence of impact.[12] Currently, evidence is lacking to support accurate predictions of the force required to cause intracranial injury. Most young children with non-accidental head injury have associated serious injuries, suggesting they have been victim to considerable violence. Although Geddes *et al.*[15] suggest that acceleration–deceleration injury does not have to be *severe* in shaken baby syndrome, there is currently no evidence to show that minimal shaking can cause shaken baby syndrome. The amount of force necessary to produce hypoxic brain injury, even in the absence of any other injuries, is unlikely to occur during normal childcare or play activities. These studies have significant forensic implications.

Clinical presentations of shaken babies are rather non-specific and include irritability, lethargy, fits, apneic attacks, and fluctuating levels of consciousness; they may also appear to be septic. Parents may admit to shaking the child mildly because he "stopped breathing."[18] Many victims sustain extracranial injuries although sometimes there are very few signs of abuse. Retinal examination is required, since retinal hemorrhages occur in approximately 70% cases of non-accidental head injury.[19] Retinal hemorrhages rarely result from accidental trauma (0 out of 20 cases in the above series), although small unilateral hemorrhages may occasionally be seen after severe non-inflicted brain injury.[20] Retinal hemorrhages may also rarely occur after cardiopulmonary resuscitation, convulsions, and some neurological conditions. Examination of the retina should be done by ophthalmologists to reduce the incidence of false-negative examinations. In one series of shaken baby syndrome children, non-ophthalmologists were unable, or did not attempt, visualization of the fundus in 55% of cases.[21]

Legal considerations

As stated above, careful and clear documentation of information, as well as involvement of all associated professional agencies are crucial to the care of these children. A senior pediatrician should be allocated early in the child's care to coordinate the investigations and liaise with both the family and with other agencies. Notes should contain clear details of who is involved and which agencies and individuals have been involved.

When asked for opinions on the cause of the injuries, in any case, it is important to be aware of the different levels of certainty that are needed in different situations. In the early stages of care, the issue centers around safety of the child (and, more particularly, the safety of any siblings). In this regard it is only important that NAI is more likely than not "on a balance of probability". This 51% likelihood of NAI is very different from the criminal level ("beyond reasonable doubt") needed to convict. It is essential that all professionals are both prepared to comment clearly on the issues on which they have knowledge as well as limiting themselves to such areas. Therefore, if an opinion on – for example – MRI findings is requested from an intensive care doctor, it is usually more appropriate to refer such an opinion to a neuroradiologist.

Medico-legal reports are always wanted, and should be generated clearly and in a timely manner. A senior doctor should review such reports. Finally, all PICUs should have clear guidelines clarifying local procedure to be followed in cases of suspected NAI, with phone numbers and contact details.

Learning points

- Concerns about child abuse must be investigated thoroughly.
- A vague, inconsistent or incongruous history or delay in presentation should arouse suspicion.
- Full examination and meticulous note keeping are important.
- Excessive bruising should be investigated and may require expert opinion.
- Metaphyseal–epiphyseal, humeral and rib fractures are suspicious.
- A skeletal survey can be considered and is best interpreted by a consultant pediatric radiologist with expertise in non-accidental injuries.
- Serious head injury is the commonest cause of death in abused children.
- Shaking babies may result in hypoxic–ischemic brain damage, presenting as fits, apnea or reduced conscious level.
- Ophthalmological examination is required in suspected non-accidental head injury.

Acknowledgments

The editors are grateful to Dr. Marcus Likeman, Consultant Radiologist at Bristol Children's Hospital, for providing the CT scan image used in this chapter.

References

1. Department for Education and Skills. *Referrals, Assessments and Children and Young People on Child Protection Registers. Year Ending 31 March 2003.* London, TSO, 2004
2. Lord Laming *Inquiry into the death of Victoria Climbie.* London, Stationery Office, 2003.
3. Hobbs CJ. Physical abuse. In: Hobbs CJ, Hanks HGI, Wynne JM, eds. *Child Abuse and Neglect.* Edinburgh, Churchill Livingstone, 1993.
4. Jayawant S, Rawlinsin A, Gibson F *et al.* Subdural haemorrhages in infants: population based study. *Br Med J* 1998; **317**: 1558–61.
5. Dunstan FD, Guildea ZE, Kontros K *et al.* A scoring system for bruise patterns: a tool for identifying abuse. *Arch Dis Child* 2002; **86**: 330–3.
6. Stephenson T, Bialas Y. Estimation of age of bruising. *Arch Dis Child* 1996; **74**: 53–5.
7. Vora AJ, Makris M. An approach to investigation of easy bruising. *Arch Dis Child* 2001; **84**: 488–91.
8. Worlock P, Stower M, Barbor P. Patterns of fractures in accidental and non-accidental injury in children: a comparative study. *Br Med J* 1986; **293**: 100–2.
9. Carty HML. Fractures caused by child abuse. *J Bone Joint Surg B* 1993; **75**: 849–57.

10. Mandelstam SA, Cook D, Fitzgerald M *et al.* Complementary use of radiological skeletal survey and bone scintography in detection of bony injuries in suspected child abuse. *Arch Dis Child* 2003; **88**: 387–90.
11. Lantz PE, Sinal SH, Stanton CA *et al.* Perimacular retinal folds from childhood head trauma. *Br Med J* 2004; **328**: 754–6.
12. Hadley MN, Sonntag VK, Rekate HL *et al.* The infant whiplash-shake injury syndrome: a clinical and pathological study. *Neurosurgery* 1989; **24**: 536–40.
13. Geddes JF, Plunkett J. The evidence base for shaken baby syndrome. *Br Med J* 2004; **328**: 719–20.
14. Risdon RA, Krous HF. Shaken baby syndrome. *Br Med J* 2004; **328**: 720–1.
15. Geddes JF, Vowles GH, Hackshaw AK *et al.* Neuropathology of inflicted head injury in children. *Brain* 2001; **124**: 1299–306.
16. Haviland J, Ross Russell R. Outcome after severe non-accidental head injury. *Arch Dis Child* 1997; **77**: 504–7.
17. Kemp AM, Stoodley N, Cobley C *et al.* Apnoea and brain swelling in non-accidental injury. *Arch Dis Child* 2003; **88**: 472–6.
18. Fox D, Bignall S, Marriage SC. Parental resuscitation techniques after apparent life threatening events in infancy. *Arch Dis Child* 1997; **76**: 289.
19. Ewing-Cobbs L, Kramer L, Prasad M *et al.* Neuroimaging, physical and developmental findings after inflicted and non-inflicted traumatic brain injury in young children. *Pediatrics* 1998; **102**: 300–7.
20. Betz P, Puschel K, Miltner E *et al.* Morphometrical analysis or retinal hemorrhages in the shaken baby syndrome. *Forensic* 1996; **78**: 71–80.
21. Morad Y, Kim YM, Mian M *et al.* Nonophthalmologist accuracy in diagnosing retinal hemorrhages in the shaken baby syndrome. *J Pediatr* 2003; **142** (4): 431–4.

Chapter 6

Management of a 3-year-old child with drowning

Margrid Schindler

Introduction

The definition of drowning agreed by the task force of the First World Congress on drowning in 2003 is: "the process of experiencing respiratory impairment from submersion or immersion in a liquid."[1] Drowning is an important cause of childhood morbidity and mortality, with 27% of deaths from unintentional injury in the United States being due to drowning at age 1–4 years. Males are more commonly involved than females. The majority of drownings occur in fresh water. Of infant (<1 year) drownings, 55% were in bathtubs; among children between the ages of 1 and 4 years, 56% of drownings were in artificial pools; and among older children, 63% of drownings were in natural collections of fresh water.[1] The sequelae of global hypoxic–ischemic brain injury are the most devastating outcome of drowning.[2]

Presentation

During a large family gathering, the 3-year-old grandson was noted to be missing. A search of the house and back garden ensued and eventually the boy was located face down and lifeless in the neighbor's swimming pool. He was removed from the water and basic Cardiopulmonary Resuscitation (CPR) was immediately commenced by a cousin, a trained nurse. On arrival of the ambulance team 10 minutes later, the child was still lifeless with absent pulse and respiration. CPR was continued in the ambulance, which arrived at the hospital emergency department 8 minutes later.

Initial assessment and management

On arrival, he was still flaccid with no palpable pulse and absent respiration. He was immediately intubated and ventilated with 100% O_2. Chest compressions were continued and an intra-osseous needle was inserted into the left tibia and adrenaline 1.4 ml 1:10 000 administered. He was cold to touch and the rectal temperature was 30 °C. All wet clothing was removed, and a heat and moisture exchanger was placed at the end of the endotracheal tube. A nasogastric tube was inserted, the stomach aspirated, and gastric lavage was commenced with warmed saline. A 14 G cannula was inserted into the peritoneum and connected to a three-way tap and 200 ml of warmed saline (44 °C) was instilled in the peritoneum.

After a further 10 minutes of CPR and another 1.4 ml adrenaline and vasopressin 0.4 mcg kg^{-1} by intra-osseous injection, a pulse returned. A femoral arterial line was inserted and arterial blood pressure (BP) was 70/50 (mean 60) mmHg, heart rate (HR) 140 b min^{-1}, capillary refill >4 seconds. With hand ventilation at 25 breaths min^{-1} with peak inspiratory pressures of 30 cmH$_2$O, the arterial blood gas (ABG) showed a pH 6.8, PaCO$_2$ 70 mmHg, PaO$_2$ 100 mmHg, bicarbonate 9 mmol l^{-1}, BE −22, lactate 15 mmol l^{-1}, Na 139 mmol l^{-1}, K 7.2 mmol l^{-1}, Hct 33%, Glu 14 mmol l^{-1}. The rectal temperature had risen to 33 °C, and his pupils were large but sluggishly reactive. He was making occasional gasping respiration, but

Case Studies in Pediatric Critical Care, ed. Peter. J. Murphy, Stephen C. Marriage, and Peter J. Davis. Published by Cambridge University Press. © Cambridge University Press 2009.

not responding to painful stimuli. A chest X-ray showed bilateral hazy opacification of the lung fields. 30 ml of 4.2% sodium bicarbonate was given via an intra-osseous needle. The BP drifted to 55/42 (mean 47) and a femoral central venous line was inserted; the central venous pressure measured through this line was 22 mmHg. An adrenaline infusion was commenced at 0.2 mcg kg^{-1} per min with good effect. A repeat ABG showed pH 7.1, PaCO$_2$ 50 mmHg, PaO$_2$ 120 mmHg, bicarbonate 14 mmol l^{-1}, BE −18, lactate 14 mmol l^{-1}, Na 144 mmol l^{-1}, K 6.4 mmol l^{-1}, Hct 33%, Glu 18 mmol l^{-1}. A further 15 mmol of sodium bicarbonate, IV, was given and he was transferred to PICU.

Progress in the pediatric intensive care unit

In the pediatric intensive care unit, he was sedated and muscle relaxed with morphine and vecuronium infusions and he was kept cooled to 34 °C for 24 hours. Cardiovascularly his perfusion improved and acidosis resolved, but he continued to require inotropic support for 24 hours. His respiratory status deteriorated with poor oxygenation, and further widespread infiltrates and left lower lobe consolidation were evident on chest X-ray. His initial ventilator settings were pressure control ventilation, with peak inspiratory pressures (PIP) of 28 cmH$_2$O and positive end expiratory pressure (PEEP) of 6 cmH$_2$O, ventilator rate of 25 breaths per minute and 80% O$_2$. On this his ABG showed pH 7.2, PaCO$_2$ 60 mmHg, PaO$_2$ 70 mmHg, bicarbonate 18 mmol l^{-1}, BE −10. The PIP and PEEP were increased to 30/8 cmH$_2$O, ventilator rate increased to 30 breaths min^{-1}, 100% O$_2$ and the inspiratory time was lengthened to 50% to increase the mean airway pressure and improve oxygenation. In view of the deteriorating chest X-ray, he was also commenced on cefuroxime 25 mg kg^{-1}, 8 hourly.

The blood glucose concentration remained high at 15 mmol l^{-1} and he was commenced on an insulin infusion 0.1 U kg^{-1} per h, which reduced the blood glucose level to 8.

Twenty-four hours later, he was becoming increasingly edematous with poor urine output, and so was commenced on furosemide infusion at 0.2 mg kg^{-1} per h. Cooling was discontinued and he was allowed to passively rewarm. An electroencephalogram (EEG) was performed, which showed generalized slow wave activity, which may have been due to hypoxic ischemia or the effect of the sedation drugs. No epileptiform discharges were seen.

This result was explained to the parents and they were told of the worrying neurological prognosis in view of the prolonged cardiac arrest on presentation, but that it was too early to predict the outcome with certainty, and that the plan was to stop the muscle relaxants and reduce the sedation to allow clinical examination of his neurological status. A neurological consultation was also requested.

Seventy-two hours after admission, he was cardiovascularly stable off inotropic support, and his respiratory status was improving with the ventilator pressures having been reduced to 26/8 and 60% oxygen. He was beginning to make some spontaneous respiratory effort. Neurologically, he was no longer muscle relaxed but remained on a morphine infusion at 20 mcg kg^{-1} per h. His pupils were reactive and equal. Corneal and occulocephalic reflex were present. Deep pain induced by supraorbital nerve pressure resulted in decerebrate posturing (flexor upper limb response, and extensor lower limb response). There was no gag reflex and he had a poor cough on deep endotracheal suctioning. A repeat EEG showed persistent slow wave responses, and a magnetic resonance image scan (MRI) of brain performed earlier that morning showed evidence of widespread hypoxic ischemic changes, and basal ganglia infarcts (Fig. 16.1).

The PICU and neurology consultants explained to the parents that he had sustained severe neurological injury, which if he survived, would result in severe disability and he

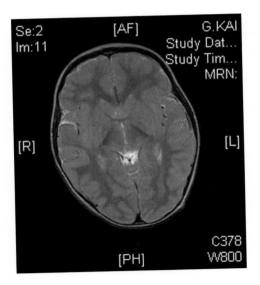

Fig. 16.1. Magnetic resonance image scan (MRI) of brain showing evidence of widespread hypoxic ischemic changes and basal ganglia infarcts.

would require assistance with basic needs, and that one of the possible options to consider was withdrawal of intensive care support to allow him to die. The parents stated that they had read on the internet that hypothermia at the time of drowning results in miraculous survivors despite long resuscitation times. The PICU consultant explained that these were special circumstances where the patient had fallen through ice and had inhaled and swallowed ice cold water resulting in very rapid and severe cooling, and that this was not the case with their son, who was most likely hypothermic on arrival due to prolonged exposure during resuscitation. The parents refused to accept this and said that they wanted everything possible done.

Over the next 48 hours, the morphine infusion was discontinued, and the ventilation was gradually weaned to pressure support 6 cmH$_2$O on a PEEP of 5 and 40% oxygen, and extubation was attempted. Unfortunately, he developed severe stridor and respiratory distress and was re-intubated 1 hour later with a smaller endotracheal tube and was commenced on dexamethasone 0.25 mg kg^{-1} 6-hourly. Neurologically, he continued to have a weak cough and gag, but was making spontaneous non-purposeful movements with the left arm and occasionally semi-purposeful movements with his right arm. His mother was convinced that he squeezed her hand to command, but the nurses were unconvinced.

The PICU and neurology consultant again met with the parents and explained the likely poor neurological outcome, that despite the presence of stridor at extubation, his neurological state had most likely contributed to the failed extubation, and that subsequent attempts might also be unsuccessful due to poor secretion clearance. The parents still felt that he would get better and that the PICU team had extubated him to early, as he had had increased tracheal secretions that morning. Extubation was again attempted 72 hours later when the secretions had decreased and he had developed a small leak around the endotracheal tube. The PICU team recommended that he not be re-intubated if he failed again, but the parents refused to accept this and said they wanted everything possible done. He was successfully extubated to BiPAP via face mask at pressures of 15/8 cm H_2O, and continued to require physiotherapy and deep suctioning to aid secretion clearance. BiPAP support was gradually weaned off over the next 3 days, and he was discharged to the ward on nasogastric feeds and ongoing physiotherapy.

Two weeks later he developed severe respiratory distress and right lower lobe pneumonia on the ward requiring readmission to the intensive care unit for mechanical ventilation. A pH study and upper gastrointestinal contrast study showed evidence of moderate gastro-esophageal reflux, and a fundoplication and insertion of gastrostomy tube was performed. He was again weaned and successfully extubated, and discharged to the ward. He was discharged home 6 weeks later. Six months later when reviewed in outpatient clinic, he continued to require gastrostomy feeds and suffered frequent chest infections, and was unable to sit or stand independently. However, he smiled and interacted with his mother and reached out and grasped toys, and his mother felt he was making progress.

Discussion

Pathophysiology of submersion injury

During the initial minutes of submersion, there is panic and struggle to surface. Small amounts of water are aspirated often triggering laryngospasm, and large volumes of water are swallowed. The laryngospasm abates and the victim aspirates water, and there may also be vomiting and aspiration of gastric contents. Evolving hypoxia causes neuronal injury and eventually circulatory collapse, with further ischemic brain injury.[2]

Possible associated factors in drowning include prolonged QT syndrome induced arrhythmias, epilepsy, drug intoxication, and trauma. A review of submersion victims found a low prevalence of cervical spine injury (0.5%), and all those who sustained cervical spine injury had clinical signs of serious injury and a history of high-impact trauma before submersion. Thus, without a history of trauma or signs of injury, there is little evidence supporting cervical spine immobilization in drowning victims.[2]

Initial assessment, resuscitation, and management

There are a number of factors associated with unfavorable outcome that are listed in Table 16.1, but none, either individually or in combination have been shown to have absolute

Table 16.1. *Factors associated with unfavorable outcome*

Male[23]
Water temperature >10 °C[8]
Duration of submersion >10 minutes[9]
Time to effective basic life support >10 minutes[24]
Absent pulse on arrival in emergency department[5]
Minimum blood pH <7.1[24]
Blood glucose >11 mmol l^{-1} [23]
Absent pupillary responses[23]
GCS <5 in emergency department or intensive care[3]

predictive significance. Therefore, full resuscitation should be attempted, at least briefly, in all drowning patients arriving in emergency departments.[3]

The outcome of cardiac arrest in children is dependent first and foremost on the duration of the cardiac arrest, but is also influenced by the location and cause of the arrest. The worst outcomes occurs following out-of-hospital cardiac arrest. Sirbaugh[4] reviewed 300 pediatric out-of-hospital cardiac arrests and only found a 2% survival to discharge, all with significant neurological sequelae. Similarly, Schindler[5] reviewed 80 out-of-hospital cardiac arrests and found a 7% survival to 12 months after discharge, with 50% of survivors being in a persistent vegetative state and the remainder had moderate disability. A 10-year literature review of studies where resuscitation times had been analyzed after an out-of–hospital cardiac arrest (6 studies involving 198 children) showed that there were no survivors to hospital discharge if greater than 20 minutes of resuscitation was required following out-of-hospital arrest.[5]

After submersion, Corneli[6] found no hypothermic protection if the core temperature was warmer than 30–32 °C. The survivors of prolonged submersion (>15 minutes) all had an initial temperature of <25 °C. This strongly suggests that, if there is no return of spontaneous circulation following 20 minutes of effective cardiopulmonary resuscitation (CPR) and the core temperature is >32 °C after an out-of-hospital cardiac arrest, then resuscitation should be discontinued. In the case presented, the duration of submersion was unknown, and the child had 18 minutes of basic life support prior to arrival in the hospital emergency department. If hypothermia had not been present, then resuscitation could safely have been limited to 10 minutes in this case, as 93% of survivors of a pediatric out-of-hospital cardiac arrest were resuscitated within 11 minutes of arrival in hospital.[5]

Full resuscitation should be attempted and efforts made to rewarm the child to 32–33 °C.[7] Temperatures less than 31 °C are associated with decreased or absent systemic blood pressure, bradycardia, arrythmias, and temperatures less than 25 °C are associated with apnea, asystole and clinical appearance of death.[6]

Diagnosis of hypothermia requires a high index of suspicion and a low-reading thermometer (ordinary thermometers do not record less than 34 °C). Core temperature can be measured at the tympanic membrane, esophagus, bladder, and deep rectal (thermometer should be inserted at least 10 cm into the rectum).[6]

Rewarming methods are listed in Table 16.2. First, further heat loss should be prevented by removing wet clothing and avoiding contact with cold surfaces. Elevating room temperature to 21–23 °C, overhead heaters and warm dry blankets allow passive rewarming in mildly hypothermic patients, while the severely hypothermic patient will require active core rewarming. The simplest of these methods is to use warmed intravenous fluids and humidified oxygen. Parenteral solutions in plastic bags can be heated in a microwave oven to 40 °C, and a heat and moisture exchanger placed at the end of the endotracheal tube will dramatically reduce evaporative heat loss from the respiratory tract.[6] It is important to ensure the warmed fluid reaches the patient by shortening the tubing or, better still, using a commercial blood warmer. Warmed gastric lavage or enemas, and bladder irrigation can also be performed easily and provides considerable heat transfer.[6] Even larger amounts of heat can be provided using peritoneal lavage/dialysis, which is also relatively easy to accomplish in most hospitals. The dialysate (or 0.9% saline in emergency situation) is warmed to 54 °C so that it enters the peritoneal cavity at 43 °C and hourly cycles are preferred.[7] In this case, a large bore IV cannula placed in the peritoneum was initially used to instil the first 10–20 ml kg^{-1} warmed peritoneal fluid, to achieve rapid heat transfer and avoid possible delays, while trying to locate specialized peritoneal dialysis catheter sets. Closed pleural lavage also transfers large amounts of heat. In

Table 16.2. *Rewarming methods*

Passive:	Warm room (21–23 °C)
	Remove wet clothing
	Avoid cold surfaces
	Dry blankets
Active External:	Warmed blankets
	Chemical hot packs
	Radiant overhead heaters
	Bear Hugger warm air blanket
	Warm water mat under patient
Core:	Warm IV fluids 37–40 °C
	Heated humidified oxygen (40–44 °C)
	Warmed gastric lavage
	Warmed bladder lavage
Core, high heat transfer:	Warmed pleural lavage
	Peritoneal dialysis
	Haemodialysis
	Extracorporeal circulation (cardiopulmonary bypass)

severe cases cardiopulmonary bypass has been used, but this is only available in tertiary centers providing pediatric cardiac surgery.[6]

Orlowski[8] noted that water colder than 10 °C accounts for all reported cases of survival after prolonged (>15 minutes) submersion, and 16 of 17 cases probably involved water colder than 5 °C. Even in ice-water drowning, hypothermia by no means guarantees survival. Unless cooling occurs quickly, before hypoxia becomes severe, little useful cerebral protection is provided. Rapid cooling of body temperature due to pulmonary cooling by rapid breathing in and out of ice-cold water, gastric cooling from swallowed cold water in addition to surface cooling (especially from scalp, where blood vessels do not constrict) is required to offer protection.[1] Cooling that occurs during rescue and transport to hospital is of little benefit and may render deep body temperature on arrival in hospital an unreliable prognostic indicator.[7,9] Hyperkalemia in severely hypothermic patients is usually indicative of asphyxial cardiac arrest before significant cooling occurred.[7] Even in cases with rapid cooling, broad cognitive learning difficulties are often detected on longer-term neurological follow-up.[10]

It has been suggested that vasopressin may have a role in pediatric cardiac arrest, and it was used in this case. In a randomized trial of 1219 adults after an out-of-hospital cardiac arrest, vasopressin had similar effects to adrenaline in the management of ventricular fibrillation and pulseless electrical activity, but was superior to adrenaline in patients with asystole. Vasopressin followed by adrenaline was more effective than adrenaline alone in the treatment of refractory cardiac arrest.[11] Use of vasopressin has been reported in four children during cardiac arrest in the PICU and was thought to be beneficial.[12]

Table 16.3. *Complications of drowning*

Decreased cardiac index
Hypothermic cardiac arrhythmia
Pulmonary edema
Aspiration
Acute Respiratory Distress Syndrome (ARDS)
Pneumonia
Sepsis
Disseminated Intravascular Coagulation (DIC)
Rhabdomyolysis
Acute tubular necrosis
Hypoxic ischemic encephalopathy
Cerebral edema
Basal ganglia and "water shed" cerebral infarcts

Ongoing management of drowning and its complications

Table 16.3 gives a list of complications of drowning. The early literature on drowning stressed different hemodynamic and electrolyte effects, dependent on whether drowning was in fresh or salt water. In dogs, inhalation of hypertonic and hypotonic solutions produced, respectively, a rise and a fall in the serum sodium but not of a magnitude to be clinically significant.[13] Subsequent studies of human drowning victims showed that electrolyte abnormalities were minimal, hemoglobin concentrations were minimally altered, and there may be slight increased intravascular volume after fresh water drowning and hypovolemia after salt water drowning, but these are transient and not usually clinically significant.[2] In animal studies, the cardiovascular effect of drowning was an abrupt fall in cardiac index and a sudden rise in pulmonary capillary wedge pressure, central venous pressure, and pulmonary vascular resistance, most likely as a direct result of anoxia, rather than the tonicity of the water.[13]

Hypoxia, hypercarbia, and metabolic acidosis are likely to be present in victims of drowning.[1] Close monitoring with pulse oximetry, repeated blood gases, and a chest X-ray are required. Aspiration of water and gastric contents (drowning probably never occurs without aspiration to some degree) results in surfactant disruption, alveolar collapse, atelectasis, and intrapulmonary shunting.[1] Severe pulmonary dysfunction after drowning often progresses to Acute Respiratory Distress Syndrome (ARDS) and high positive end-expiratory pressures are frequently required. Pulmonary edema is common, for which diuretics may be required.[1] While pneumonia is also a common sequela, prophylactic antibiotics have not been shown to be beneficial. However broad-spectrum antibiotics should be instituted if there is any evidence of infection. Corticosteriods also do not improve outcome and may increase infection rates.[1]

The primary cerebral insult during drowning is from hypoxia. With cardiovascular compromise, cerebral blood flow falls, resulting in additional ischemic injury. High ICP correlates with poor neurologic outcome, but ICP <20 mmHg does not indicate good outcome.[2] Also, aggressive treatment of intracranial hypertension has not proven to be beneficial to victims of near-drowning.[2] Thus, ICP monitoring is not recommended following near-drowning.

Repeated clinical neurologic examination including Glasgow Coma Score (GCS) and brainstem reflex testing is the most accurate and reproducible method available early in the course of the injury for predicting outcome in children who have suffered hypoxic ischemic brain injury.[2] In particular, the presence of coma on admission and a Glasgow Coma Score of <5 at 24 hours after admission are associated with unfavorable outcome.[14] Adjunctive investigations such as magnetic resonance imaging or neurophysiological testing may be useful if there is clinical doubt or if the child's caregivers request confirmatory testing.[2]

The role of electroencephalography (EEG) early following drowning is often limited due to the use of sedatives and analgesics in the intensive care unit. A flat or severely attenuated EEG or burst suppression during the initial 24 hours reflects the initial insult. A persistently attenuated record without medications, however, is predictive of a poor neurologic prognosis.[2] Mandel[14] found that, in children with hypoxic ischemic encephalopathy, a discontinuous EEG, the presence of spikes or epileptiform discharges were associated with an unfavorable outcome.

Brainstem auditory-evoked responses can be altered by both central and peripheral auditory disorders, and are particularly vulnerable to hypoxia in young patients.[2] Fisher[15] found that, drowning patients who were declared brain-dead or died, exhibited abnormal brainstem auditory-evoked response measurements on admission and until death; however wave V could not be detected on admission in 61% of these patients.

Somatosensory-evoked potentials may be more accurate in predicting outcome in children who have suffered hypoxic ischemic cerebral injury[2]; however, no studies on its use in pediatric submersion victims have yet been published. In children with hypoxic ischemic encephalopathy from other causes, the bilateral absence of the N20 wave on short-latency sensory evoked potentials had a positive predictive value for unfavourable outcome of 100% (sensitivity 63%).[14] Thus, an early clinical assessment in the first 24 hours, combined with an EEG and somatosensory evoked potentials, may allow an early prediction of the prognosis of children with hypoxic ischemic encephalopathy.

Although computer tomography of the brain and neck is indicated in the hospital emergency department if there is a history or signs suggestive of trauma, the role of computer tomography in the early evaluation of hypoxic–ischemic injury in the drowning victim is limited.[2] Dubowitz[16] performed serial brain magnetic resonance imaging and quantitative magnetic resonance spectroscopy on 22 children admitted to the ICU after drowning and found excellent predictive value of magnetic resonance imaging when performed on day 3 or 4 (100% positive predictive value and 100% negative predictive value). Generalized or occipital edema and basal ganglia T2 hyperintensity correlated with poor outcome. Patchy high T2 signal in the cortex or subcortical lines were specific but insensitive for poor outcome as were brainstem infarcts.

Management of hypoxic–ischemic encephalopathy

The primary hypoxic–ischemic injury is irreversible, and the main aim of cerebral resuscitation is to prevent secondary neuronal damage. In the past, hyperventilation, hypothermia, barbiturate coma, and glucocorticoids were advocated, but later prospective studies failed to show any improvement from this approach.[1] Good supportive care with optimum oxygenation,[16] normocarbia,[17] and normal systemic blood pressure[16] are recommended.

Increased blood glucose concentrations after ischemic injury may impair neurological recovery, and a recent randomized controlled trial in critically ill adults has suggested that close glycemic control (maintaining blood glucose level between 4–6 mmol l^{-1}) is associated with improved outcome.[19] Thus, careful attention should be paid to glucose control in these patients, and hence an insulin infusion was used in the early stages of this child's illness.

A recent adult randomized control trial showed a better neurological outcome with induced hypothermia (32–34 °C) after cardiac arrest due to ventricular fibrillation,[20] and, assuming that the pathophysiology of anoxic injury after submersion is the same, this would suggest that perhaps drowning victims who have suffered a cardiac arrest should be cooled to 34 °C, or at least not actively rewarmed above 34 °C. However, no pediatric data on the use of hypothermia post-cardiac arrest is available at present.

The degree of hypoxic–ischemic injury varies in different regions of the brain following drowning, with vascular end zones ("watershed" areas), the hippocampus, insular cortex, and the basal ganglia are particularly susceptible[2] with resultant impaired memory and learning, depressed visual motor skills, extending to more moderate and severe neurologic sequelae in some children.[2]

Bratton[21] found that all survivors with good neurological outcome had spontaneous purposeful movements within 24 hours after submersion. A Glasgow Coma Score (GCS) of >5 on arrival in the hospital emergency department or ICU was also highly predictive of a good neurologic outcome and no patients admitted to the ICU with a GCS of 3 had a good outcome.[22] Lavelle and Shaw[3] found that unreactive pupils in the emergency room and a GCS <5 on arrival were the best independent predictors of poor neurologic outcome. Children do not have a better outcome than adults.[9] Of 72 children who were comatose on admission following drowning, there were 38 deaths, 14 remained in a vegetative state, 3 had severe impairment requiring dependent care, 6 had mild impairment and 11 were discharged normal.[23]

No outcome predictor available at present is absolute, making accurate prediction very difficult. Perceptions of a "good outcome" may vary among different parents and medical teams, but overall the outcome from pediatric drowning victims who are comatose on admission is poor, with death or moderate to severe neurodisability the most likely outcomes.

Learning points

- Global hypoxic–ischemic brain injury is the most devastating outcome of drowning.
- Factors associated with unfavourable outcome do not have absolute predictive significance. Full resuscitation should be attempted in all drowning patients arriving in emergency departments, at least briefly.
- Initial core temperatures warmer than 30–32 °C offer no hypothermic protection.
- No return of spontaneous circulation following 20 minutes of effective cardiopulmonary resuscitation (CPR) in the hospital emergency department and the core temperature is >32 °C after an out-of-hospital cardiac arrest, then resuscitation should be discontinued.
- Hypothermic patients should be rewarmed to 32 °C, with warmed IV fluids, humidified oxygen, and peritoneal dialysis using warmed fluids being the most effective and widely available methods.
- Acute respiratory distress syndrome (ARDS), pulmonary edema, and pneumonia are common sequelae. Positive end-expiratory pressure is frequently required.

- Routine prophylactic antibiotics or corticosteroids are not recommended.
- Initial clinical neurological assessment on arrival in the hospital emergency department or ICU including brainstem reflexes and Glasgow Coma Score and a subsequent MRI scan of brain performed on day 3–4 are useful outcome predictors.
- Generalized supportive measures and prevention of any secondary hypoxic, hypotensive, or metabolic complications are the key to the management of the hypoxic–ischemic encephalopathy.
- Submersion >10 minutes, the need for continued CPR in the hospital emergency department, presence of coma or fixed dilated pupils on admission, initial pH <7.1 and seizures continuing >24 hours are suggestive, but not 100% predictive, of a poor neurological outcome.

References

1. Salomez F, Vincent JL. Drowning: a review of epidemiology, pathophysiology, treatment and prevention. *Resuscitation* 2004; **63**: 261–8.
2. Ibsen LM, Koch T. Submersion and asphyxial injury. *Crit Care Med* 2002; **30** (Suppl.): S402–8.
3. Lavelle JM, Shaw KN. Near drowning: is emergency department cardiopulmonary resuscitation or intensive care unit cerebral resuscitation indicated? *Crit Care Med* 1993; **21**: 368–73.
4. Sirbaugh PE, Pepe PE, Shook JE *et al.* A prospective, population-based study of the demographics, epidemiology, management and outcome of out-of-hospital pediatric cardiopulmonary arrest. *Ann Emerg Med* 1999; **33**: 174–84.
5. Schindler MB, Bohn D, Cox PN *et al.* Outcome of out-of-hospital cardiac or respiratory arrest in children. *N Engl J Med* 1996; **335**: 1473–9.
6. Corneli HM. Accidental hypothermia. *J Pediatr* 1992; **120**: 671–9.
7. Golden F, Tipton MJ, Scott RC. Immersion, near-drowning and drowning. *Br J Anaesthesia* 1997; **79**: 214–25.
8. Orlowski JP. Drowning, near-drowning and ice-water submersions. *Pediatr Clin North Am* 1987; **34**: 75–92.
9. Suominen P, Baillie C, Korpelia R, Rautanen S, Ranta S, Olkkola KT. Impact of age, submersion time and water temperature on outcome in near-drowning. *Resuscitation* 2002; **52**: 247–54.
10. Hughes SK, Nilsson DE, Boyer RS *et al.* Neurodevelopmental outcome for extended cold water drowning: a longitudinal case study. *J Int Neuropsychol Soc* 2002; **8**: 588–95.
11. Wenzel V, Krismer AC, Arntz HR *et al.* A comparision of vasopressin and epinephrine for out-of-hospital cardiopulmonary resuscitation. *N Engl J Med* 2004; **350**: 105–13.
12. Mann K, Berg RA, Nadkarni V. Beneficial effects of vasopressin in prolonged pediatric cardiac arrest: a case series. *Resuscitation* 2002; **52**: 149–56.
13. Orlowski JP, Abulleil MM, Phillips JM. The hemodynamic and cardiovascular effects of near-drowning in hypotonic, isotonic, or hypertonic solutions. *Ann Emerg Med* 1989; **18**: 1044–9.
14. Mandel R, Martinot A, Delepoulle F *et al.* Prediction of outcome after hypoxic-ischemic encephalopathy: a prospective clinical and electrophysiologic study. *J Pediatr* 2002; **141**: 45–50.
15. Fisher B, Peterson B, Hicks G. Use of brainstem auditory-evoked response testing to assess neurological outcome following near drowning in children. *Crit Care Med* 1992; **20**: 578–85.
16. Dubowitz DJ, Bluml S, Arcinue E, Dietrich RB. MR of hypoxic encephalopathy in children after near drowning: carrelation with quantitative proton MR spectroscopy and clinical outcome. *AJNR Am J Neuroradiol* 1998; **19**: 1617–27.
17. Aggarwal R, Deorari AK, Paul VK. Post-resuscitation management of asphyxiated neonates. *Indian J Pediatr* 2001; **68**: 1149–53.

18. Vannucci RC, Brucklacher RM, Vannucci SJ. Effect of carbon dioxide on cerebral metabolism during hypoxic ischemia in the immature rat. *Pediatr Res* 1997; **42**: 24–9.
19. Van den Berghe G, Wouters P, Weekers F *et al*. Intensive insulin therapy in the critically ill patients. *N Engl J Med* 2001; **345**: 1359–67.
20. Mild therapeutic hypothermia to improve the neurologic outcome after cardiac arrest. *N Engl J Med* 2002; **346**: 549–56.
21. Bratton SL, Jardine DS, Morray JP. Serial neurologic examinations after near drowning and outcome. *Arch Pediatr Adolesc Med* 1994; **148**: 167–70.
22. Allman FD, Nelson WB, Pacentine GA, McComb G. Outcome following cardiopulmonary resuscitation in severe pediatric near drowning. *Am J Dis Child* 1986; **140**: 571–5.
23. Graf WD, Cummings P, Quan L, Brutocao D. Predicting outcome in pediatric submersion victims. *Ann Emerg Med* 1995; **26**: 312–19.
24. Orlowski JP. Prognostic factors in pediatric cases of drowning and near drowning. *JACEP* 1979; **8**: 176–9.

Child with dengue hemorrhagic fever

Adrian Y. Goh

Introduction

Dengue is the most common and important mosquito-borne viral infection[1] and can manifest as Dengue Fever (DF), which is often a self-limiting febrile illness or less commonly dengue hemorrhagic fever (DHF). The major pathophysiologic hallmarks that distinguish DHF from DF and other diseases are increased vascular permeability leading to plasma leakage and circulatory collapse (Dengue Shock Syndrome/DSS). Management involves close monitoring and early detection of shock, with prompt and judicious use of appropriate fluids to correct hypovolemia, yet prevent fluid overload. Blood transfusions may be indicated in patients with refractory shock or shock in the presence of falling hematocrit.

Case history

An 8-year-old girl presented to her local district hospital with 5-day history of continuous fever. She became more unwell on the day of admission with recurrent bouts of vomiting, abdominal pain, and reduced urine output. Further discussion showed that her neighbor had a similar illness requiring admission to the hospital a week ago. Her history, physical examination and initial investigations are as summarized in Table 17.1.

Examination

On examination she was noted to be conscious but slightly confused and was mildly tachypneic. Her non-invasive blood pressure reading was normal at 100/80 mmHg but her pulse was rapid (148 beats min^{-1}) and felt thready with a sluggish capillary refill time of 4–5 seconds. She had a mild petechial rash over her antecubital fossa. Her Glasgow Coma Score (GCS) was assessed as 14/15 (E4, M6, V4) as she was somewhat agitated and confused as to her whereabouts. Oxygen was administered via a face mask at 15 l min^{-1} and a large bore 18G cannula was inserted. Blood was sent for full blood count (including hematocrit), electrolytes, glucose, and a blood culture. A 300 ml bolus of 0.9% saline was administered rapidly with some improvement in the capillary refill to 3–4 seconds, but the HR remained elevated at 135 b min^{-1}. A repeat bolus of 300 ml 0.9% saline was given; her heart rate dropped to 120 b min^{-1}, with normal capillary refill time, and she became less agitated.

She was admitted to the ward where her fluid requirements for the next 24 hours were calculated. Her maintenance fluid (ongoing requirements 1800 ml over 24 hours, i.e. 70 ml/h) was commenced using 4.5% dextrose 0.9% saline with 40 mmol l^{-1} of potassium chloride added once she passed urine. As it was thought that her clinical picture was consistent with dengue infection, no antibiotics were administered. After arriving in the ward, repeat blood investigations were sent consisting of FBC and hematocrit.

Case Studies in Pediatric Critical Care, ed. Peter. J. Murphy, Stephen C. Marriage, and Peter J. Davis.
Published by Cambridge University Press. © Cambridge University Press 2009.

Table 17.1. *Clinical and investigative findings on admission*

Past medical history	Healthy and well	
Regular medications	None	
Allergies	None known	
Examination	Awake but slightly confused and agitated	
	Airway clear, face mask oxygen	
	Tachypneic respiratory rate 40/min	
	Chest clear, bilateral air entry, Sats 98% in air	
	Normal heart sounds, pulse 140/min, BP 100/80	
	Capillary refill time = 4 seconds	
	Petechial rash, Temperature 37 °C	
Investigations	Weight	30 kg
	FBC	Hb 16.8 g dl^{-1}, PCV 0.62
		Plat 80 × 109 l^{-1},
		WBC 3.8 × 109 l^{-1}
	U+Es	Na$^+$ 134 mmol l^{-1}, K$^+$ 4.1 mmol l^{-1},
		Urea 13.2 mmol l^{-1}, Creatinine 117 μmol l^{-1}
	Glucose	5.8 mmol l^{-1}
	Venous blood gas	pH 7.18, pCO_2 23 mmHg, HCO_3^- 16.5 mmol l^{-1}, BE −8

Her repeat blood investigations showed: full blood count: Hb 15.4 g dl^{-1}, PCV 0.55, platelet 76 × 109 l^{-1}, TWC 5.7 × 109 l^{-1}, blood glucose 7 mmol l^{-1}, Na 135 mmol l^{-1}, K 4.3 mmol l^{-1}. As her clinical status was thought to be stable with normal blood pressure of 100/90 mmHg, a pulse rate of 108 b min^{-1} and a capillary refill of 2–3 seconds, she was maintained on her current rate of infusion. Hourly pulse and blood pressure monitoring was done. It was planned to repeat her blood investigations at 06 00 h in the morning. Her non-invasive blood pressure remained stable, between 110/90 mmHg to 100/80 mmHg. However, there was an unnoticed gradual rise in her HR from 95 b min^{-1} to 138 b min^{-1} over the next 4–6 hours.

At 06 00 h when the registrar came to take her blood she was becoming drowsier and less responsive. Her PR was 155 b min^{-1} with a sluggish capillary refill time of 4–5 seconds. Pulses were thready with only a systolic blood pressure recorded at 80 mmHg. There was no conjunctival pallor. A repeat 600 ml bolus of normal saline was administered fast and the regional pediatric intensive care unit was contacted for possibility of transfer. Blood was taken for venous blood gas and cross match for fresh whole blood, plasma, cryoprecipitate, and platelets and plans were made for immediate transfer. An attempt to site a radial arterial line failed, resulting in a large hematoma on her left wrist requiring continuous pressure to stop the bleeding. The repeat blood tests showed a HB of 17.0 g dl^{-1}, PCV 0.68, platelet 12 × 109 l^{-1}, TWC 4.2 × 109 l^{-1}, Na 131 mmol l^{-1}, K 5.6 mmol l^{-1}, pH 7.1 pCO_2 35 mmHg, HCO$_3$ 8.3, BE −20, lactate 2.8 mmol l^{-1}. The district hospital registrar wanted to prophylactically transfuse platelets to improve the platelet count but was advised against it by the regional PICU consultant. On advice from the regional PICU a further 600 ml of normal saline was administered. She was transferred by the district hospital registrar via road

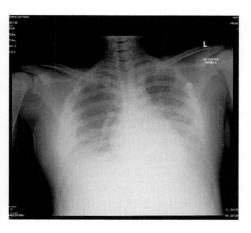

Fig. 17.1. Chest radiograph on admission to pediatric intensive care.

ambulance as there was no retrieval system in place in Malaysia. The PR remained between 140 to 145 b min^{-1} and blood pressure was barely recordable. Her saturation was 98% on high flow face mask of 10 l min^{-1}. A 600 ml bolus of Gelafundin (a synthetic colloid) was administered during the journey. The 60-minute journey was otherwise uneventful.

Progress in the pediatric intensive care unit

In the PICU she remained encephalopathic with a GCS of 9/12 (E 2, M 4, V 3) and a PR of 160 b min^{-1}, capillary refill of 4 seconds, BP of 90/43 mmHg. She was now increasingly tachypnic with a respiratory rate of 50 min^{-1}. Examination revealed decreased breath sounds in the whole right lung with stony dull percussion note. A radiograph was obtained (Fig. 17.1), which confirmed a large right sided effusion. Her repeat blood investigations on arrival showed a HB of 12.8 g dl^{-1}, PCV 0.47, Platelet 13 × 109 l^{-1}, pH 7.12, HCO$_3$ 10.2 mmol l^{-1}, BE −16, lactate 3.9 mmol l^{-1}. As she remained in a state of refractory shock and there was a significant fall in the hematocrit (although the hematocrit remained within the normal range for age), it was suspected that she has bled significantly and 600 ml of fresh whole blood (recently donated 3 days ago) was transfused rapidly which raised her BP to 100/80 mmHg.

A decision to intubate was made, because she remained in a state of refractory shock with encephalopathy. Furthermore, this would facilitate insertion of central venous access and monitoring. She was intubated orally with a size 6.0 cuffed endotracheal tube, using ketamine 2 mg kg^{-1}, atropine 0.02 mg kg^{-1}, midazolam 0.1 mg kg^{-1} and atracurium 1 mg kg^{-1}. There was a fall in the blood pressure to 88/55 mm Hg, which improved with further transfusion of 500 ml of fresh whole blood. A 7.0 French gauge triple lumen central venous catheter was inserted in the right femoral vein and an arterial line was inserted, with some difficulty, in the left femoral artery. An orogastric tube was inserted, which showed fresh bleeding. Ventilation was not problematic initially using pressure controlled ventilation with a ΔPIP of 14 cmH$_2$O and PEEP of 6 cmH$_2$O, rate of 30 min^{-1}, Ti 0.8 seconds, FiO$_2$ of 0.35. Although her arterial pressure improved to 100/45 mm Hg, her peripheries remained ice cold and there was hardly any urine produced. Her repeat set of bloods showed a Hb of 9.8 g dl^{-1}, PCV 0.30, platelets 22 × 109 l^{-1}, pH 7.28 HCO$_3$ 17 mmol l^{-1}, BE −3, lactate 2.8 mmol l^{-1},

Prothrombin ratio (PTr) 2.6, partial thromboplastin time (pTT) 135 s, control 36 s, D-dimer positive, urea 19.6 mmol l^{-1}, creatinine 183 μmol l^{-1}. Over the next 4 hours 400 ml of fresh frozen plasma and 4 units of cryoprecipitate was transfused.

Twelve hours following admission to PICU her arterial pressure remained borderline low at 90/45 mm Hg with continuing tachycardia, despite massive transfusions of crystalloids and blood products. It was difficult to differentiate whether the ongoing shock was attributable to blood loss or plasma leakage. A 3-D echocardiogram showed good cardiac function (ejection fraction 77%, fraction shortening 45%, LVIDd 3.5 cm, LVPWs 1.9 cm). Low-dose dopamine infusion was started at 5 mcg kg^{-1} per min. It was decided to keep her hematocrit between 0.38 and 0.40. In the presence of shock higher values of HCT was attributed to hemoconcentration and the patient received transfusion of Gelafundin/crystalloid. Conversely, low values of hematocrit were attributed to blood loss and she would receive a blood transfusion. She also received several units of fresh frozen plasma, cryoprecipitate and platelets in an attempt to correct the coagulopathy. After 24 hours of admission she had received a total of 5500 ml of crystalloid, colloid, and blood products. Her abdomen became increasingly distended and her lung compliance worsened requiring increasing ventilation with ΔPIP of 20 cmH_2O and PEEP of 14 cmH_2O and FiO_2 0.55. She also appeared noticeably edematous. Her gas exchange remained acceptable with PaO_2 in the range of 60 to 65 mm Hg (PaO_2/FiO_2 150). Her blood pressure stabilized with warmer peripheries and her HR was less tachycardic (110–120 b min^{-1}). By 36 hours after admission she no longer required large boluses of fluids/blood to maintain her hemodynamic status. Her hematocrit stabilized at 0.36, and platelet between 20 to 30 × 109 l^{-1}. Melenic stools became evident now once she opened her bowels. Her dengue serology (dengue IgM) was positive.

Her urine output remained poor throughout admission (<0.5 ml kg^{-1} per h), with a rising trend of blood urea and creatinine from 17.4 to 26.4 mmol l^{-1} and 194 to 467 μmol l^{-1}, respectively, by 36 hours of admission. Other organ dysfunction included liver dysfunction with a rise of AST/ALT from 111/828 IU l^{-1} to a maximum of 895/5348 IU l^{-1} by 48 hours of admission, and a serum ammonia of 179 mmol l^{-1}. Her conscious level remained depressed even after cessation of sedative drugs, but a cerebral CT scan did not show any evidence of hemorrhage or cerebral edema. In view of her gross fluid overload, oligo-anuric acute renal failure, generalized edema, CNS obtundation (probable renal, hepatic, and possible post-ischemic), she was started on continuous renal replacement therapy (CRRT) at 36 hours after admission using continuous veno-venous hemodiafiltration (CVVHDF). A bicarbonate buffered solution (hemosol) was used because of her significant liver dysfunction. No anti-coagulation was used because of her coagulopathy, with filter life being increased with hourly 100 ml flushes of 0.9% saline. Fluid extraction was gradually increased from 200 ml h^{-1} to 700 ml h^{-1} aiming for a cumulative negative balance between 1000 and 1500 ml 24 h^{-1}. It was carefully titrated to her hemodynamic status and was gradually increased as stability was achieved. Mechanical ventilation became easier at this point, ΔP was reduced gradually to 12 cmH_2O and PEEP to 8 cmH_2O with an accompanying improvement in oxygenation (PaO_2/FiO_2 >250). The use of CRRT also allowed the use of parenteral nutrition by 72 hours of admission. Enteral feeding was commenced the following day. Her urea and creatinine gradually normalized and dialysis was stopped after 7 days. Her urine output improved but had to be maintained with a frusemide infusion of 1 mg kg^{-1} per h for the following 48 hours before spontaneous diuresis occurred. She was extubated after 6 days of ventilation. She was now more conscious and opening her eyes, but made incomprehensible sounds and was occasionally restless. There were concerns about hypoxic–ischemic encephalopathy, but magnetic resonance imaging with diffusion-weighted imaging (MRI-DWI) revealed no abnormality after 10 days of admission. She was transferred to the general ward for continued care, where she was discharged after a total hospital stay of 17 days. On follow-up after 2 months she had returned to her normal pre-illness functional level.

Discussion

Dengue is the most common and widespread arthropod-borne arboviral infection in the world today.[1] The geographical spread, incidence and severity of dengue fever (DF) and dengue haemorrhagic fever (DHF) are increasing in the Americas, South-East Asia, the Eastern Mediterranean and the Western Pacific. Some 2500 million to 3000 million people live in areas where dengue viruses can be transmitted. It is estimated that each year 50 million infections occur, with 500 000 cases of DHF and at least 12 000 deaths.[2] There are four serotypes of dengue virus (DEN 1, DEN 2, DEN 3, DEN 4), which are antigenically similar but different enough to elicit only transient cross protection after infection by one of them. All four serotypes may circulate concurrently, but one may predominate depending on the susceptibility or immunity of the population. There are two distinct host serological responses, namely primary and secondary. Primary response occurs in non-immune individuals undergoing their first dengue infection, whilst a secondary (anamnestic) response occurs in individuals having memory cells from previous dengue infection. Secondary infection is a risk factor for DHF, including passively acquired antibodies in infants.[3] Other risk factors include virus strain and age of the patients.[4] Although DHF/DSS can occur in adults, most cases are in children <15 years, with circumstantial evidence suggesting that certain population groups are more susceptible to vascular leak syndrome.

Initial assessment and management

Dengue virus infection may be asymptomatic, cause undifferentiated febrile illness, dengue fever (DF) or dengue hemorrhagic fever (DHF).[5] DF is often an acute biphasic fever, with headaches, myalgia, arthralgia, rash, and leukopenia. It is commonly benign but may occasionally present with atypical hemorrhage (Fig. 17.2). The clinical features of DHF/DSS are rather stereotyped, with acute onset of high (continuous) fever, haemorrhagic diathesis (most frequently on the skin), hepatomegaly, and in some cases circulatory disturbance (in the most severe form as shock) and should be suspected in any child from an endemic area

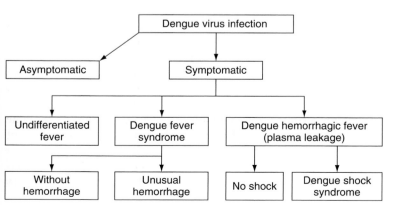

Fig. 17.2.
Manifestations of the
Dengue syndrome.

Table 17.2. *WHO classification of dengue hemorrhagic fever (DHF) and dengue shock syndrome (DSS)*

DHF grade	Hemorrhage	Thrombocytopenia: Platelets × 10^9 l^{-1}	Increased vascular permeability
I	Positive tourniquet test only	≤100	Plasma leakage[a]
II	Spontaneous bleeding[b]	≤100	Plasma leakage[a]
III (DSS)	Positive tourniquet test and /or Spontaneous bleeding[b]	≤100	Plasma leakage[a] and circulatory failure with pulse pressure ≤ mmHg or hypotension for age
IV (DSS)	Positive tourniquet test and /or Spontaneous bleeding[b]	≤100	Plasma leakage[a] and profound shock with undetectable pulse and blood pressure

[a] As evidenced by any of the following: elevation of the admission hematocrit to ≥20% above the expected mean for age, sex and population, reduction of the hematocrit to ≥20% of the baseline value after resuscitation, and clinical signs of plasma leakage such as pleural effusion or ascites.
[b] Example skin petechiae, bruising or mucosal/gastrointestinal bleeding.

Table 17.3. *Ranges of hematocrit for age*

Age	Range (%)	Mean (%)
2 weeks	42–66	50
3 months	31–41	36
6 months – 6 years	33–42	37
7 years – 12 years	34–40	38
Adult		
Male	42–52	47
Female	37–47	42

From *Nelson Textbook of Pediatrics*, 15th edn, p. 1379.

with prolonged fever of >3 days. It is thus possible to make an early and yet accurate clinical diagnosis of DHF before the critical stage or before shock occurs, by using the pattern of clinical presentation together with thrombocytopenia and *concurrent hemoconcentration*, which represent abnormal hemostasis and plasma leakage, respectively.[6]

It would be prudent to admit all suspected cases of childhood dengue, as there are no definitive risk factors that predict the development of shock or bleeding. Using degree of thrombocytopenia as admission criteria is flawed as it is poorly predictive for the development of DSS/bleeding.[7,8] The severity of DHF can be divided into four grades (Table 17.2). Thrombocytopenia with concurrent hemoconcentration (defined as an increase in >20% from baseline or evidence of increased capillary permeability) differentiates Grade I and II DHF from DF. However, this differentiation can be difficult because of variations in normal baseline hematocrit in the pediatric population (Table 17.3).

Management of grade I and II dengue hemorrhagic fever

All cases should be admitted for monitoring. Oral intake should be encouraged and in those who are drinking poorly intravenous fluids at maintenance rates of 4–5 ml kg^{-1} per h using D5% 0.45% saline or D5% 0.9% saline (in older children) should be administered. Vital signs, urine output, and conscious level should be closely monitored. Hematocrit should be monitored at least once a day or more often if required. Non-steroidal drugs or aspirin should be avoided as it has been shown to aggravate platelet dysfunction and predispose to severe and refractory bleeding.[9] It is important to recognize that, in the majority, deterioration occurs at the time of fever defervescence. In mild cases this might be accompanied by mild changes in pulse rate and blood pressure, together with peripheral coolness and congestion, suggesting a degree of hypovolemia secondary to plasma leakage (often with mild elevations of hematocrit). This might recover spontaneously or after fluid therapy. Hematocrit levels should return to normal accompanied by improvement in circulation once appropriate fluids are given. There is no role for the prophylactic transfusion of blood products such as platelets to correct thrombocytopenia. Preventive transfusions with plasma and platelets in an attempt to correct coagulopathy and thrombocytopenia does not produce sustained improvements in coagulation and platelet levels during the plasma leakage phase of DHF/DSS. Adequate management of shock prevented development of bleeding, even in those who were not transfused.[10] Reduce or discontinue intravenous fluids after 24–48 hours after fever defervescence, due to the relatively short period of increased capillary permeability. Continuing intravenous fluids at such rates is likely to lead to pulmonary edema or gross edema. Convalescence is usually uncomplicated with gradual recovery of the platelet counts.

Management of dengue shock syndrome

In severe cases the patient's condition suddenly deteriorates a few days after onset of fever, with signs of circulatory collapse similar to our patient. Although this often happens between day 3 and day 7 after onset of fever and whilst the fever is settling, 44% of children with DSS have been found to be febrile (temperature 38–39 °C) at the time of shock.[11] One of the earliest sign is narrowing of the pulse pressure to ≤20 mmHg. Patients whose pulse pressure is ≤10 mmHg are those who are more likely to have prolonged shock and experience subsequent episodes of shock after initial resuscitation. DSS is a medical emergency: prompt and adequate fluid replacement is necessary to expand plasma volume. Rapid infusions of 20 ml kg^{-1} of crystalloids are given until circulation is restored. Positive pressure may be required for rapid push of fluids. The infusion rate should be returned to normal once hemodynamics are normalized and continuously adjusted based on frequent micro-hematocrit assessments. The example in our patient would be as follows:

Following initial bolus of 600 ml 0.9% saline (20 ml kg^{-1}), calculate intravenous fluids for mild to moderate isotonic dehydration (usually between 5 and 10%) based on 30 kg body weight.

Maintenance fluid $= (10 \times 100) + (10 \times 50) + (10 \times 20) = 1700$ ml
5% deficit $= (5 \times 30\,\text{kg} \times 1000)/100 = 1500$ ml
Total fluids over 24 hours $= 1700 + 1500 = 3200$
$= 130\,\text{ml h}^{-1} - 1$ of D5% 0.45% saline

Although the patient was deemed to be "stable" worrying signs remained, including a narrow pulse pressure, tachycardia and an elevated hematocrit. Frequent assessment of hematocrit would have detected a rise, which would have preceded the shock. In the event of a rise in hematocrit with stable hemodynamics 300 ml of colloids could have been administered over 2–3 hours. It could have been possible that earlier administration of appropriate fluids would have reversed or avoided development of irreversible shock with resulting bleeding and end-organ failure.

From a state of compensated shock patients may pass rapidly into a profound state of shock with imperceptible pulse and blood pressure, which may lead to a more complicated course of tissue acidosis, gastrointestinal bleeding and end-organ failure. In these cases larger volumes are required rapidly. An average of 134 ml kg^{-1} over 36–48 hours was required in 222 patients during a randomized trial of fluid resuscitation in DSS.[12] This is in contrast to the American College of Critical Care Medicine guidelines for resuscitation in pediatric and neonatal septic shock which recommended the use of inotropes or pressors once >60 ml kg^{-1} of fluids is required.[13] Inotropes are rarely required in DSS as the main pathophysiology of shock is hypovolemia from massive capillary leak. The choice of fluids, however, remains unclear. It would be reasonable to use 0.9% saline as initial resuscitation fluid and consider colloids if volumes >40 ml kg^{-1} are required to correct shock. Ringer's lactate, which was the World Health Organization recommended fluid for resuscitation in DHF, performed the least well in the aforementioned trial with the longest recovery time. A comparison of colloid and crystalloid suggested benefits in children presenting with lower pulse pressures (i.e. those in more severe states of shock) who received colloids.[12]

Management of intractable shock and transfusion of blood

In cases of persistent shock after adequate initial resuscitation with crystalloids and colloids, despite a decline in the hematocrit level, significant concealed internal bleeding (most often gastrointestinal) should be suspected and fresh whole blood transfused. The amount transfused should just be sufficient to raise the red blood cell concentration to normal. Hemoconcentration often masks the degree of internal hemorrhage. The hematocrit (and hemoglobin) would appear normal despite large GI bleeding. Vice versa, ongoing blood loss and subsequent transfusion of whole blood would make assessment of plasma loss using hematocrit difficult. In a patient with refractory shock/bleeding who has been transfused we often choose a cut-off hematocrit (usually in the range of 0.4 to 0.45 depending on age), above which we would transfuse colloids/crystalloids, below which we would transfuse red cells. Transfusion of other blood products like cryoprecipitate, plasma, and platelets might be needed at this time to correct the disseminated intravascular coagulopathy (DIC). Promising treatment modalities in this subgroup include the use of recombinant activated factor VII.[14] Factors that would make one suspect internal bleeding would be prolonged duration of shock and low-normal hematocrit at diagnosis of shock. Additional factors would be the presence of significant organ dysfunction at time of shock (suggesting prolonged shock) such as elevated creatinine, hyperlactatemia, and DIC. Mechanical ventilation may be required due to increasing respiratory distress from pleural effusion/ascites. Once the hematocrit has stabilized in the region of 0.4, we would continue intravenous fluids, which should be reduced within 24 to 48 hours after onset of shock. Reabsorption of extravasated plasma occurs 2 to 3 days after, and may cause hypervolemia, hypertension, and pulmonary edema in those still receiving fluids, or in those who are in an oliguric phase of acute renal failure like our patient. This may require diuretics or renal replacement, respectively.

Additional points

1. Insertion of nasogastric tube and endotracheal tube carries the risk of trauma and hemorrhage to nasal passages and stomach. If it is necessary, the oral route is preferable.

2. Insertion of intercostal drains carries the risk of trauma and hemorrhage to the lung. Careful titration of intravenous fluids to achieve stable vital signs, with reduction of intravenous fluid intake once stable vital signs are achieved, will limit the accumulation of large pleural effusions, ascites, and positive fluid balance in children. Large pleural effusions during the recovery phase after 48 hours may need small doses of frusemide.

3. Insertion of central venous line carries the risk of hemorrhage and should not be routinely inserted.

4. The use of corticosteroids in the treatment of shock has failed to show any benefits.[15]

5. Echocardiogram assessment is recommended in cases of profound shock as a small percentage have decreased function requiring inotropes and may also be useful to assess volume status.[16,17]

Learning points

1. A child from an endemic area with high fever, flushing without coryza and petechiae should be suspected to have dengue infection.

2. Presence of thrombocytopenia and concurrent hemoconcentration is essential to the clinical diagnosis of DHF/DSS.

3. The critical period is during fever defervescence, with a rising hematocrit (by ≥20 %) indicating significant plasma loss and need for IV fluid therapy. Be wary that a percentage might still be febrile during the critical period. Early and appropriate IV replacement can prevent shock and modify severity.

4. Assessment of patient's clinical state, together with micro-hematocrit assessment, can guide treatment before the critical stage of shock occurs.

5. DSS is a state of hypovolemic shock secondary to large plasma losses. Replacement with isotonic fluids like 0.9% saline and/or colloids is life-saving. Colloids may have advantages over crystalloids.

6. Volume replacement should be guided by the rate of plasma leakage (clinical state, hematocrit, urine output). There is no role of prophylactic transfusion of blood products.

7. Significant bleeding is often the result of prolonged shock, leading to tissue acidosis, disseminated intravascular coagulopathy, and end-organ failure. Bleeding can be suspected in patients with refractory shock and those with relatively low hematocrit at diagnosis of shock.

8. The duration of plasma leakage is for a period of 24–48 hours and over-replacement with more volume and/or longer periods may lead to generalized edema and pulmonary congestion, especially when reabsorption of extravasated plasma occurs.

References

1. Rigau-Perez J G, Clark G C, Gubler D J *et al.* Dengue and dengue hemorrhagic fever. *Lancet* 1998; **91**: 2395–400.

2. World Health Organization. *Key issues in dengue vector control towards the operationalization of a global strategy: Report*

of consultation. Geneva WHO 1995. (CID/FIL (Den)/IC.96.1).

3. Kliks S C, Nimmannitya S, Nisalak A *et al*. Evidence that maternal dengue antibodies are important in the development of dengue hemorrhagic fever in infants. *Am J Trop Med Hyg* 1988; **38**: 411–19.

4. Vaughn D W, Green S, Kalayanarooj S *et al*. Dengue viremia titer, antibody response pattern, and virus serotype correlate with disease severity. *J Infect Dis* 2000; **181**: 2–9.

5. World Health Organization. *Dengue Hemorrhagic Fever: Diagnosis, Treatment, Prevention and Control*. 2nd edn, Geneva, WHO, 1997.

6. Bhamarapravati N. Pathology of Dengue infections. In: Gubler DJ, Kuno Q, eds. *Dengue and Dengue Hemorrhagic Fever*. Wallingford, UK, CAB International, 1997; 115–32.

7. Lum L C, Goh A Y, Chan P W *et al*. Risk factors for hemorrhage in severe dengue infections. *J Pediatr* 2002; **140**: 629–31.

8. Chuansumrit A, Philmothares V, Tardtong P *et al*. Transfusion requirements in patients with dengue hemorrhagic fever. *Southeast Asian J Trop Med Public Health* 2000; **3**: 10–14.

9. Mitrakul C, Poshyachinda M, Futrakul P *et al*. Hemostatic and platelet kinetic studies in dengue hemorrhagic fever. *Am J Trop Med Hyg* 1977; **26**: 975–84.

10. Lum L C, Abdel-Latif M E, Goh A Y *et al*. Preventive transfusion in dengue shock syndrome-is it necessary? *J Pediatr* 2003; **143**: 682–4.

11. Kalyanarooj S, Chansiriwongs V, Nimmanitiya S. Dengue patients at the Children's Hospital, Bangkok, 1995–1999 Review. *Dengue Bull* 2002, **26**: 33–43.

12. Nhan N T, Phuong C X, Kneen R *et al*. Acute management of Dengue Shock Syndrome: a randomized double-blind comparison of 4 intravenous fluid regimens in the first hour. *Clin Infect Dis* 2001; **32**: 204–13.

13. Carcillo J A, Fields A I, American College of Critical Care Medicine Committee Task Force Members. Clinical practice parameters for hemodynamic support of pediatric and neonatal patients in septic shock. *Crit Care Med.* 2002;**30**(6): 1365–78.

14. Chuansumrit A, Tangnararatchakit K, Lektakul Y *et al*. The use of recombinant activated factor VII for controlling life-threatening bleeding in Dengue Shock Syndrome. *Blood Coagul Fibrinolysis*. 2004 Jun;**15**(4): 335–42.

15. Tassaniyom S, Vasanawathana S, Chirawatkul A, Rojanasuphot S. Failure of high dose methylprednisolone in established dengue shock syndrome: a placebo controlled double blind study. *Paediatrics* 1993; **92**: 111–15.

16. Kabra S K, Juneja R, Madhulika *et al*. Myocardial dysfunction in children with dengue haemorrhagic fever. *Natl Med J India* 1998; **11**: 59–61.

17. Khongphatthanayothin A, Suesaowalak M, Muangmingsook S *et al*. Hemodynamic profiles of patients with dengue hemorrhagic fever during toxic stage: an echocardiographic study. *Intens Care Med* 2003; **29**: 570–4.

The child with HIV infection

Mark Hatherill

Introduction

The introduction of effective antiretroviral therapy in the last decade has changed the face of the HIV epidemic in high-income countries.[1] In "developed" regions, children with HIV infection form an enlarging cohort of clinically stable children on long-term Antiretroviral Therapy (ART), with low HIV viral loads and normal CD4 T lymphocyte counts. Although some children may develop opportunistic infections due to failure of therapy, or present with complications of antiretroviral drugs, their medium-term prognosis is good.

However, even in "developed" high-income countries, many HIV-infected children presenting for the first time to critical care services are previously undiagnosed, and have never received antiretroviral therapy.[2,3] These children commonly present in infancy with severe respiratory infections such as *Cytomegalovirus* (CMV) or *Pneumocystis jiroveci* pneumonia (PJP), which have traditionally carried a high mortality.

By contrast, the natural history of childhood HIV infection in "developing" low-income countries has changed little.[4] In these regions, with limited access to antiretroviral therapy, there is a high mortality rate in the first year of life and few children survive beyond 3 years of age. In addition, the burden of disease due to viral, bacterial, and opportunistic respiratory infections is appreciably greater in HIV-infected than HIV-uninfected children.[5]

Case history

A 6-month-old male infant was brought to casualty by his grandmother with a 5-day history of rapid breathing, dry cough, and difficulty in feeding. He had been seen 3 days previously by a primary care physician and was treated with a nasal decongestant and an antipyretic, but his symptoms had worsened. His mother had been unwell and unable to bring him to hospital.

He had been born at term weighing 2.6 kg. Mother had been counseled and offered antenatal HIV testing but had declined. There had been no immediate postnatal problems. He was exclusively breastfed until starting solids, and he now weighed 6.5 kg, having grown along the 25th centile for weight. His immunizations were up to date and he had no known tuberculosis contacts.

Initial course in hospital

In casualty he was noted to look well nourished. There was no oral or perineal candidiasis. There were a few small (<1 cm) firm inguinal and axillary lymph nodes. His temperature was 38 °C, with a tachycardia of 165 beats per minute, but he was peripherally warm, well

Case Studies in Pediatric Critical Care, ed. Peter. J. Murphy, Stephen C. Marriage, and Peter J. Davis.
Published by Cambridge University Press. © Cambridge University Press 2009.

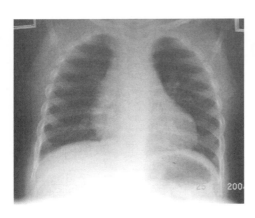

Fig. 18.1. Admission chest radiograph shows air bronchograms in both lower lobes, but no hyperinflation, atelectasis, or lobar consolidation.

perfused, with a capillary refill time of 2 seconds. He did not appear cyanosed, but his oxygen saturation (SaO$_2$) was 84% in room air, 87% in nasal cannula oxygen, and 98% in face mask oxygen. His respiratory rate was 60 per minute with nasal flaring. He had mild costal recession but no audible wheeze. Bronchial breathing was heard at both lung bases. A 1–2 cm soft liver was palpable but there was no splenomegaly. Chest radiograph showed air bronchograms in both lower lobes, but no hyperinflation, or lobar consolidation (see Fig. 18.1). He was initially assessed as a well-nourished infant with a viral or bacterial bronchopneumonia.

He was admitted to the high-dependency area of the general pediatric ward for pulse oximetry and ECG monitoring. A peripheral venous cannula was inserted and intravenous maintenance fluids were commenced. Blood was sampled for a full blood count, electrolytes, and a blood culture, and intravenous ampicillin 50 mg kg^{-1} 6-hourly and gentamicin 7.5 mg kg^{-1} daily were commenced. His serum sodium was 145 mmol l^{-1} and chloride 109 mmol l^{-1}. His total leukocyte count was 29×10^9 l^{-1}, hemoglobin 11 g dl^{-1}, and platelets 486×10^9l^{-1}. The differential blood count showed 41% neutrophils, 44% lymphocytes, and 6% immature neutrophils. The C-reactive protein was <1 mg l^{-1}. Arterial blood gas (ABG) analysis showed pH 7.34, pCO$_2$ 5.8 kPa, and pO$_2$ 12.6 kPa.

He was reviewed the following morning and noted to be "quiet," lying in a frog-like position. His SaO$_2$ was 84%, now in 80% head box oxygen, with a respiratory rate of 80 breaths per minute, grunting, and with a tachycardia of 180 b min^{-1}. Repeat chest radiograph now showed consolidation in all four quadrants, with a milky appearance suggestive of interstitial disease (see Fig. 18.2). He was assessed as being in hypoxic respiratory failure and a decision was made to intubate and ventilate prior to transfer to the PICU.

High-flow oxygen was administered via an anesthetic "T-piece" bag and mask system to provide positive end-expiratory pressure (PEEP). A nasogastric tube was placed to decompress the stomach. He was anesthetized with intravenous etomidate 0.3 mg kg^{-1} and atracurium 0.5 mg kg^{-1}, and intubated with a 3.5 mm nasal endotracheal tube secured at 12 cm at the nostril. His chest was "stiff" to hand-ventilate and SaO$_2$ remained <90%, although there was no hyper-resonance to suggest a pneumothorax, and breath sounds were equal bilaterally. Endotracheal tube position was confirmed to be 3–4 cm at the vocal cords by direct laryngoscopy. SaO$_2$ rose gradually with hand ventilation, using a manual high-PEEP recruitment maneuver.

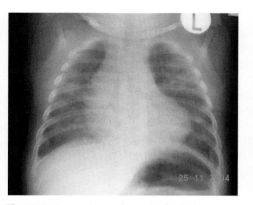

Fig. 18.2. Repeat chest radiograph after 24 hours shows consolidation in all 4 quadrants, with a milky appearance suggestive of interstitial disease.

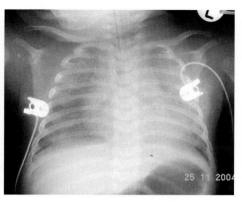

Fig. 18.3. The post-intubation chest radiograph shows a diffuse bilateral infiltrate with a ground glass appearance. The endotracheal tube is in an acceptable position, but the nasogastric tube lies in the esophagus.

Course in PICU

He was nursed prone, sedated with intravenous morphine by infusion at 20 mcg kg^{-1} per h and oral clonidine 5 mcg kg^{-1} 8-hourly. He was initially ventilated using an SIMV rate of 25 per minute, pressures of 24/8, and FiO$_2$ 0.6. Repeat ABG analysis showed pH 7.39, pCO$_2$ 4.9 kPa, pO$_2$ 8.3 kPa, and base deficit −1.6 mmol l^{-1}, with SaO$_2$ 96%. The pO$_2$ (mm Hg)/FiO$_2$ ratio was calculated as 104 and the oxygenation index (OI) was 11.

$$\text{Oxygenation index (OI)} = \text{MAP} \times \text{FiO}_2 \times 100/p\text{O}_2(\text{mm Hg})$$

It was planned to reduce both ventilatory rate and peak pressure, tolerating hypercapnia and SaO$_2$ 88–92%. The post-intubation chest radiograph showed a diffuse bilateral infiltrate with a ground glass appearance (see Fig. 18.3). The endotracheal tube was in an acceptable position, but the nasogastric tube lay in the esophagus and was advanced. The possibility of PJP was raised in view of the worsening hypoxic respiratory failure, and both intravenous co-trimoxazole 7.5 mg kg^{-1} 6-hourly and oral prednisone 2 mg kg^{-1} daily were commenced. An arterial cannula was inserted for continuous arterial blood pressure monitoring and blood sampling. Artificial milk feeds were started and total fluid intake was restricted to 60 ml kg^{-1} per day. Urine output was 1.3 ml kg^{-1} per h.

The family were counselled and consented to testing for HIV. Blood was sampled and an HIV ELISA was requested. Additional investigations included a serum albumin 24 g l^{-1}, total protein 59 g l^{-1}, and LDH 1169 U l^{-1}. The leukocyte count had fallen to 20 × 10^9 l^{-1}, with 31% neutrophils, and 35% immature neutrophils, although the serum procalcitonin level was <0.5 mcg l^{-1}. A non-directed bronchoalveolar lavage (BAL) was performed and lavage fluid sent to microbiology for microscopy, culture, and *Pneumocystis jiroveci* immunofluorescence, and to virology for immunofluorescence and viral culture. An echocardiogram showed a structurally and functionally normal heart.

On day 2, the admission BAL sample was confirmed positive for *Pneumocystis jiroveci* fluorescent antibody. Scanty neutrophils were noted, but no bacteria or acid-fast bacilli.

The HIV ELISA was also reported as positive. The parents were counseled that the ELISA test suggested perinatal exposure to HIV, and although not diagnostic in infants, the presence of an opportunistic infection (PJP) was highly suggestive of HIV infection. A polymerase chain reaction (PCR) test for HIV was sent and both parents were offered testing.

On day 3, SaO_2 fell below 88% in FiO_2 0.75, with ventilatory pressures of 20/8. He was turned prone again and pressures were increased to 24/10, which allowed a gradual reduction of the FiO_2 to 0.5, with SaO_2 92%.

By day 4, attempts to wean ventilation had been unsuccessful. SaO_2 was 88% in FiO_2 0.6, with pressures of 23/10, and an SIMV rate of 25. The pO_2 was 6.5 kPa, and despite pH 7.36 and pCO_2 4.9 kPa, he appeared sweaty and tachypneic, with a spontaneous respiratory rate of 50 per minute. The pO_2/FiO_2 ratio was 82 and OI was 14.

No growth had been reported from the admission blood culture at 72 hours and temperature had remained <38 °C. Total leukocyte count had fallen to 8×10^9 l^{-1}, with 57% neutrophils and 19% immature neutrophils. Hemoglobin was 7.4 g dl^{-1} and a blood transfusion was ordered. The trough gentamicin level was appropriate at 0.6 mg l^{-1}, but the peak was sub-therapeutic at 6.0 mg l^{-1} and the dose was increased. The HIV qualitative PCR was reported to be positive, confirming the diagnosis of HIV infection. The BAL and blood culture were repeated, and blood was sampled for cytomegalovirus pp65 antigen.

On day 6 the blood culture was reported to be growing a methicillin-sensitive *Staphylococcus aureus* at 48 hours. There was discussion as to whether this organism is a contaminant or a pathogen. In view of the lack of improvement and immunodeficiency, antibiotic therapy was changed to piptazobactam and amikacin in order to cover methicillin-sensitive *S. aureus* and provide broader Gram-negative cover.

On day 7 the leukocyte count was 15×10^9 l^{-1}, with 56% neutrophils and 20% immature neutrophils, although he remained apyrexial with a serum procalcitonin level <0.5 mcg l^{-1}. The serum albumin had fallen to 18 g l^{-1}. The cytomegalovirus pp65 antigen was negative. There was no bacterial or fungal growth from the second BAL, and the repeat *Pneumocystis jiroveci* immunofluorescence was negative. Both peak and trough amikacin levels were therapeutic.

Since he was tolerating enteral feeds and had been hemodynamically stable with single organ system (respiratory) failure, the infectious diseases team were consulted about starting antiretroviral therapy. The family were counseled about the risks and benefits of antiretroviral therapy and they agreed to consider starting ART. Blood was sampled for CD4 T lymphocyte count and HIV viral load. Liver enzymes were within the normal range and serum lactate was 0.8 mmol l^{-1}.

On the morning of day 8, FiO_2 had risen to 1.0 in order to maintain SaO_2 >88%. The pH was 7.36 and pCO_2 6.2 kPa, with ventilatory pressures of 24/12 and SIMV rate of 20 per minute. The pO_2/FiO_2 ratio had fallen to 49 and the OI had risen to 28.

High frequency oscillatory ventilation was commenced, with initial settings of mean airway pressure (MAP) 29 cmH$_2$O, amplitude 50 cmH$_2$O, frequency 11 Hz, and FiO_2 0.7. Chest radiograph showed good lung expansion, but with features of early honeycombing, suggestive of lung fibrosis secondary to ventilator-induced volutrauma (see Fig. 18.4). The endotracheal tube appeared too high and was advanced by 1 cm. ABG analysis showed pH 7.33, pCO_2 8.4 kPa, pO_2 7.9 kPa, and base excess 6.8 mmol l^{-1}.

The absolute CD4 T lymphocyte count was reported as 188×10^6 l^{-1} (range 500×10^6 – 2010×10^6 l^{-1}), with a CD4 T lymphocyte percentage of 11.7%. The HIV viral load was

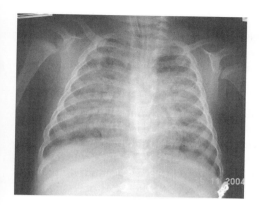

Fig. 18.4. Chest radiograph on HFOV shows good lung expansion. There are features of early honeycombing, suggestive of lung fibrosis secondary to volutrauma. The endotracheal tube appears too high.

1.6×10^6 RNA copies per ml. The family agree to start ART and stavudine $1 \, \mathrm{mg \, kg}^{-1}$ 12-hourly, lamivudine $4 \, \mathrm{mg \, kg}^{-1}$ 12-hourly, and ritonavir $250 \, \mathrm{mg \, m}^2$ 12-hourly were commenced.

That afternoon, the virology laboratory reported that the shell vial culture from the second BAL sample was positive for CMV. There was some discussion about whether the CMV was a pathogen or not, since the pp65 antigen was negative, but the steroid therapy was thought to pose an additional risk factor and intravenous ganciclovir $5 \, \mathrm{mg \, kg}^{-1}$ 12-hourly was commenced.

Over the following 5 days MAP and amplitude were gradually weaned to MAP 14 cm H_2O, amplitude 30 cm H_2O, and FiO_2 0.4. The pO_2/FiO_2 ratio was 190 and OI was 7. He was converted to conventional mechanical ventilation at pressures of 20/8 on day 14. The piptazobactam and amikacin were stopped after 7 days.

Conventional ventilatory pressures were weaned rapidly and he was successfully extubated onto nasal cannula oxygen on day 15. The co-trimoxazole was converted to an oral dose to complete 21 days of treatment, and the prednisone and ganciclovir were continued, as was the ART regimen. He was discharged to the general pediatric ward on day 17 under the care of the infectious diseases team.

Discussion

Pediatric HIV infection is associated with apoptosis of CD4 T lymphocytes, defective IL-2 and interferon-gamma production, defects of B lymphocyte function, natural killer cell activity, neutrophil bactericidal activity, and defective antigen-specific immunoglobulin production.[6] These defects in the host response lead to susceptibility to viral and intracellular organisms, as well as bacterial sepsis, particularly due to encapsulated bacteria such as *Pneumococcus*.

In "developing" countries, particularly in Sub-Saharan Africa where HIV prevalence is high, there is a correspondingly high index of suspicion for opportunistic infections such as PJP. For this reason, infants presenting with pneumonia who have clinical stigmata of HIV infection (oropharyngeal or perineal candidiasis, generalized lymphadenopathy, hepatosplenomegaly, or failure to thrive) are often treated empirically for PJP until a diagnosis can be made. This approach is reasonable, given the probable benefit of early steroid therapy in preventing hypoxic respiratory failure.

In "developed" countries, where antenatal diagnosis of maternal HIV infection is routine, the success of perinatal prophylaxis has dramatically reduced the incidence of vertically transmitted HIV infection.[1,7] The unintended consequence is that an increasing proportion of children newly infected with HIV have not been diagnosed antenatally. These antiretroviral-naïve children are at risk of life-threatening opportunistic infections such as PJP, but live in a healthcare environment where the level of suspicion for such infections is low. This factor underlines the importance of early diagnosis of HIV infection when effective therapy is available.

In this setting, signs and symptoms of maternal illness may alert the clinician to a possible immunodeficiency. The classical clinical stigmata of HIV infection, such as failure to thrive, lymphadenopathy, hepatosplenomegaly, and oropharyngeal candidiasis, may not yet have developed in early infancy. A high serum total protein, due to a disproportionately raised globulin fraction, is often found in HIV infection. Similarly, a markedly raised Lactate Dehydrogenase (LDH) is a non-specific indicator of severe pneumonia such as PJP.

The definitive diagnosis of HIV infection in children older than 18 months of age may be made on the basis of two positive ELISA tests for HIV.[8] If maternal HIV infection is present, maternally transmitted HIV antibody may persist, giving rise to a positive HIV ELISA up to the age of 18 months. Such children may be termed HIV antibody exposed. Therefore, in order to confirm a diagnosis of HIV infection in children under the age of 18 months who have a positive HIV ELISA, or documented maternal infection, an HIV polymerase chain reaction (PCR) test is required. In a non-breastfeeding population, the HIV PCR is positive in more than 90% of HIV infected infants by 2 weeks of age, and in almost 99% of infants by 6 weeks of age.

Other bacterial infections

Respiratory infections, particularly PJP, are the major cause of morbidity and mortality in HIV-infected infants.[9] It is important to note that undiagnosed HIV-infected infants would not have received co-trimoxazole prophylaxis against PJP, which presents commonly between the ages of 2–6 months[2,10]. Although a low CD4 T lymphocyte percentage and high viral load are associated with a greater risk for PJP, a normal CD4 count is not necessarily protective.

The clinical and radiological features of PJP are often non-specific in the early stages and may be complicated by the presence of viral or bacterial co-infection. Classically, infants with PJP present with tachypnea, alar flaring, grunting, and hypoxia. In the absence of significant lower airway obstruction, the lack of marked costal recession may lead the inexperienced clinician to underestimate the severity of the pneumonia. Radiological features may be disarmingly unimpressive in the early stages of disease, but progress rapidly to a bilateral diffuse interstitial pattern with small lung volumes. Histologically, the alveoli are packed with an acellular exudate and microatelectasis leads to reduced lung compliance.[11]

Prompt diagnosis of PJP is vital, since early intervention may prevent the development of hypoxia and avert the need for mechanical ventilation. An induced sputum sample may be useful, but if facilities are available, urgent diagnostic bronchoscopic lavage may be required. Mechanically ventilated children may undergo a non-directed bronchoalveolar lavage (BAL). Fluorescent antibody stains for *Pneumocystis jiroveci* cysts and trophozoites have improved sensitivity compared with silver stains, to the extent that diagnostic lung biopsy, once a gold standard, is now rarely performed. Modern quantitative PCR techniques are even more sensitive and able to detect very low numbers of organisms.

Treatment should not be delayed if early diagnostic BAL is not possible, since rapid progression to hypoxic respiratory failure may be imminent. Intravenous co-trimoxazole should be started with a 10–15 mg kg^{-1} loading dose (trimethoprim component), followed by 5.0–7.5 mg kg^{-1} 6 hourly for 21 days, plus oral prednisone 2 mg kg^{-1}/ dose daily for 10–14 days. Although prospective pediatric randomized controlled trials do not exist, the adult evidence and retrospective pediatric studies suggest that early steroid therapy reduces the risk of progressive hypoxia and the need for mechanical ventilation.[12,13]

Our experience has been that children who require mechanical ventilation for PJP fall into two categories with a bimodal response to therapy. Some children, including those who meet ARDS criteria for severity of lung injury (pO_2/FiO_2 ratio <200) respond rapidly to treatment and are often weaned and extubated after 3–4 days of mechanical ventilation. Other children respond very slowly, or not at all, and remain hypoxic, requiring high PEEP or mean airway pressure into the second and third week of the illness. Many of these children are subsequently diagnosed as having co-infections, such as CMV or adenovirus, nosocomial bacterial sepsis, including Gram-negative organisms, or pulmonary candidiasis.

Antimicrobial therapy for PJP is controversial.[11] Since the trimethoprim component is probably ineffective against *Pneumocystis*, co-trimoxazole may be considered sulphonamide monotherapy. Failure to respond to therapy may be due to sulphonamide resistance, but since it is not possible to culture the organism routinely, true drug resistance is difficult to assess. However, mutations in the gene coding for DHPS, a sulphonamide target enzyme, are common in adults and are associated with prior co-trimoxazole prophylaxis. Whether such mutations are clinically significant is less clear, since many patients carrying this mutation respond appropriately to co-trimoxazole therapy.[11]

A number of alternatives to co-trimoxazole have been used in adult practice, including dapsone, which has a mechanism of action similar to co-trimoxazole, the anti-malarial atovaquone, or a combination of clindamycin and primaquine. Pentamidine is effective against *Pneumocystis*, although it has significant side effects, including neutropenia, thrombocytopenia, and hepatitis. There are no data to suggest that outcome is improved by changing to pentamidine in the face of lack of response to co-trimoxazole. In this situation, the emphasis should be on investigating for viral, bacterial, and fungal co-infections, particularly in the setting of secondary deterioration.

Evidence of cytomegalovirus is found frequently in the presence of PJP.[2,10] It may be difficult to decide whether this organism is causing disease or not. However, it has been suggested that steroid therapy for PJP is a risk factor for the development of CMV pneumonitis.[14] It might be reasonable to treat any evidence of CMV with an agent such as ganciclovir, particularly if there has been poor response to appropriate therapy against *Pneumocystis*.

HIV-infected children have a greater burden of disease due to non-opportunistic bacterial pathogens, such as *Streptococci*, *Staphylococci*, *Haemophilus*, and Gram-negative bacilli, particularly in developing regions.[5] These organisms may be responsible for community-acquired co-infection, or nosocomial super-infection, and lead to delayed or inadequate response to therapy. HIV-infected children are also more likely to carry antimicrobial-resistant strains of these organisms, such as methicillin-resistant *Staphylococcus*. In areas where *Mycobacterium tuberculosis* is endemic, pulmonary tuberculosis should always be considered. Since HIV-infected children may not respond to tuberculin testing, diagnosis may be made by demonstration of acid-fast bacilli in the BAL sample.

HIV-infected children are also at risk for other fungal infections, such as *Candida albicans* and other *Candida* species, which may involve the esophagus, trachea, and lungs. *Candida* may be isolated from the BAL specimen and nosocomial candidemia is associated with central venous cannulae. Note that widespread use of fluconazole prophylaxis has resulted in an increase in fluconazole-resistant non-albicans species, which would require amphotericin as a first-line agent.

ICU Management of PJP infected children

The prognosis of children who develop hypoxic respiratory failure due to PJP has improved considerably since the early days of the HIV epidemic, when >80% of children died.[15] Besides high-dose co-trimoxazole and steroid therapy, general improvements in pediatric intensive care, including meticulous attention to fluid balance, avoidance of pulmonary volutrauma, the use of high PEEP/low tidal volume ventilatory strategies and high-frequency oscillatory ventilation, may all have contributed to this improvement in outcome.

The fluid and energy needs of these children deserve continuous attention. The true metabolic requirements of sedated, ventilated children may be a fraction of what was commonly supposed. There is rarely an indication to withhold enteral feeds, and even if feed intolerance occurs, jejunal tube feeding is usually successful. The maintenance fluid requirements of an infant with net insensible fluid loss of 35 ml kg^{-1} per day and urine output of 1 ml kg^{-1} per h (approximately 25 ml kg^{-1} per day) should rarely exceed 60 ml kg^{-1} per day. If larger volumes are required for caloric requirements, a diuretic may be added.

Ventilatory strategies are aimed at avoiding pharmacologic paralysis where possible, allowing permissive hypercapnea and permissive hypoxia (SaO$_2$ 85%–92%), and avoiding ventilator-induced lung injury. Conventional tidal volumes should be reduced to 6–7 ml/kg. PEEP of 8–15 cm H$_2$O, or more, is often needed to maintain adequate oxygenation. Although HFOV has not been shown to improve outcome in these children, HFOV may be useful to the intensivist by allowing gradual recruitment of "solid", small volume, poorly compliant lungs.

Organ-specific complications of HIV infection may complicate the clinical course. Anemia, neutropenia, and thrombocytopenia are common. In the setting of acute illness, the cardiovascular complications of HIV infection are relevant.[16] Although HIV cardiomyopathy is common in older children, and often associated with HIV encephalopathy, reduced Left Ventricular (LV) fractional shortening and increased LV mass may be demonstrated in early infancy. If cardiomegaly is detected, it is important to exclude the presence of a pericardial effusion, and early echocardiography is recommended.

ICU survival of infants ventilated for PJP is now greater than 75%, even without early antiretroviral therapy. It is to be expected that availability of ART will improve the hospital survival and medium- to long-term outcome of HIV-infected children who present with PJP or CMV pneumonitis.[1,2,10]

The exact composition of the antiretroviral regimen may vary between centers, and is likely to change rapidly as new drugs become available. At present, several antiretroviral agents are associated with hepatic and mitochondrial dysfunction leading to lactic acidosis.[17] On this basis, ART would rarely be commenced in the setting of multi-organ failure or severe sepsis. However, in the setting of single system respiratory failure in a child tolerating enteral feeds, ART might be started in the PICU. However, it is unclear whether early ART is beneficial during the acute respiratory illness, since both HIV viral load and CD4 % may take several weeks, or even months, to return to normal.

Learning points

- The incidence of vertically acquired HIV infection has declined rapidly in developed countries.
- Undiagnosed HIV infection still presents with life-threatening opportunistic infections during infancy.
- The early clinical and radiological features of PJP may be non-specific.
- The cardinal clinical feature of PJP is hypoxia.
- Early steroid therapy may avert hypoxic respiratory failure in PJP.
- Co-trimoxazole is first-line therapy for PJP.
- Co-infection with viral, bacterial, and fungal organisms is common and may delay response to therapy.
- Severity of lung disease may be assessed by serial calculation of oxygenation index.
- PICU survival of children with PJP who require mechanical ventilation has improved substantially.
- Medium-term outcome of HIV-infected infants who survive PJP to be established on ART is relatively good.

References

1. Sharland M, Gibb DM, Tudor-Williams G. Advances in the prevention and treatment of paediatric HIV infection in the United Kingdom. *Arch Dis Child* 2002; **87**: 178–80.
2. Williams AJ, Duong T, McNally LM *et al.* Pneumocystis carinii pneumonia and cytomegalovirus infection in children with vertically acquired HIV infection. *AIDS* 2001; **15**: 335–9.
3. Gibb DM, Duong T, Tookey PA *et al.* Decline in mortality, AIDS, and hospital admissions in perinatally HIV-1 infected children in the United Kingdom and Ireland. *Br Med J* 2003; **327**: 1019.
4. Taha TE, Graham SM, Kumwenda NI *et al.* Morbidity among HIV-infected and uninfected African children. *Pediatrics* 2000; **106**: E77.
5. Madhi SA, Petersen K, Madhi A, Khoosal M, Klugman KP. Increased disease burden and antibiotic resistance of bacteria causing severe community-acquired lower respiratory tract infections in human immunodeficiency virus type 1-infected children. *Clin Infect Dis* 2000; **31**: 170–6.
6. Tudor-Williams G, Pizzo PA. Pediatric human immunodeficiency virus infection. In Steihm ER ed. *Immunologic Disorders in Infants and Children*, 4th edn. Philadelphia, WB Saunders Company.
7. Thorne C, Newell ML. Prevention of mother-to-child transmission of HIV infection. *Curr Opin Infect Dis* 2004; **17**: 247–52.
8. Lyall EGH. Paediatric HIV in 2002 – a treatable and preventable infection. *J Clin Virol* 2002; **25**: 107–19.
9. Graham SM, Gibb DM. HIV disease and respiratory infection in children. *Br Med Bull* 2002; **61**: 133–50.
10. Cooper S, Lyall H, Walters S *et al.* Children with human immunodeficiency virus admitted to a paediatric intensive care unit in the United Kingdom over a 10-year period. *Intensive Care Med* 2004; **30**: 113–18.
11. Kovacs JA, Gill VJ, Meshnick S, Masur H. New insights into transmission, diagnosis, and drug treatment of Pneumocystis carinii pneumonia. *J Am Med Assoc* 2001; **286**: 2450–60.
12. McLaughlin GE, Virdee SS, Schleien CL, Holzman BH, Scott GB. Effect of corticosteroids on survival of children with acquired immunodeficiency syndrome and Pneumocystis

carinii-related respiratory failure. *J Pediatr* 1995; **126**: 821–4.

13. Montaner JS, Lawson LM, Levitt N, Belzberg A, Schechter MT, Ruedy J. Corticosteroids prevent early deterioration in patients with moderately severe *Pneumocystis carinii* pneumonia and the acquired immunodeficiency syndrome (AIDS). *Ann Intern Med* 1990; **113**: 14–20.

14. Nelson MR, Erskine D, Hawkins DA, Gazzard BG. Treatment with corticosteroids: a risk factor for the development of clinical cytomegalovirus disease in AIDS. *AIDS* 1993; **7**: 375–8.

15. Notterman DA, Greenwald BM, Di Maio-Hunter A, Wilkinson JD, Krasinski K, Borkowsky W. Outcome after assisted ventilation in children with acquired immunodeficiency syndrome. *Crit Care Med* 1990; **18**: 18–20.

16. Starc TJ, Lipshultz SE, Easley KA et al. Incidence of cardiac abnormalities in children with human immunodeficiency virus infection: the Prospective P^2C^2 HIV Study. *J Pediatr* 2002; **141**: 327–35.

17. McComsey G, Lonergan JT. Mitochondrial dysfunction: Patient monitoring and toxicity management. *J Acquir Immune Defic Syndr* 2004; **37**: S30–5.

Recommended reading

1. UNAIDS. *Report on the global AIDS epidemic.* www.unaids.org.

Refractory narrow complex tachycardia in infancy

Trevor Richens

Introduction

Narrow complex tachycardias occur frequently in patients on pediatric intensive care units (PICU). Although the myocardial substrate for supraventricular tachycardias (SVT) may exist prior to PICU admission, SVTs are more likely to occur in this setting for a number of reasons. Electrolyte imbalance, hypoxia, catecholamine drive (exogenous or endogenous), and indwelling intracardiac lines may precipitate episodes of arrhythmia, whereas any child undergoing cardiac surgery will be at risk by the very nature of the procedure. [1]

All medical staff working in the PICU setting should be able to accurately diagnose a narrow complex tachycardia and offer the appropriate management. This chapter aims to provide some understanding of the underlying electrophysiological mechanisms and to suggest a logical way of diagnosing and managing SVT.

Case history

A baby girl was born at term with an antenatal diagnosis of ventricular septal defect. Early electrocardiogram showed a short PR interval and delta wave consistent with Wolff–Parkinson–White syndrome (WPW) and echocardiogram demonstrated a large perimembranous ventricular septal defect with non-compaction of the myocardium.

She deteriorated, at home, on day 8 and presented moribund, requiring intubation, ventilation, and inotrope support using dopamine, dobutamine, and milrinone. An ECG (ECG 1 (Fig. 19.1(a)), Rhythm Strip 1 (Fig. 19.1(b))) showed sinus rhythm and an echocardiogram showed poor biventricular function. The inotropes were weaned over the next 72 hours as her ventricular function improved. Because of the defect morphology, she underwent pulmonary artery banding rather than complete repair on day 14 of life. During the procedure, the heart was extremely irritable with the rhythm switching in and out of narrow complex tachycardia on several occasions. Initially, sinus rhythm returned spontaneously; however, towards the end of the procedure a single 3J DC shock was required and the child was started on intravenous amiodarone at 25 mcg kg^{-1} per min to prevent further arrhythmias. A 12-lead ECG was not possible in theater. No inotropes were required post-operatively and the amiodarone was weaned to 15 mcg kg^{-1} per min and then gradually off, whilst digoxin was started 24 hours after returning from theater. Two further episodes of narrow complex tachycardia occurred in the first 48 hours post-surgery, both during chest physiotherapy. These episodes responded to vagal maneuvers. After these episodes she remained stable off amiodarone and on digoxin with a digoxin level of 3.5 nmol l^{-1}. The 12-lead electrocardiograms during the tachycardias showed loss of delta wave, deeply inverted P waves in the inferior leads and long RP interval with the P wave position in the cycle being confirmed by a trans-esophageal wire. She was extubated at 72 hours and returned to the ward 4 days later.

Case Studies in Pediatric Critical Care, ed. Peter. J. Murphy, Stephen C. Marriage, and Peter J. Davis.
Published by Cambridge University Press. © Cambridge University Press 2009.

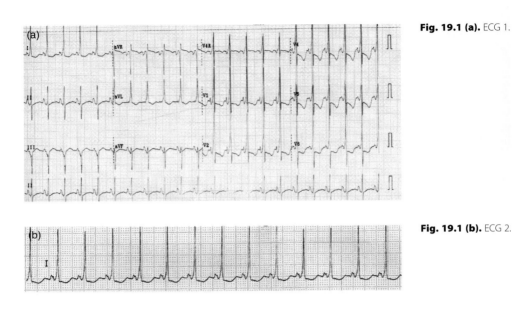

Fig. 19.1 (a). ECG 1.

Fig. 19.1 (b). ECG 2.

Fig. 19.2. Rhythm Strip 1.

Her admission in a moribund state remained unexplained; however ongoing problems with narrow complex tachycardias raised concerns that an arrhythmia might have precipitated the deterioration in ventricular function. Given further episodes of tachycardia on digoxin, with a measured high plasma level, she was switched to amiodarone. She was eventually discharged home at 6 weeks of age after her parents were given instruction on counting her heart rate twice daily.

Four weeks later she re-presented having been generally miserable for 48 hours but breathless, pale, and sweaty for 4 hours. On examination, she was grey, clammy, tachypnoic, her heart rate was too fast to count, and her liver was enlarged. Her electrolytes were normal, Her ECG (ECG 2 (Fig. 19.2)) demonstrated a narrow complex tachycardia at 290 b min^{-1} with loss of delta wave, and echocardiogram showed mild impairment of ventricular function.

The tachycardia was terminated using facial immersion in icy water for 5 seconds and her amiodarone dose was increased. Five days later she was again discharged home after a normal 24 ECG recording.

Two days later she again presented with palor and tachypnea. Electrolytes were normal (Table 19.1), ECG showed a narrow complex tachycardia rate 300 b min^{-1} with loss of delta wave, and echo showed poor ventricular function. After facial immersion was attempted twice without effect, she received two IV boluses of adenosine 0.1 mg kg^{-1} then 0.3 mg kg^{-1}, again without a response. Amiodarone infusion, 25 mcg kg^{-1} per min, was commenced,

Table 19.1. *Early vital signs and blood results*

	Ventilated	Pre-ECMO	On ECMO
Heart rate	255	200	119
BP	80/45	65/45	90/81
SaO2	98	78	100
RR	28	22	15
Toe core gap	1	6	3.5
pO_2	197	142	580
pCO_2	30	35	35
pH	7.43	7.31	7.5
BE	− 3.6	− 7.4	− 3.5
Lactate	3		
Na (mmol l^{-1})	136	135	138
K (mmol l^{-1})	5.6	4.4	3.8
Cl (mmol l^{-1})	101	97	98
U (mmol l^{-1})	13.7	16.4	14.7
Cre (µmol l^{-1})	51	54	46
Ca (mmol l^{-1})	1.04	1.12	
PO_4(mmol l^{-1})	2.39		1.56
Mg (mmol l^{-1})	1.08		1.25

digoxin started, and she was intubated and ventilated prior to DC cardioversion. One, 2, and 5 J kg^{-1} synchronized, DC shocks were tried, again without effect and her tachycardia rate persisted at 300 b min^{-1}. Her cardiac output started to deteriorate with falling blood pressure, dwindling urine output, progressive acidosis and rising lactate. Inotrope support with dopamine was commenced, central venous, and arterial access secured through the femoral site, and she was electively cooled to a core temperature 34–35 °C. A temporary right ventricular pacing lead was inserted as backup whilst the cooling and antiarrhythmic agents slowed the tachycardia rate to 198 b min^{-1}. Despite this, her cardiac output remained poor and she progressed to mechanical support with extra-corporeal membranous oxygenation (ECMO) (isolated ventricular assist techniques were not available). She was placed on veno-arterial ECMO without incident. Through an open incision, a 10FG Biomedicus arterial cannula was inserted into the common carotid and a 10FG Biomedicus venous cannula into the internal jugular vein. She was commenced on 300 ml min^{-1} flows (30% estimated cardiac output) using a roller pump circuit and instantly reverted to sinus rhythm on initiation of bypass, although her myocardium rapidly stunned (a frequent occurrence on veno-arterial ECMO) (Table 19.1). Amiodarone and digoxin were continued and the flows were weaned as her function improved until, after 72 hours of support, her flows were down to 20% of predicted cardiac output. At this point she had a brief recurrence of narrow complex tachycardia coupled with a fall in her mixed venous saturation suggesting significant reduction in cardiac output. Subsequently, her flows were increased, flecainide

2 mg kg^{-1} was added, and she was taken to the catheter laboratory for electrophysiological studies and possible radiofrequency ablation of the culprit accessory pathway.

At catheter, a right posteroseptal pathway was identified which ceased to conduct after three "burns" with concurrent loss of delta wave on the ECG. The amiodarone, digoxin, and flecainide were stopped and ECMO support weaned off over the next 24 hours. Forty-eight hours later she underwent elective repeat cardiac electrophysiological studies that showed no evidence of accessory pathway conduction and no inducible arrhythmia. She was extubated and discharged from intensive care within 7 days and had elective VSD closure and pulmonary artery debanding 2 months later. She has had no recurrence of arrhythmias in 5 years of subsequent follow-up.

Discussion

This child had the substrate for SVT prior to entering PICU, with obvious pre-excitation (WPW) on the surface ECG. In addition, she had structural heart disease, a separate risk factor for narrow complex tachycardia found in 25% of patients.[2] She underwent no intracardiac procedure that might have resulted in scar formation or conduction damage, but developed arrhythmias in the acute post-operative phase when catecholamine levels would have been particularly high. The arrhythmias persisted and became more refractory with time. Although overt WPW was present on the ECG, the incessant and refractory nature of the arrhythmia made the diagnosis less straightforward and the possibility that more than one abnormality may be present required consideration.

The delta wave, present on the sinus rhythm ECG, represented a manifest accessory pathway. Loss of the delta wave during the tachycardia implies that ventricular depolarization occurred via the AV node rather than the accessory pathway, either because the accessory pathway was not involved or because it constituted the retrograde limb of the re-entrant circuit during SVT (Fig. 19.3).

The incessant nature of the arrhythmia, the deeply inverted P waves in the inferior leads, and long RP interval in this child were strongly suggestive of the Permanent

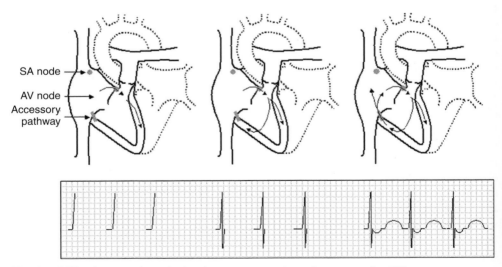

SA node
AV node
Accessory pathway

Fig 19.3. AVRT with retrograde conduction along accessory pathway. P wave seen after QRS.

form of Junctional Reciprocating Tachycardia (PJRT). However, in PJRT there is classically no pre-excitation in sinus rhythm, mitigating against this being the underlying mechanism.

The refractory nature of the arrhythmia in this child suggests an Atrial Ectopic Tachycardia (AET). An ectopic focus, located low in the atrial septum, will produce a P wave axis similar to PJRT and the accessory pathway may not be involved in the arrhythmia. This arrhythmia had a long RP interval (opposed to a long PR), which was confirmed by trans-esophageal ECG. This again supports a diagnosis of PJRT or AET, and therefore questions the relevance of the accessory pathway. Amiodarone was started early in this child and achieved rhythm stability, but was switched to digoxin because of concerns about ventricular function. It was felt safe to use digoxin in a child with a manifest accessory pathway because of her age. Breakthrough of the arrhythmia, despite adequate digoxin levels, prompted a switch back to amiodarone, a more effective antiarrhythmic agent. This also failed and flecainide was added for synergy, despite the concerns of its use in a child with structural heart disease and impaired ventricular function.

Ultimately, we were unable to control the arrhythmia pharmacologically. As her hemodynamic state worsened, her arrhythmia became more refractory, presumably either driven by endogenous and exogenous catecholamines or by wall stresses in the cardiac chambers. Initiation of mechanical support coincided with stopping inotropes, either or both of which resulted in reversion to sinus rhythm. Because weaning of support triggered further SVT, further pharmacological therapy was felt unlikely to be successful. Radiofrequency ablation, although not without risk, proved extremely effective. Interestingly, there was a loss of the delta wave after RFA suggesting possible involvement in the tachycardia mechanism.

Specific arrhythmias

Mechanisms underlying SVT can be split into two types: re-entry and automatic, ectopic tachycardias, re-entry being more common in children.

Re-entry tachycardias

Re-entry tachycardias tend to have a high rate (>230 b min^{-1}, but up to 300 b min^{-1} in infancy), are often paroxysmal in nature, with abrupt initiation and termination, and are mediated by the existence of a re-entry circuit. A re-entry circuit involves an electrical loop with one area of slow, and another of unidirectional, electrical conduction. This combination permits initiation and perpetuation of the abnormal rhythm (Fig. 19.3). The different anatomical substrates forming this circuit give rise to the various types of re-entry tachycardia and usually involve an accessory pathway, myocardial scar or other anatomical anomaly. The commonest form in childhood is Atrioventricular Re-entry Tachycardia (AVRT), whereas in adults it is Atrioventricular Nodal Re-entry Tachycardia (AVNRT). More unusual forms include Intra-Atrial Tachycardias (ART) and the PJRT.

AVRT, WPW, and AVNRT

AVRTs are a heterogenous group of arrhythmias involving a re-entry circuit comprising an anterograde limb through the AV node and a retrograde limb through an accessory pathway. This mechanism underlies 55% of all childhood SVTs. Many accessory pathways conduct only retrograde and are referred to as concealed pathways. Others conduct both anterograde

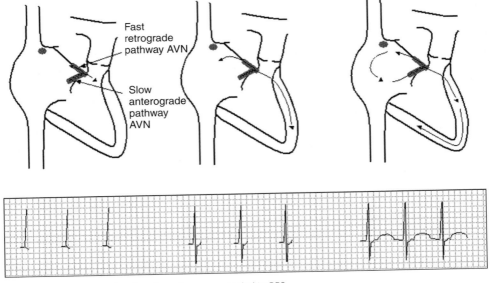

Fig 19.4. AVNRT – typical or slow-fast – P wave concealed in QRS.

and retrograde, the former producing the characteristic delta wave and short PR interval of WPW, and are referred to as manifest.

Rapid retrograde conduction through a concealed or manifest accessory pathway is relatively common and underlies most forms of AVRT. This is a relatively benign phenomenon and in practice is diagnosed by the existence of a retrograde P wave in the ST segment, resulting from retrograde conduction of the impulse through the accessory pathway to the atria. This retrograde P wave depolarizes the atrium in turn before conducting back down the AV node to the ventricle once more, initiating the re-entrant circuit (Fig 19.3.). Of greater concern is the capacity of the manifest accessory pathway present in WPW to conduct rapidly anterograde. Such pathways have the capacity to conduct atrial fibrillation directly to the ventricular myocardium resulting in a very fast rate with risk of ventricular fibrillation and sudden death. Many manifest accessory pathways; however, they will not conduct rapidly anterograde as shown by the disappearance of the delta wave above a particular heart rate.

AVNRT in contrast has a re-entry circuit over fast and slow pathways within the AV node and the perinodal tissue (Fig. 19.4).

The surface ECG may show no P wave activity as atrial depolarization is concealed by the QRS. In atypical AVNRT the atrial depolarization will be delayed by slow retrograde conduction, so the P wave can be seen just after the QRS. Because atrial systole occurs simultaneously with ventricular systole in AVNRT, it may be recognized clinically by cannon waves in the jugular veins and by neck pounding. Acutely, most re-entrant forms of SVT are susceptible to termination by adenosine. If the diagnosis is correct, and termination is not achieved, it is likely that the method of administration has been ineffective rather than the arrhythmia resistant to adenosine. If, after successful cardioversion, the child rapidly reverts back into the tachycardia, then additional "prophylactic" therapy is indicated, assuming other contributing factors such as electrolyte imbalance and proarrhythmic drugs have been addressed. Digoxin, historically well established in the treatment of narrow complex tachycardia, is not without problems. Accidental overdosing is not unusual, sinus bradycardia occurs frequently and ventricular fibrillation has been reported even in the absence of a manifest accessory pathway.[15] Close monitoring of levels in unstable patients minimizes these problems.[16] Its modest efficacy as a single agent [15,17,18,19] improves in combination with a beta-blocker to 70%.[18,20] Digoxin (and verapamil) should be avoided in children over 1 year, where a manifest accessory pathway exists (delta wave on ECG) unless it has been shown not to conduct at high rates. This is because shortening of the refractory period of the accessory pathway may facilitate rapid conduction of atrial flutter/fibrillation to the ventricle. Beta-blockers can be used either alone or in combination with digoxin to prevent recurrence of SVT. Most agents have a similar efficacy [21,22] and are generally well tolerated in children in the absence of significant cardiac dysfunction or reversible airways disease. Sotalol possesses class III antiarrhythmic activity, together with weak beta-blocking ability. It is better tolerated in children with impaired ventricular function or reversible airways disease and has a lower arrhythmia recurrence rate.[23,24] Unfortunately, proarrhythmic episodes including bradycardia, heart block, and torsades can occur early after initiation, but are less of a problem long term.[25] Amiodarone is another class III agent with the advantage of minimal effects on ventricular function when given orally (although a significant negative inotrope intravenously). It is better tolerated in children than adults with a lower incidence of hypothyroidism, corneal microdeposits, hypotension, bradycardia, QT prolongation, and Torsades de Pointes. There are several potential interactions with other antiarrhythmic agents; amiodarone blocks removal of digoxin, quinidine, flecainide, and verapamil elevating serum levels.[26] It lengthens the QT interval in common with the class I antiarrhythmics lidocaine and procainamide so concurrent administration should be avoided. It is highly effective at preventing recurrence of re-entrant arrhythmias,[27] particularly in combination with a beta-blocker or flecainide.[28–30]

Flecainide is a class Ic antiarrhythmic with a colourful past because of safety concerns, particularly in patients with structural heart disease.[31] The main concerns in childhood relate to widening of the QRS and ventricular arrhythmias, although such proarrhythmic events are rare in children.[32] Flecainide is highly effective in controlling re-entrant tachycardias [31–33], and co-administration with either sotalol [36] or amiodarone [30] can be used in refractory arrhythmias.

Propafenone is a Ic class antiarrhythmic agent with additional beta blocking and weak calcium channel blocking activity. Its proarrhythmia problems appear similar to flecainide and again are more common in children with structural heart disease.[35] Propafenone blocks retrograde conduction through accessory pathways and, as such, is particularly effective in tachycardias reliant on this mechanism such as AVRT, PJRT, and WPW. Its longer duration of action compared with adenosine makes it useful in intravenous form for termination of arrhythmias that have a high early recurrence rate.[36] Orally, it is very effective at preventing recurrence,[37] although in patient groups with concealed accessory pathways safer agents are generally used as first-line therapy.

PJRT

PJRT is an uncommon but incessant form of tachycardia, causing 1% of childhood SVT. It is mediated by a concealed accessory pathway situated in the posterior septum near the tricuspid valve/coronary sinus annulus conducting at a slow rate. This results in an incessant narrow complex tachycardia at a rate of 120 b min^{-1} to 250 b min^{-1} with characteristic

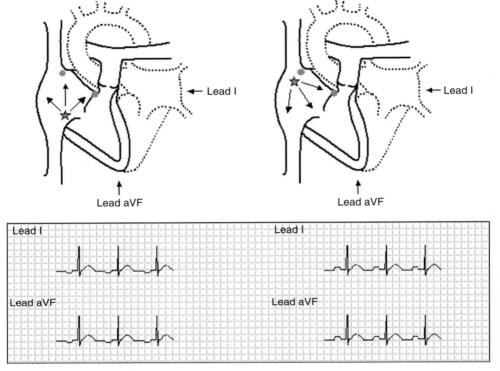

Fig 19.5. Atrial ectopic tachycardia – P wave axis shift.

ECG findings of deep inverted P waves in the inferior leads together with a long RP interval (Fig 19.5.).

The tachycardia rate becomes slower and less incessant with increasing age, so greater hemodynamic compromise is found in younger patients.[3] The incessant nature of the tachycardia can result in the development of a dilated cardiomyopathy if the arrhythmia goes unnoticed. This is often the mode of presentation, particularly in younger children, and may necessitate inotropic support in PICU.

In contrast to AVRT and AVNRT, PJRT is rarely terminated for more than a few beats after cardioversion. One report has shown that intravenous propafenone can terminate PJRT without adverse events and also maintain sinus rhythm in four out of five children.[36] Longer-term PJRT is chronically refractory to most anti-arrhythmic agents, ultimately requiring radiofrequency ablation;[3] however, a combination of oral digoxin and propafenone seems effective in maintaining sinus rhythm or at least controlling rate of the arrhythmia in 88% of children, thus delaying or avoiding ablation.[38]

ART

ART comprises approximately 12.5% of SVTs in childhood. The majority occur where a re-entry circuit exists around a surgical scar after procedures such as the Mustard, Senning, or Fontan operations where extensive atrial suturing takes place. Atrial flutter, another form of ART, is rare in children, occurring primarily in otherwise well infants where a re-entrant circuit forms around the tricuspid valve.[4] The flutter rate changes with age; in neonates it may be as fast as 400 b min^{-1}; however, during infancy and childhood this slows to the adult flutter rate of 300 b min^{-1}. Most AV nodes will not conduct at such rates and the transmitted ventricular response is typically half the atrial rate, i.e. 2:1 block. Uncommonly in infants, the AV node conducts the atrial flutter rate to the ventricle without block resulting in ventricular rates in excess of 300 b min^{-1}. A typical ECG finding of saw tooth flutter waves is seen where 2:1 block occurs.

Antiarrhythmic agents are rarely successful at terminating ART and the favored approach is DC cardioversion or overdrive pacing.[4] Atrial flutter in neonates rarely recurs after the first year,[39] so the need for prophylactic pharmacological therapy is questionable.[40] ART related to surgical scars generally occurs in older children and is often refractory to medical treatment requiring revision of the surgical repair and concurrent interventional treatment (surgical or transcatheter) of the arrhythmia substrate.[41] Amiodarone is effective in some children with post-operative atrial arrhythmias, although in the long term tolerance is limited by side effects. This can be offset by the addition of a beta-blocker allowing a reduction in amiodarone dose.[42] An obvious alternative is sotalol, which has shown favorable results in children with a lower side effect profile than amiodarone.[43]

Ectopic tachycardias

Atrial ectopic tachycardia (AET)

AET is uncommon, comprising 5–10% of pediatric narrow complex tachycardias and arising as a result of increased automaticity of small areas of atrial tissue. These tachycardias are commonly incessant, producing few symptoms in infants until the chronic high rate results in a dilated cardiomyopathy.[5] Rarely, they are paroxysmal and relatively benign. The rate usually varies between 150 and 300 but usually over 200 b min^{-1}, and the site of the ectopic focus within the atrium determines the P wave morphology. If located near the SA node, the P wave may be difficult to distinguish from sinus tachycardia; however, when located more inferiorly the P wave axis will shift becoming negative in leads II, III, and aVF. (Fig. 19.6).

Typically, these arrhythmias are catecholamine sensitive and undergo "warm up" and "cool down" periods unlike re-entry arrhythmias, which tend to start and stop abruptly. Usually idiopathic in childhood, atrial tachycardia is associated with viral infections such as respiratory syncytial virus and is a feature of digoxin toxicity particularly in the presence of hypokalemia, where 2:1 block is often present.

Idiopathic AET is often resistant to pharmacological therapy, although for children under 3 years the chances of spontaneous cessation are good and a conservative approach should be pursued. Digoxin, beta-blockers, and propafenone are poorly effective as monotherapy, but in combination they are successful in 60–90% of children, and the substitution of amiodarone or flecainide improves control in more refractory cases.[44,45] Above 3 years of age the arrhythmia is unlikely to resolve, medical treatment is difficult, and ablation may need to be considered early.[44] In patients with congenital heart disease, who develop AET in the immediate post-operative period, the arrhythmia is likely to be transient. Electrolyte correction (particularly potassium), digoxin and/or beta-blockers will control the rhythm in most children, and amiodarone maybe effective as a second-line agent where required.[46]

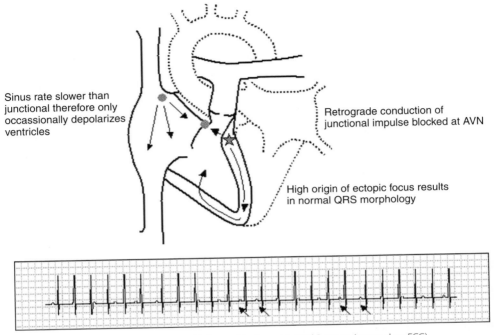

Sinus rate slower than junctional therefore only occassionally depolarizes ventricles

Retrograde conduction of junctional impulse blocked at AVN

High origin of ectopic focus results in normal QRS morphology

Fig 19.6. JET – complete AV dissociation with intermittently conducted P waves (arrowed on ECG).

Junctional ectopic tachycardia (JET)

JET is an incessant tachycardia, rare outside the immediate post-operative setting. The congenital form presents in the first 6 months of life, often with a dilated cardiomyopathy.[6]

More commonly, JET is seen in the immediate post-operative period after congenital heart surgery, where bruising or damage to the junctional area results in a transient increased automaticity of the conduction tissue with a resulting incessant narrow complex tachycardia.

The area of increased automaticity is located just below the AV node and ventricular depolarization follows a normal pattern with a narrow QRS. Usually, retrograde AV block is present and there is atrio-ventricular dissociation with P waves seen "marching through" the QRS complexes (Fig. 19.7).

Less commonly, retrograde conduction to the atria occurs through the AV node or a concealed accessory pathway and P waves will be found in the ST segment in a similar way to AVRT.

In the post-surgical patient JET is a self-limiting phenomenon where the object of treatment is rate control and establishment of atrio-ventricular synchrony until the tachycardia abates. A staged approach has been advocated,[47] although aggressive early control avoids further hemodynamic compromise. Minimalizing inotrope use, controlled central cooling to 35 °C, and intravenous amiodarone[48] for 48 to 72 hours is usually successful, although occasionally adequate rate control can be achieved by cooling to 37 °C alone, thus avoiding the potential complications of hypothermia. Once the rate has dropped adequately (usually <160 b min^{-1}), atrio-ventricular synchrony can be established by atrial or dual

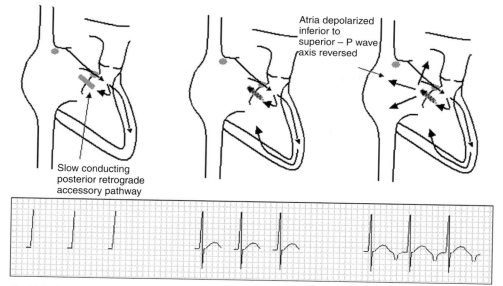

Fig 19.7. PJRT – slowed retrograde conduction delays results in long RP interval.

chamber pacing at just over the tachycardia rate. Flecainide and procainamide[49,50] can be used as alternatives to amiodarone.

In the congenital form of JET, success is defined as rate control with alleviation of symptoms and improvement in ventricular function rather than conversion to sinus rhythm. Children often present with a dilated poorly functioning left ventricle, which will improve with sufficient rate control. Digoxin has no beneficial effect on JET and may induce ventricular arrhythmias;[51] however it is still controversially used as an adjunct to treat ventricular dysfunction.[52] Rhythm control is often difficult to achieve, requiring a combination of agents. Whilst propafenone was found to be successful in one study,[53] others have found it less so and suggest the combination of amiodarone and flecainide.[54] Overall, it would seem that persistence with different regimens is likely to gain rate control eventually.

Broad complex SVT

Some broad complex tachycardias are supraventricular. Importantly, the general rule that all broad complex tachycardias are ventricular in origin should apply in children, as it does in adults; however the exceptions need to be understood. Many children with congenital heart disease have partial or complete right bundle branch block, particularly after right heart surgery or in right heart volume loading situations. More rarely, left bundle branch block may be seen, usually after left heart surgery. Pre-existing bundle branch block will result in a broad QRS complex SVT, and comparison of sinus rhythm and tachycardia QRS morphologies may help in the diagnosis. In addition, either the right or left bundle branches may fail to conduct above a certain heart rate. Beyond this, conduction is blocked and the ECG will take on a bundle branch morphology, again resulting in a broad complex tachycardia, a situation known as aberrance. Unfortunately, the recognition of a right or left bundle branch block pattern on the 12-lead ECG does not necessarily confirm a supraventricular origin; right ventricular dysplasia, for instance, can present with a left bundle branch block morphology ventricular tachycardia. If in doubt, a pediatric cardiac electrophysiologist should be asked to review.

General management

Investigation

A 12-lead ECG of the tachycardia should be obtained, if possible with a recording of any termination mechanism. Esophageal and/or epicardial recordings may be needed. Electrolytes should be normalised. A full medication history should be checked and consideration given to possible ingestion/administration of other proarrhythmic agents. Inotrope infusions should be reviewed as several types of SVT, particularly automatic tachycardias, are catecholamine sensitive. An echocardiogram should be obtained to identify any underlying structural abnormality and assess ventricular size and function.

ECG

The clinical setting must be considered when interpreting the ECG. Sinus tachycardia is common and can be paroxysmal, particularly in the paralyzed ventilated patient. Inadequate sedation, seizures, drugs, fever, and fluid shifts are just a few of the reasons why this might occur. Distinction can be difficult, particularly when relying on a single ECG lead such as a patient monitor. In general, if a child is hemodynamically tolerating the tachycardia, a 12-lead ECG should be obtained before any attempt at cardioversion. In addition, multiple leads should be recorded during any electrical or pharmacological attempts at restoring sinus rhythm, as the pattern of termination may provide the diagnosis.[7] In some cases the 12-lead surface ECG is not adequate, and further investigations such as transesophageal or, in the post-operative cardiac patient, epicardial ECGs, may be required. In other situations pharmacological trials, particularly with adenosine, can provide vital information. Rarely, more advanced techniques such as programed atrial pacing or full electrophysiological studies may be required.

Many algorithms exist to facilitate the accurate diagnosis of SVT. All rely on the identification of the P wave, its relation to the QRS, and its electrical axis. Many split tachycardias into short RP and long RP groups.

Short RP

Where the P wave is closest to the preceding R wave (RP <50% RR interval), it is said to be a short RP tachycardia. This group includes AVRT, AVNRT, forms of atrial tachycardia where AV block is present, and atypical JET where AV association persists. Position of the P wave relative to the QRS helps in distinguishing between the different causes. In AVNRT and atypical JET the P wave is usually within the QRS, whereas in AVRT and in atypical AVNRT it is in the ST segment.

Long RP

Long RP includes all tachycardias where RP >50% RR interval. Sinus tachycardia, atrial tachycardias with little or no AV block, atypical AVNRT, and PJRT all have long RP intervals. Because the PR interval is often reasonably short, the P wave can be identified around the terminal portion of the T wave. The P wave axis is key in diagnosis. Sinus

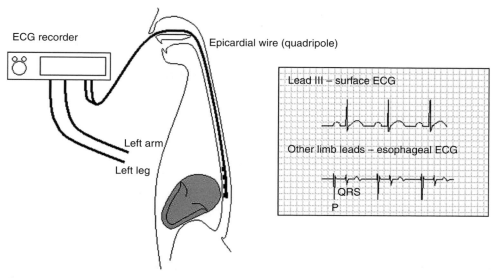

Fig 19.8. Pacing of transesophageal electrode and ECG traces recorded.

tachycardia and AET arise near the SA node and have a normal P wave axis, i.e. positive in all limb leads other than aVR. Atrial tachycardias arising from the inferior portion of the atria, PJRT, and atypical AVNRT depolarize the atria in a reverse direction, with consequent P wave inversion in the inferior leads II, III, and aVF.

Adjuncts to the surface ECG

In some instances careful analysis of the 12-lead ECG may not allow an accurate diagnosis to be made and atrial cardiograms, from esophageal or epicardial leads are extremely helpful. Another way of obtaining more diagnostic information is the diagnostic use of adenosine.

Transesophageal ECG

Specialized transesophageal pacing wires are now produced for adults and children that are well suited to recording electrocardiograms.[8] If these are not available either a straightforward temporary pacing wire or quadripolar electrophysiology, electrodes make very good substitutes. The wire is introduced like a nasogastric tube. The distance can be measured against the child prior to insertion by estimating a point in the mid-axillary line level with the nipple. Once in position, the wire is connected to a 12-lead ECG machine (Fig. 19.8).

Pacing leads have two electrodes allowing acquisition of a bipolar cardiogram, although it is possible to connect up just one of the electrodes and obtain a unipolar cardiogram. The bipolar trace will provide a better atrial recording and can be obtained by substituting the two pacing lead electrodes for the right arm and right leg electrodes. Lead III will show the surface ECG, whilst the other limb leads will show the esophago-atrial ECG. Alternatively, a unipolar trace can be obtained by substituting one of the pacing lead electrodes with V1, displaying the esophago-atrial ECG on V1 and the rest of the ECG will be a normal surface ECG. The advantage of a quadripole electrode is that two leads can be used to record a bipolar atrial cardiogram, whilst the other two can be used to pace if needed. With the wire in position, it can be moved up and down the esophagus until an optimal recording is obtained (Fig. 19.8).

Complications of esophageal lead placement are rare, although esophageal ulceration has been reported in adult and pediatric patients with long term use (>60 hours). Mild pressure necrosis related to electrode placement rather than electrical stimulation has also been reported.

The placement of an esophageal electrode also allows the use of programed stimulation as a diagnostic tool or as a way of cardioverting some types of SVT.

Epicardial ECG

Patients returning from cardiac theater after open heart procedures frequently have epicardial pacing leads attached to the surface of the atria. These are brought out of the skin on the right side of the sternum and can be used in a similar way to the esophageal lead to record the atrial cardiogram. Acquisitions of unipolar or bipolar recordings are obtained by substituting the pacing wires for the ECG leads as outlined above. As with esophageal pacing, the electrode can also be used for stimulation to help diagnose and treat some forms of SVT.

The advantage of obtaining bipolar rather than unipolar recordings by these techniques is the amplification of the atrial signal relative to the QRS complex. In difficult diagnostic cases such as AVNRT, this may facilitate distinction of the P wave from the QRST complex.

Adenosine

Narrow complex tachycardias differ in their response to AV node slowing or block. This can be achieved by vagal maneuvers such as valsalva, carotid sinus massage, or face immersion in cold water. In an intensive care setting the preferred way to block AV node conduction is adenosine, a short-acting nucleotide that blocks AV node conduction and suppresses automaticity of the sinoatrial node as well as atrial and Purkinje tissue, although has no effect on ventricular tissue at pharmacologic doses.[9] In awake patients physical side effects such as chest discomfort, flushing, and a feeling of impending doom are common but short lived. Reported cardiac adverse effects, most notably atrial fibrillation, occur in approximately 2.7% of adult patients,[10] although it is likely to be less common in children.[11] Although some caution has been expressed over its use in patients with asthma because of problems with inhaled adenosine, with intravenous use this is more a theoretical concern. Adenosine may also be affected by pre-existing drug treatment; dipyridamole (Persantin) is occasionally used as an anti-platelet agent, although rarely in children and potentiates the actions of adenosine by inhibiting cellular uptake. Aminophylline and other methylxanthines in contrast attenuate the effects of adenosine, and carbamazepine can result in higher degrees of AV block.

Adenosine is inactivated rapidly in blood and needs to be administered by rapid intravenous bolus injection through a central or proximal vein immediately followed by a large volume flush. Successful administration has also been reported using the interosseous route where no venous access is possible.[12] Care must also be taken not to withdraw any blood into the syringe, as this will inactivate the adenosine *ex vivo*. The recommended starting dose is 0.05 mg kg^{-1}, although this is rarely effective and 0.1 mg kg^{-1} is more appropriate increasing up to a maximum of 0.4 mg kg^{-1}. Of note children with poor cardiac function or with Fontan-type circulations will have delayed venous return requiring higher doses to ensure an effective amount remains in the circulation by the time it reaches the coronary circulation. Equally, children with obligatory right to left shunts such as Tetralogy of Fallot will have rapid transit from venous to coronary circulation and may require less.

From a diagnostic point of view, adenosine will block AV node and accessory pathway conduction and therefore terminate re-entry tachycardias such as AVRT, AVNRT, and PJRT. Patients with sinus tachycardia will show AV node block and slowing of the sinus rate, both of which will be transient. Adenosine terminates up to 58% of AET but only 30% of re-entry and 25% of atrial tachycardia related to surgical scars.[9,13] If tachycardia termination is only transient, analysis of the mechanism of termination may help determine the type of arrhythmia. Termination with a P wave after the final QRS suggests AVRT or AVNRT, whereas termination with a QRS suggests atrial tachycardia. AV node block may allow visualization of the underlying atrial rhythm and confirmation of diagnosis in atrial tachycardia and atrial flutter. JET will slow transiently and the dissociated, sinus-mediated P waves may be revealed, however the tachycardia will not terminate.[9]

Treatment strategy

Acute management is dependent on how the arrhythmia is tolerated by the child and its underlying mechanism. In well-tolerated tachycardias, time can be taken to make an accurate diagnosis before instituting targeted therapy. If poorly tolerated, termination or rate control of the arrhythmia may be the paramount concern.

Cardioversion

The best way to terminate the tachycardia will depend on the underlying mechanism. AVRT, AVNRT, and PJRT may terminate with vagal stimulation alone, although intravenous adenosine will often be required. Although verapamil has been used for this purpose, it is best avoided since it is profoundly negatively inotropic, has caused refractory electro-mechanical dissociation in infants, and has a prolonged duration of action, all of which make it an unsuitable agent for any seriously ill child. Automatic atrial tachycardias are unlikely to respond to vagal maneuvers, adenosine, overdrive pacing, or DC shock and will usually require pharmacologic intervention before restoration of sinus rhythm can be maintained. Sinus tachycardia and JET will not terminate with adenosine, although the rate of sinus tachycardia will transiently slow and AV block may be seen. If adenosine fails to achieve cardioversion, however transiently, a decision must be made as to the urgency of restoring sinus rhythm. If hemodynamic compromise is present, cardioversion can be attempted either by external DC shock at $1-2\,\mathrm{J\ kg^{-1}}$ or, in the case of atrial re-entrant tachycardia, by transesophageal, or if available epicardial overdrive pacing.

Overdrive pacing

In intensive care, overdrive pacing is particularly useful in terminating atrial re-entry tachycardias, where the chance of acute termination by adenosine is low. If atrial epicardial wires are *in situ*, or if an esophageal wire can be introduced, then overdrive pacing can be attempted as an alternative to DC shock. Overdrive pacing works by using rapid atrial paced stimuli to "capture" the atria and interrupt the re-entrant circuit, a process called entrainment. A series of 4–10 paced beats at a rate of $400\,\mathrm{min^{-1}}$ (RR interval 150 ms) has been shown to be effective in 70–80% of children with various forms of atrial re-entry tachycardia.[4,14] Many standard temporary pacing boxes have the facility to pace at such rates; however, a specialized programmable stimulator may be preferred. The main potential complication of this technique is the induction of atrial fibrillation; however, this is rare and usually transient.[4]

Table 19.2. *Suggested approach to treatment*

AVRT/AVNRT

Acute termination: IV adenosine

First line: beta-blocker ± digoxin if no WPW

Second line: flecainide or propafenone if no structural heart disease, amiodarone if structural heart disease present

PJRT

Acute termination: IV propafenone

Maintenance: digoxin and propafenone

ART

Acute termination: DC shock or overdrive pacing

Maintenance neonatal flutter: none

Maintenance scar-related: amiodarone and beta-blocker

AET

First line: beta-blocker and digoxin

Second line: substitute propafenone or amiodarone for beta-blocker

Post-operative JET

Cool to 35–37 °C, amiodarone, cardiac pacing

Congenital JET

Amiodarone and propafenone, digoxin if ventricular dysfunction

Pharmacological therapy

Unfortunately, many forms of tachycardia are resistant to cardioversion or will rapidly recur after restoration of sinus rhythm. In such cases commencing an antiarrhythmic agent may pharmacologically cardiovert the rhythm, maintain sinus rhythm after cardioversion by another means, or provide rate control of the tachycardia. The choice of antiarrhythmic agent will vary according to the specific type of arrhythmia concerned, and a suggested approach to treatment is outlined in Table 19.2, with doses listed in Table 19.3.

Radiofrequency Ablation (RFA) in PICU

RFA refers to the interruption of accessory pathways and ectopic foci by using radiofrequency energy to heat the tip of an intracardiac catheter positioned against the endocardial surface at the target area. The thermal energy produced at the tip causes local tissue destruction, effectively blocking electrical activity at the site of the "burn." Because of concerns regarding the effect of such endocardial scarring on the developing heart and the natural tendency for many arrhythmias to resolve in the first years of life, ablation is generally avoided in infancy. In children, it is used where symptoms are poorly controlled by first-line medical therapy. The success rate in children is similar to that in adults, with cessation of the tachycardia in 91% of accessory pathways and 87% of ectopic foci.[55]

It is rare, but recognized, for a child in intensive care to require RFA as the vast majority of SVT can be controlled with medical therapy. In those where cardioversion cannot be accomplished such as atrial ectopic tachycardias, adequate rate control is usually possible,

Table 19.3. *Recommended drug doses*

Drug	Loading/Acute termination	Maintenance
Adenosine	0.1–0.4 mg kg^{-1} bolus	
Amiodarone	5–7 mg kg^{-1} over 30–60 min, or 25 mcg kg^{-1} min^{-1} for 4 hours	5–15 mcg kg^{-1} per min IV 5–10 mg kg^{-1} per day PO
Atenolol		1–2 mg kg^{-1} per day PO
Digoxin	15 mcg kg^{-1} then 5 mcg kg^{-1} after 6 hours	5 mcg kg^{-1} PO or IV BD
Flecainide	0.5–2 mg kg^{-1} over 5 min	3–12 mg kg^{-1} per day PO
Nadolol		1–5 mg kg^{-1} per day PO
Propafenone	1.5–2 mg kg^{-1} over 3 min	200–600 mg m^{-2} per day
Propranolol	0.1 mg kg^{-1} over 10 min (repeat if needed up to 3x)	0.1–0.3 mg kg^{-1} 3-hourly 0.5–1 mg kg^{-1} PO QDS
Sotalol	0.5–2 mg kg^{-1} over 10 min	2–8 mg kg^{-1} per day PO

and its need may be transient. For the small numbers that have a refractory SVT with significant hemodynamic compromise, RFA may provide the best way of controlling the arrhythmia. Such patients are often extremely unwell with precarious hemodynamics, and may not tolerate the rhythm manipulations involved in RFA. Hemodynamic stability can be obtained by supporting the cardiac output using Extracorporeal Support (ECS). In some cases, where the cardiac function is largely responsible for perpetuation of the arrhythmia, cardioversion can occur spontaneously as support is initiated; however, SVT may return when the support is weaned.[56] The time on ECS can therefore be used to treat the underlying cause, wait for it to resolve, optimize the antiarrhythmic treatment, or, as in this child, use RFA to modify the conduction system to affect a "cure."

Learning points

- SVTs are more likely to occur in children on the PICU due to the potential for electrolyte imbalance, hypoxia, indwelling intracardiac lines, and enhanced catecholamine drive.
- Mechanisms underlying SVTs can be split into two types: re-entry tachycardias and automatic/ectopic tachycardias.
- Re-entry tachycardias are more common, tend to have a high rate, and are often paroxysmal in nature.
- Types of ectopic tachycardia include atrial ectopic tachycardia and junctional ectopic tachycardia.
- Acute management of an SVT is dependent both on how the arrhythmia is tolerated by the child and on the underling mechanism of the SVT.
- For the very few children who have refractory SVT with significant hemodynamic compromise radiofrequency ablation (RFA) may provide the optimal way of controlling the arrythmia. Extracorporeal support e.g. ECMO, Ventricular Assist, may also be required to support cardiac output, as affected patient may not tolerate the rhythm manipulations involved in RFA.

References

1. Trohman RG. Supraventricular tachycardia: implications for the intensivist. *Critical Care Med* 2000; **28**(10): N129–35.
2. Pfammatter JP, Bauersfeld U. Safety issues in the treatment of paediatric supraventricular tachycardias. *Drug Safety* 1998;18(S): 345–56.
3. Dorostkar PC, Silka MJ, Morady F, Dick M. Clinical course of persistent junctional reciprocating tachycardia. *J Am Coll Cardiol* 1999; **33**(2): 366–75.
4. Brockmeier K, Ulmer HE, Hessling G. Termination of atrial reentrant tachycardia by using transoesophageal atrial pacing. *J Electrcardiol* 2002; **35**: 159–63.
5. Paker DL, Bardy GH, Worley SJ *et al.* Tachycardia-induced cardiomyopathy: a reversible form of left ventricular dysfunction. *Am J Cardiol* 1986; **57**: 563–70.
6. Sarubbi B, Musto B, Ducceschi V *et al.* Congenital junctional ectopic tachycardia in children and adolescents: a 20 year experience based study. *Heart* 2002; **88**(2): 188–90.
7. Engelstein ED, Lippman N, Stein KM *et al.* Arrhythmias/EP Intervention/pacing: mechanism-specific effects of adenosine on atrial tachycardia. *Circulation* 1994; **89**(6): 2645–54.
8. Hessling G, Brockmeier K, Ulmer H. Transoesophageal electrocardiography and atrial pacing in children. *J Electrocardiol* 2002; **35**: 143–9.
9. Glatter KA, Cheng J, Dorostkar P *et al.* Electrophysiological effects of adenosine in patients with supraventricular tachycardia. *Circulation* 1999; **99**: 1034–40.
10. Pelleg A, Pennock RS, Kutalek SP. Proarrhythmic effects of adenosine: one decade of clinical data. *Am J Ther* 2002; **9**: 141–7.
11. Sherwood MC, Lau KC, Sholler GF. Adenosine in the management of supraventricular tachycardia in children. *J Paediatr Child Health* 1998; **34**(1): 53–6.
12. Friedman FD. Interosseous adenosine for the termination of supraventricular tachycardia in an infant. *Ann Int Med* 1996; **28**(3): 356–8.
13. Engelstein ED, Lippman N, Stein KM, Lerman BB. Arrhythmias/EP intervention/pacing: mechanism-specific effects of adenosine on atrial tachycardia. *Circulation* 1994; **89**(6): 2645–54.
14. Rhodes LA, Walsh EP, Saul JP. Conversion of atrial flutter in pediatric patients by transoesophageal atrial pacing: a safe, effective, minimally invasive procedure. *Am Heart J* 1995; **130**: 323–7.
15. Villain E, Bonnet D, Acar P *et al.* Recommendations for the treatment of supraventricular tachycardia in infants. *Arch de Ped* 1998; **5**(2): 133–8.
16. Pfammatter JP, Stocker FP. Role of digoxin in the long term treatment of supraventricular tachycardias in infancy. *Eur J Pediatr* 1998; **157**: 101–6.
17. Sreeram N, Wren C. Supraventricular tachycardia in infants: response to treatment. *Arch Dis Child* 1990; **65**(1): 127–9.
18. Weindling SN, Saul JP, Walsh EP. Efficacy and risks of medical therapy for supraventricular tachycardia in neonates and infants. *Am Heart J* 1996; **131**: 66–72.
19. O'Sullivan JJ, Gardiner HG, Wren C. Digoxin or flecainide for prophylaxis of supraventricular tachycardia in infants. *J Am Coll Cardiol* 1995; **26**: 991–4.
20. Tortoriello TA, Snyder CS, Smith EO *et al.* Frequency of recurrence among infants with supraventricular tachycardia and comparison of recurrence rates among those with and without preexcitation and among those with and without response to digoxin and/or propanolol therapy. *Am J Cardiol* 2003; **92**(9): 1045–9.
21. Mehta AV, Subrahmanyam AB, Anand R. Long-term efficacy of atenolol for supraventricular tachycardia in children. *Pediatr Cardiol* 1996; **17**(4): 231–6.
22. Mehta AV, Chidambaram. Efficacy and safety of oral and intravenous nadolol for supraventricular tachycardia in children. *J Am Coll Cardiol* 1992; **19**(3): 630–5.
23. Celiker A, Ayabakan C, Ozer S, Ozme S. Sotalol in treatment of pediatric cardiac arrhythmias. *Pediatr Int* 2001; **43**: 624–30.
24. Maragnes P, Tipple M, Fournier A. Effectiveness of oral sotalol for the treatment of pediatric arrhythmias. *Am J Cardiol* 1992; **69**(8): 751–4.
25. Pfammater JP, Paul T, Lehman C *et al.* Efficacy and pro-arrhythmia of oral sotalol

in pediatric patients. *J Am Coll Cardiol* 1995; **26**: 1002–7.

26. Koren G. Interaction between digoxin and commonly co-administered drugs. *Pediatrics* 1985; **75**(6): 1032–7.

27. McKee MR. Amiodarone – an "old" drug with new recommendations. *Curr Opin Pediatr* 2003; **15**: 193–9.

28. Etheridge SP, Craig JE, Compton SJ. Amiodarone is safe and highly effective therapy for supraventricular tachycardia in infants. *Am Heart J* 2001; **141**: 105–10.

29. Drago F, Mazza A, Guccione P *et al.* Amiodarone used alone or in combination with propanolol; a very effective therapy for tachyarrhythmia in infants and children. *Pediatr Cardiol* 1998; **19**(6): 445–9.

30. Fenrich AL, Perry JC, Friedman RA. Flecainide and amiodarone: combined therapy for refractory tachyarrhythmias in infancy. *JACC* 1995; **25**(5): 1195–8.

31. Cockrell JL, Scheinman MM, Titus C *et al.* Safety and efficacy of oral flecainide therapy in patients with atrioventricular re-entrant tachycardia. *Ann Int Med* 1991; **114**: 189–94.

32. Perry JC, Garson A. Flecainide acetate for treatment of tachyarrhythmias in children: review of world literature on efficacy, safety and dosing. *Am Heart J* 1992; **124** (6): 1614–21.

33. O'Sullivan JJ, Gardiner HM, Wren C. Digoxin or flecainide for prophylaxis or supraventricular tachycardia in infants? *JACC* 1995; **26**(4): 991–4.

34. Price JF, Kertesz NJ, Snyder CS *et al.* Flecainide and sotalol: a new combination therapy for refractory supraventricular tachycardia in children <1 year of age. 2002; **39**(3): 517–20.

35. Janousek J, Thomas P. Safety of oral propafenone in the treatment of arrhythmias in infants and children. *Am J Cardiol* 1998; **81**(9): 1121–4.

36. Hessling G, Brockmeier K, Ruediger H, Herbert E. Electrophysiological efficacy of intravenous propafenone in terminating atrioventricular reentrant tachycardia in children. *Am J Cardiol* 2001; **87**(6): 802–4.

37. Musto B, D'Onofrio A, Cavallaro C, Musto A. Electrophysiological effects and clinical efficacy of propafenone in children with recurrent paroxysmal supraventricular tachycardia. *Circulation* 1988; **78**(4): 863–9.

38. Van Stuijvenberg M, Beaufort-Krol GC, Haaksma J, Bink-Boelkens MT. Pharmacological treatment of young children with permanent junctional reciprocating tachycardia. *Cardiol Young* 2003; **13**(5): 408–12.

39. Etheridge SP, Judd VE. Supraventricular tachycardia in infancy: evaluation, management and follow up. *Arch Pediatri Adolesc Med* 1999; **153**(3): 267–71.

40. Lisowski LA, Verheijen PM, Benatar AA *et al.* Atrial flutter in the perinatal age group: diagnosis, management and outcome. *J Am Coll Cardiol* 2000; **35**(3): 771–7.

41. Balaji S, Johnson TB, Sade RM *et al.* Management of atrial flutter after the Fontan procedure. *J Am Coll Cardiol* 1994; **23** (5): 1209–15.

42. Lucet V. Late atrial tachycardia after Fontan-type procedure. Cooperative study of 52 cases. *Arch de Mal du Co Vaiss* 2002; **95** (5): 447–52.

43. Beaufort-Krol G, Bink-Boelkens M. Effectiveness of sotalol in children after surgery for congenital heart disease. *Am J Cardiol* 1997; **79**(1): 92–4.

44. Salerno JC, Kertesz NJ, Friedman RA, Fenrich AL. Clinical course of atrial ectopic tachycardia is age-dependent: results of treatment in children <3 or >3 years of age. *J Am Coll Cardiol* 2004; **43** (3): 438–44.

45. Bauersfeld U, Gow R, Hamilton RM, Izukawa T. Treatment of atrial ectopic tachycardia in infants <6 months old. *Am Heart J* 1995; **129**: 1145–8.

46. Rosales AM, Walsh EP, Wessel DL, Triedman JK. Postoperative ectopic atrial tachycardia in children with congenital heart disease. *Am J Cardiol* 2001; **88** (10): 1169–72.

47. Walsh EP, Saul JP, Sholler GF *et al.* Evaluation of a staged treatment protocol for rapid automatic junctional tachycardia after operation for congenital heart disease. *J Am Coll Cardiol* 1997; **29**(5): 1046–53.

48. Laird WP, Snyder CS, Kertesz NJ *et al.* Use of intravenous amiodarone for postoperative junctional ectopic tachycardia. *Ped Cardiol* 2003; **24**(2): 133–7.

49. Bronzetti G, Formigari R, Giardini A *et al.* Intravenous flecanide for the treatment of junctional ectopic tachycardia after surgery for congenital heart disease. *Ann Thorac Surg* 2003; **76**(1): 148–51.

50. Mandapati R, Byrum CJ, Kavey RE *et al.* Procainamide for rate control of postsurgical junctional tachycardia. *Pediatr Cardiol* 2000; **21**(2): 123–8.

51. Villain E, Vetter VL, Garcia JM *et al.* Evolving concepts in the management of congenital junctional tachycardia. A multicentre study. *Circulation* 1990; **81**: 1544–9.

52. Cilliers AM, du Plessis JP, Clur SB *et al.* Junctional ectopic tachycardia in six paediatric patients. *Heart* 1997; **78**(4): 413–15.

53. Paul T, Reimer A, Janouesek J, Kallfelz HC. Efficacy and safety of propafenone in congenital junctional ectopic tachycardia. *J Am Coll Cardiol* 1992; **20**(4): 911–14.

54. Sarubbi B, Musto B, Ducceschi V *et al.* Congenital junctional ectopic tachycardia in children and adolescents: a 20 year experience based study. *Heart* 2002; **88**(2): 188–90.

55. Scheinman M, Calkins H, Gillette P *et al.* NASPE policy statement on catheter ablation: personnel, policy, procedures and therapeutic recommendations. *PACE* 2003; **26**: 789–99.

56. Walker GM, McLeod K, Brown KL *et al.* Extracorporeal life support as a treatment for supraventricular tachycardia in infants. *Ped Crit Care Med* 2003; **4**(1): 52–4.

Further reading
Books
Practical Management of Pediatric Cardiac Arrhythmias, eds. P C. Gillette and V L. Zeigler. U.S.A, Futura Publishing Co Inc..

Clinical Pediatric Arrhythmias, eds. P C. Gillette and, A. Garson. USA, W.B. Saunders Ltd

Websites
http://www.childsdoc.org/fall98/st/svt.asp.
http://www.emedicine.com/ped/topic2535.htm.

http://www.emedicine.com/med/topic2417.htm.

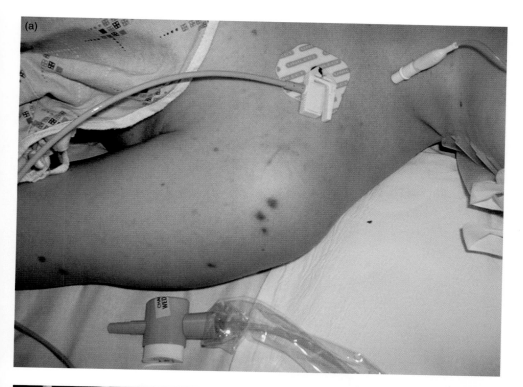

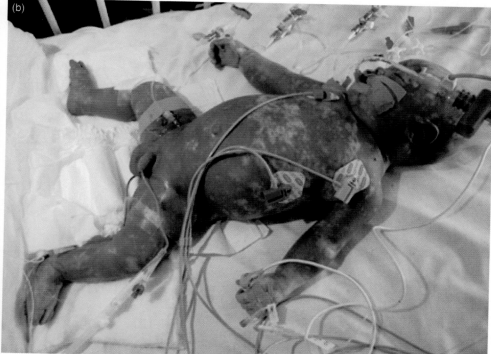

Fig. 2.1. (a) and (b): Petechial rash, purpura fulminans.

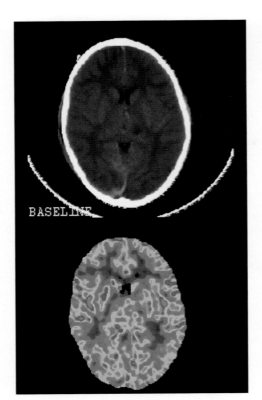

Fig. 5.2. CT scan of head and Xenon perfusion study demonstrating average cerebral blood flows in the range of 50–70 ml/100 g per min. No areas of ischemia or oligemia could be identified.

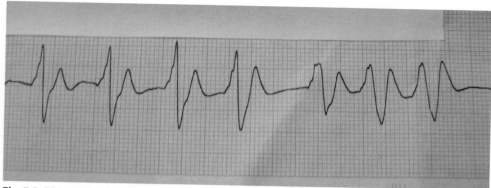

Fig. 7.3. ECG on arrival in PICU. Rate 90–120, QRS 0.12–0.132 s, QTc 0.549 s (normal <0.45).

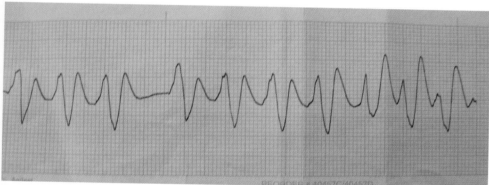

Fig. 7.4. ECG 1 hour later showing polymorphous QRS complexes leading to ventricular tachycardia.

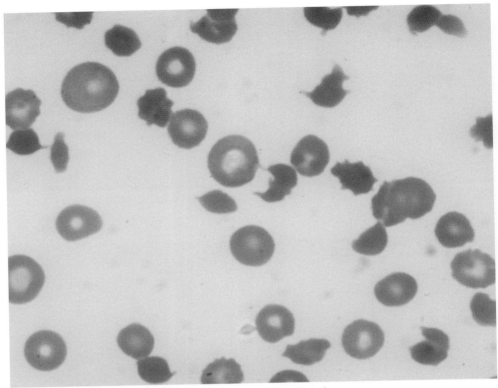

Fig. 8.1. Blood smear showing schistocytes (red blood cell fragmentation).

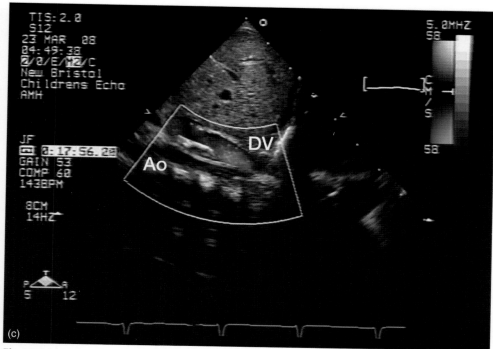

Fig. 10.2 (c).

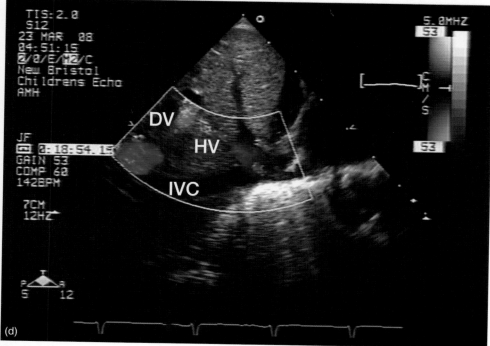

Fig. 10.2 (d).

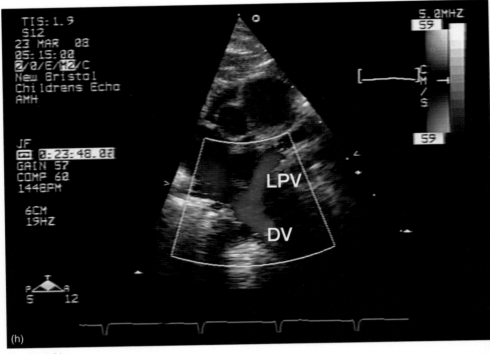

Fig. 10.2 (h).

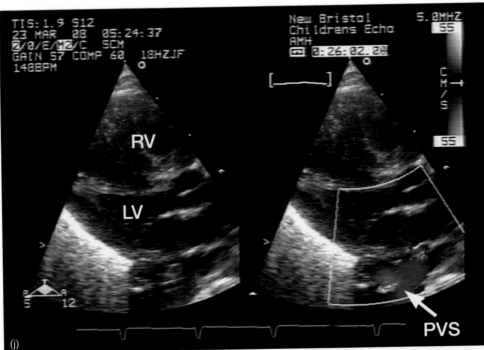

Fig. 10.2 (j). Series of echocardiograph images of obstructed TAPVC. RV = Right Ventricle, LV = Left Ventricle, IVC = Inferior Vena Cava, Ao = Aorta, DV = Descending Vein, LPV = Left Pulmonary Vein, HV = Hepatic Vein, PVS = Pulmonary Veins.

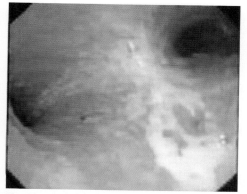 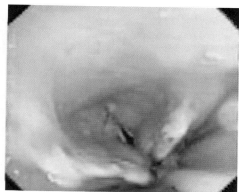

Fig. 23.5 and Fig. 23.6. Edema, ulceration, sloughing of airway mucosa at the level of carina and larynx as seen on fiberoptic bronchoscopy. (Images courtesy of Lee Woodson, MD, Ph.D.; University of Texas Medical Branch, Shriners' Burns Hospital; Galveston, TX.).

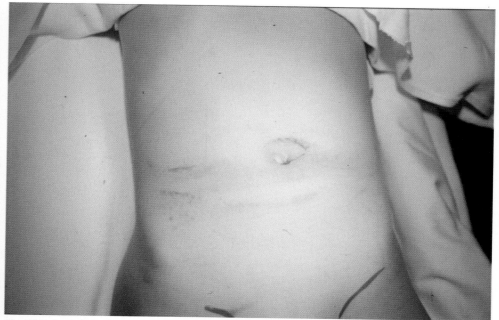

Fig. 24.7. Seatbelt Syndrome.

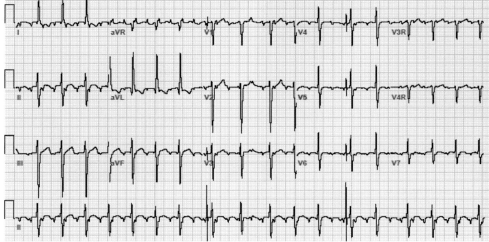

Fig. 25.2. Intra-atrial re-entrant tachycardia (IART) with 2:1 conduction.

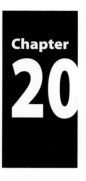

Chapter

20 The neonate with hyperammonemia

Stephen D. Playfor and Andrew A. M. Morris

Introduction

Ammonia is formed primarily during the degradation of amino acids in the liver (Fig. 20.1). This occurs whenever the diet contains more amino acids than are needed for protein synthesis, because amino acids cannot be stored. Amino acids are also degraded at times of stress, when they are released from proteins for use as fuel. Other sources of ammonia include the purine–nucleotide cycle and absorption from the intestine, where it is formed by bacteria. Ammonia is toxic and plasma concentrations are normally kept below about 35 μmol l^{-1}. Ammonia is converted to urea by the urea cycle in the periportal hepatocytes of the liver. Urea is relatively harmless and circulates at concentrations of several mmol l^{-1} before being excreted in the urine. The conversion of dietary nitrogen to urea increases with age, with a term infant excreting around 19% of their dietary nitrogen as urea nitrogen whilst children over the age of 6 years may excrete 50% of their dietary nitrogen as urea nitrogen.

Hyperammonemia occurs in many inborn errors of metabolism, including primary disorders of the urea cycle and organic acidemias, in which the urea cycle is inhibited by the accumulating metabolites. Moderately elevated levels of ammonia are relatively common in neonates and may be caused by acquired problems, such as sepsis or perinatal asphyxia. High plasma levels of ammonia are very toxic to the central nervous system and can result in death and permanent neurologic deficit.

Case history

A baby boy was born at term by spontaneous vaginal delivery, after an uneventful pregnancy, weighing 2.7 kg. He required no resuscitation at birth and fed well from the breast, being discharged home at 24 h of age. From day 2 of life, the baby became less interested in feeding and increasingly lethargic. On day 3, his parents noted that he was difficult to rouse and took him to the accident and emergency department of their local hospital.

Presentation

On arrival in the accident and emergency department, the baby was breathing spontaneously but shallowly and at a rapid rate of 85 breaths per minute. Pulse oximetry revealed saturations of 97% in air and 15 l min^{-1} of oxygen was administered by face mask. Heart rate was 130 beats per minute and his capillary refill time was 3 seconds, femoral pulses were easily palpable. The child was profoundly hypotonic and responsive only to pain. He was hypothermic with a tympanic temperature of 34.7 °C. Intravenous access was secured and blood was sent for full blood count, urea and electrolytes, glucose and blood culture. A fluid bolus of 50 ml of 0.9% saline was given intravenously. A fingerprick blood glucose estimation showed a blood glucose level of 5.7 mmol l^{-1} and a capillary blood gas revealed a marked

Case Studies in Pediatric Critical Care, ed. Peter. J. Murphy, Stephen C. Marriage, and Peter J. Davis. Published by Cambridge University Press. © Cambridge University Press 2009.

Table 20.1. *Findings on admission*

Examination	Airway clear, sats 97% in air, face mask oxygen	
	Respiratory rate 85 min^{-1}	
	Chest clear, bilateral air entry	
	Heart rate 130 min^{-1}, Capillary refill time = 3 seconds	
	Normal heart sounds, BP 95/60, femoral pulses palpable	
	Temperature 34.7 °C	
Investigations	Weight	2.3 kg (Birth weight 2.7 kg)
	FBC	Hb 16.2 g dl^{-1}, Plat 355 × 10^9 l^{-1}, WBC 13.4 × 10^9 l^{-1}
	U+Es	Na$^+$ 143 mmol l^{-1}, K$^+$ 4.3 mmol l^{-1}, Urea 15.9 mmol l^{-1}, Creatinine 157 μmol l^{-1} Mg^{2+} 1.1 mmol l^{-1}, Cl$^-$ 110 mmol l^{-1} Ca^{2+} 2.1 mmol l^{-1}
	Glucose	6.5 mmol l^{-1}
	Capillary blood gas	pH 7.01, pCO$_2$ 15.2 mmHg, HCO$_3^-$ 4.9 mmol l^{-1}, BE−25.2
	Lumbar	CSF glucose 3.9 mmol l^{-1}, CSF protein 2.2 g l^{-1}
	Puncture	WBC 1.2 × 10^6 l^{-1}, RBC 2.0 × 10^9 l^{-1} No organisms seen
	Supra-pubic	WBC 0, RBC 0
	aspirate	No organisms seen

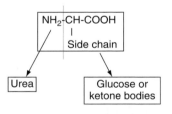

Fig. 20.1. Amino acid degradation. Urea cycle disorders interfere with the conversion of the amino group to urea. Defects in the conversion of the carbon skeleton to glucose, or ketone bodies give rise to organic acidemias.

metabolic acidosis as summarized in Table 20.1 along with other laboratory results. An intravenous dose of cefotaxime 125 mg was administered along with 3 ml of 8.4% sodium bicarbonate solution.

The child was commenced on an intravenous infusion of 10% dextrose/0.9% saline at a rate of 100 ml kg^{-1} per day. A lumbar puncture and a supra-pubic urine aspirate were obtained and sent to the laboratory (Table 20.1).

The child was transferred to the pediatric ward and reassessed by the consultant pediatrician. A plasma ammonia and lactate specimen were taken along with a repeat capillary blood gas specimen: pH 7.14, pCO$_2$ 19.8 mmHg, HCO$_3^-$ 5.7 mmol l^{-1}, BE − 20.6. As the blood gas result was being telephoned back to the ward the child began to have abnormal movements of his legs; bilateral, rhythmical clonic jerking of the legs was noted and on closer inspection his eyes were deviated to the left. A repeat fingerprick blood glucose estimation showed a blood glucose level of 6.1 mmol l^{-1}. The child was administered intravenous phenobarbital at a dose of 50 mg over 10 minutes. Ten minutes after the phenobarbital had been administered, the abnormal movements ceased but the child was noted to be unresponsive and pulse oximetry showed a saturation of 87% despite 15 l min^{-1} of oxygen. Bag valve mask ventilation was commenced and the duty anesthetist urgently summoned. Endotracheal intubation was carried out with a 3.0 mm oral endotracheal tube without the need for anesthetic drugs. The endotracheal tube was secured and the child was transferred to the neonatal intensive care unit where mechanical ventilation was instigated; intermittent mandatory ventilation, pressures 18/4, rate 40 breaths per minute, inspiratory time 0.7 second, FiO_2 0.3. The biochemist telephoned the most recent results back to the unit at this point: plasma ammonia 970 μmol l^{-1}, lactate 2.6 mmol l^{-1}.

The regional pediatric intensive care unit was contacted by telephone and the child was referred for further management. The pediatric intensive care retrieval team was mobilized and the regional metabolic disease consultant notified. According to established clinical guidelines, the referring hospital was advised to administer sodium benzoate 250 mg kg^{-1} together with sodium phenylbutyrate 250 mg kg^{-1} and arginine hydrochloride 200 mg kg^{-1} made up to a volume of 30 ml kg^{-1} with 10% dextrose and administered intravenously over 90 minutes. After the completion of this bolus, a similar intravenous infusion containing sodium benzoate 250 mg kg^{-1}, together with sodium phenylbutyrate 250 mg kg^{-1}, arginine hydrochloride 200 mg kg^{-1} and L-carnitine 100 mg kg^{-1} made up to a volume of 30 ml kg^{-1} with 10% dextrose and administered over 24 hours.

When the retrieval team arrived, the oral endotracheal tube was exchanged for a nasal one and an intravenous infusion of morphine was commenced at 15 mcg kg^{-1} per h. A 22G arterial line was inserted into the right radial artery to allow for invasive blood pressure monitoring and blood gas monitoring. Intravenous maintenance fluid was changed to 10% dextrose without saline. The return ambulance journey of 2 hours was uneventful and the child remained clinically stable.

Progress in the pediatric intensive care unit

On arrival at the regional center a full metabolic screen was sent to the reference laboratory including a repeat ammonia level which was 950 μmol l^{-1}. A 6.5F, 10 cm double lumen central line catheter was inserted into her right femoral vein under sterile conditions, using the Seldinger technique. Continuous veno-venous hemofiltration (CVVH) was commenced using a neonatal hemofilter and neonatal lines primed with blood with an initial blood flow rate of 10 ml h^{-1} which was increased up to 25 ml h^{-1} over the first 20 minutes. Fluid loss was programed to account only for the intravenous drugs being administered, leaving the child in a neutral balance excluding urine output and unmeasured losses. Replacement fluid flow rate was started at 100 ml h^{-1} and this was rapidly increased up to 400 ml h^{-1}. Intravenous cefotaxime 125 mg, 6-hourly was continued, as was intravenous phenobarbital at a dose of 10 mg 12-hourly. Six hours after admission the child was still unresponsive and the intravenous morphine infusion was discontinued. A repeat plasma ammonia was found to be 750 μmol l^{-1} and the acidosis had improved on analysis of the arterial blood gases; pH 7.30, pO_2 98.6 mmHg, pCO_2 28.7 mmHg, HCO_3^- 13.3 mmol l^{-1}, BE −11.4. The blood glucose level had risen to 14.3 mmol l^{-1} with ketonuria. An intravenous insulin infusion was commenced at 0.05 units kg^{-1} per h and close monitoring over the next few hours saw the blood glucose level stabilize between 7.7–9.5 mmol l^{-1}. The pediatric intensivist and the metabolic disease consultant met with the family of the child along with the nurse looking after the patient. The family were counseled as to the likely diagnosis of an inherited metabolic disorder and of the uncertainty surrounding the child's prognosis, in particular, the possibility of some degree of handicap as a consequence of the elevated ammonia levels.

After 24 hours of CVVH the plasma ammonia had fallen to 424 µmol l^{-1} and the arterial blood gas had improved further: pH 7.34, pO_2 101 mmHg, pCO_2 41.6 mmHg, HCO_3^- 20.4 mmol l^{-1}, BE −4.9. Given that the child's modified Glasgow Coma Score remained 3/15 with 4 mm-sized, sluggishly reactive pupils and a tense anterior fontanelle, a cranial ultrasound was carried out, which revealed a slightly compressed ventricular system sugges-tive of raised intracranial pressure. There was no suspicion of further seizure activity. Analysis of the urine organic acids established the diagnosis of Methylmalonic Acidemia (MMA) and this was discussed with the family by the metabolic team.

After 36 hours of CVVH the plasma ammonia had fallen further to 147 µmol l^{-1} and the arterial blood gas remained stable; pH 7.34, pO_2 121 mmHg, pCO_2 37.2 mmHg, HCO_3^- 21.3 mmol l^{-1}, BE −3.6. CVVH was discontinued and nasogastric feeds were introduced using expressed breast milk. With the tolerance of enteral feeds the intravenous fluids were discontinued as was the intravenous insulin infusion. The child was also found to be more responsive, was reacting to painful stimuli and was making efforts to breathe.

Despite the discontinuation of CVVH, the plasma ammonia continued to fall to 98 µmol l^{-1} at 48 hours of admission. The child was increasingly responsive and the mechanical ventilation was weaned accordingly to synchronised intermittent mandatory ventilation, pressures 16/4, rate 5 breaths per minute, inspiratory time 0.7 second, FiO_2 0.24.

At 72 hours of admission to PICU with the plasma ammonia at 73 µmol l^{-1}, the child was successfully extubated. He remained on PICU for a further 6 hours before being discharged onto the high dependency unit attached to PICU.

Discussion

Hyperammonemia has toxic effects on several organs, including the liver, but it is particularly damaging to the central nervous system. The mechanism of neurotoxicity is uncertain, but it is thought to be mediated in part by increased extracellular levels of glutamate in the brain and activation of N-methyl D-Aspartate (NMDA) receptors. Cerebral edema is the main cause of death in hyperammonemia, and survivors of coma have a high incidence of permanent neuro-logical disability. Even mild cases of hyperammonemia may result in a degree of cognitive impairment.[1] In a study of 216 patients with urea cycle disorders, 18 of the 20 long-term survivors who had a neonatal onset of disease had moderate to severe neurodevelopmental deficits.[2] Another finding of this study was that the neurodevelopmental outcome correlated with the peak blood ammonia concentration during presentation. Blood ammonia levels below 180 µmol l^{-1} were not associated with severe neurodevelopmental deficits, whereas levels above 350 µmol l^{-1} were associated with death or severe neurodevelopmental deficit.

Plasma ammonia concentrations are always low immediately after delivery, even in neonates with severe urea cycle disorders, because ammonia crosses the placenta and is disposed of by the mother. The same is true for other small molecules such as organic acids. Thus, babies with urea cycle disorders or organic acidemias are well initially for a period of 12–48 hours. As the ammonia level rises, the baby becomes symptomatic with poor feeding, lethargy, irritability, and vomiting. These symptoms correlate with an ammonia level of

$150–250$ µmol l^{-1}. This may be followed by grunting and hyperventilation due to direct stimulation of the respiratory centre in the medulla by the ammonium ion. As the ammonia level rises further, seizures may occur and the baby becomes comatose.

There are no specific physical findings associated with hyperammonemia. Affected neonates usually present with lethargy, hypotonia, and a reduced level of consciousness. Tachypnea may be caused directly by hyperammonemia or (inorganic acidemias), it may be respiratory compensation for a metabolic acidosis. Dehydration is common, sometimes secondary to vomiting but sometimes because an accumulating metabolite (such as methylmalonic acid) acts as an osmotic diuretic. Occasionally, physical examination will reveal a finding specific to an underlying inborn error of metabolism, such as the odor of "sweaty feet" in isovaleric acidemia. Some patients with argininosuccinic aciduria develop abnormal fragile hair but this is not noticeable in neonates.

Causes of hyperammonemia

Severe hyperammonemia (>350 µmol l^{-1}) is usually caused by an inborn error of the urea cycle or a "branched-chain organic acidemia" (Fig. 20.2). Urea cycle disorders result from defects in genes coding for enzymes or membrane transport systems involved in the production of urea. In the absence of newborn screening, estimation of the prevalence of urea cycle defects is difficult, but the total prevalence may be around $1:10\,000$ live births. Ornithine transcarbamoylase (OTC) deficiency is the commonest urea cycle disorder and it is inherited as an X-linked trait (unlike the other urea cycle disorders, which are autosomal recessive). Most male patients present with severe neonatal hyperammonemia and the prognosis is poor. Many female carriers are asymptomatic, but they may be affected to a variable degree depending on the X-inactivation pattern in the liver. (In each cell, one X chromosome is inactivated and the patient will be symptomatic if the chromosome with the normal OTC gene is inactivated in most hepatocytes.)

Branched-chain organic acidemias are caused by defects in the breakdown of branched-chain amino acids (leucine, isoleucine, and valine). Methylmalonic, propionic, and isovaleric

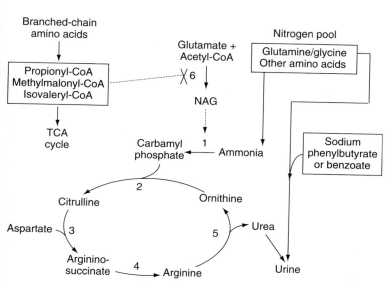

Fig. 20.2. The urea cycle and the cause of hyperammonemia in branched-chain organic acidemias. NAG = N-acetylglutamate. Enzymes 1 = carbamoyl phosphate synthetase; 2 = ornithine transcarbamoylase; 3 = argininosuccinate synthase; 4 = argininosuccinate lyase; 5 = arginase; 6 = NAG synthetase.

acidemias are the commonest of these disorders. All can cause severe hyperammonemia, probably by inhibiting N-acetylglutamate synthetase (Fig. 20.2). Most of these patients have a metabolic acidosis, but this may not be present in the early stages. Other features may include hypoglycemia, hypothermia, hypocalcemia, and leukopenia or thrombocytopenia due to bone marrow suppression. As mentioned above, patients with Methylmalonic Acidemia (MMA) may be dehydrated due to an osmotic diuresis.

Other inherited metabolic diseases that may be associated with hyperammonemia include fatty acid oxidation defects, congenital lactic acidoses, and lysinuric protein intolerance (Table 20.2). Plasma ammonia concentrations are usually less than 400 μmol l^{-1} in these disorders, and other problems dominate the clinical picture.

In neonates, mild to moderate hyperammonemia can be caused by any serious illness, including sepsis and perinatal asphyxia. In most of these cases, the plasma ammonia concentration is less than about 200 μmol l^{-1}. Other acquired causes of hyperammonemia include neonatal *Herpes simplex* infection, drugs (sodium valproate, chemotherapeutic agents, and salicylates) and liver disease. Transient hyperammonemia of the newborn is a rare but serious condition, predominantly seen in premature infants.[3] The onset of symptoms is usually on the first or second day of life and often before the introduction of any protein. Affected infants have decreased levels of consciousness and may have seizures, unreactive pupils, and loss of the occulocephalic reflex. Because of these non-specific clinical findings, hypoxic–ischemic encephalopathy and intracranial hemorrhage are frequently suspected. The hyperammonemia is usually severe and frequently warrants hemofiltration or hemodialysis. The cause is uncertain but it may be delayed maturation of the urea cycle. Mortality is 20–30% and 35–45% of affected infants suffer permanent neurological disability.

Plasma ammonia concentrations above 500 μmol l^{-1} are almost always caused by a urea cycle disorder, a branched-chain organic acidemia or transient hyperammonemia of the newborn.[4] Concentrations between 200 and 500 μmol l^{-1} suggest an inborn error, but the differential diagnosis is wider. Indeed, a number of these values are artefactual, due to the sample not being taken or processed appropriately.[4] It is, therefore, essential to send a repeat sample whenever a high ammonia value is reported.

Management of hyperammonemia

The aim of therapy in hyperammonemia should be to maintain blood ammonia levels within the normal range. The principles of treatment are as follows for a neonate with a blood ammonia level of more than 200 μmol l^{-1}.

1. Minimize endogenous ammonia production.
2. Administer substrates of the urea cycle that may be deficient.
3. Administer compounds that facilitate the removal of ammonia via alternative pathways.
4. Consider dialysis or hemofiltration for rapid reduction of ammonia levels.

Endogenous ammonia production is minimized by stopping protein administration. It is also important to prevent catabolism by providing sufficient energy in the form of carbohydrate with or without lipid. If the ammonia concentration is above 200 μmol l^{-1}, enteral feeds should be stopped and intravenous glucose (with or without lipid) should be given.

In some urea cycle disorders, the segment of the cycle that remains intact can be exploited to eliminate ammonia. Thus, arginine can be converted to citrulline, which is excreted in

Table 20.2. *Inborn errors of metabolism causing hyperammonemia*

Urea cycle defects	N-acetylglutamate (NAG) synthetase deficiency	NAG activates CPS I, the first enzyme of the urea cycle
	Carbamoyl phosphate synthetase I (CPS I) deficiency	Majority of affected infants die in the neonatal period
	Ornithine transcarbamoylase (OTC) deficiency	X-linked inheritance. The commonest urea cycle defect
	Argininosuccinate synthetase deficiency (citrullinemia)	The second most common urea cycle disorder
	Argininosuccinate lyase deficiency (argininosuccinic aciduria)	Abnormal fragile hair and chronic liver disease in some older subjects
	Arginase deficiency	Main problem is spastic diplegia. Acute hyperammonemia is unusual
	Hyperammonemia-hyperornithinemia-homocitrullinuria (HHH)	Urea cycle is interrupted by defective transport of ornithine into mitochondria
Organic acidemias	Methylmalonic acidemia (MMA) Propionic acidemia Isovaleric acidemia	Often present in the neonatal period with hyperammonemia and acidosis. Other features may include hypoglycemia, hypothermia, hypocalcemia, and bone marrow suppression
	3-Hydroxy-3-methylglutaryl (HMG)-CoA lyase deficiency	Presents with hypoglycemia, acidosis and hyperammonemia, often in neonates.
Fatty acid oxidation defects	Medium chain acyl-CoA dehydrogenase (MCAD) deficiency and other defects	Present with hypoglycemic encephalopathy ± myopathy or cardiomyopathy. During acute illness there is often moderate hyperammonemia
Congenital lactic acidoses	Pyruvate carboxylase deficiency	Presents with acidosis or neurological problems ± hyperammonemia
	Pyruvate dehydrogenase deficiency	Presents with acidosis or neurological problems. Occasionally hyperammonemia
	Mitochondrial disorders	Hyperammonemia is rare
Dibasic amino acid transport defects	Lysinuric protein intolerance	Post-prandial hyperammonemia in infancy leads to protein aversion and failure to thrive

argininosuccinate synthase deficiency, and to argininosuccinic acid, which is excreted in argininosuccinate lyase deficiency. In both cases, there is incorporation of carbamoylphosphate. Administration of arginine can, therefore, lead to the excretion of carbamoylphosphate. In carbamoyl phosphate synthetase I (CPS I) and OTC deficiencies, there is no equivalent beneficial action for arginine, nor for any other urea cycle substrate.

Amino acids are normally re-absorbed in the renal tubules, but they can be excreted after conjugation to another chemical. Sodium benzoate and sodium phenylbutyrate react with amino acids and allow nitrogen excretion by an alternative pathway to the urea cycle

(Fig. 20.2). Glycine N-acyltransferase catalyzes the reaction of benzoate with glycine to form hippurate, primarily in the liver and kidney. Phenylbutyrate is first activated to its CoA ester, then metabolized by β-oxidation in the liver to phenylacetyl-CoA, which is subsequently conjugated with glutamine. In some countries, sodium phenylacetate is marketed as an alternative to sodium phenylbutyrate.

In NAG synthetase deficiency, the urea cycle is intact but CPS I has low activity due to lack of its activator, NAG. N-carbamylglutamate is an analog of NAG that is active when administered enterally and it can prevent hyperammonemia in NAG synthetase deficiency. In the branched-chain organic acidemias, hyperammonemia is caused by inhibition of NAG synthetase. Treatment with N-carbamylglutamate has led to a rapid fall in plasma ammonia concentrations in a number of neonates with propionic or methylmalonic acidemia, avoiding the need for more invasive management.[5] The recommended dose is 250 mg kg^{-1} through a nasogastric tube; no intravenous preparation is available. In neonates, one cannot reliably distinguish between urea cycle disorders and organic acidemias until definitive investigations are available. We therefore suggest that N-carbamylglutamate is given in all cases of severe neonatal hyperammonemia, at the same time as starting intravenous sodium benzoate, sodium phenylbutyrate, and arginine. Hemodialysis/filtration should be made at the same time and the procedure should be started if the ammonia concentration has not improved significantly after 3 hours.

The degree of neurological damage in severe hyperammonemia is related to the duration of exposure. Dialysis reduces ammonia concentrations much faster than the measures outlined above and it has been used in hyperammonemic infants since the late 1970s. Dialysis or related procedures should be considered if the plasma ammonia concentration is greater than 500 μmol l^{-1} or when the initial plasma ammonia is greater than 350 μmol l^{-1} and it is no lower after 3 hours of intravenous drug therapy. Ammonia is a low molecular weight molecule, smaller than urea, and as such it can be cleared across a semipermeable membrane with an equal or greater clearance rate than that achieved for urea. Various modes of dialysis have been shown to be effective in reducing blood ammonia levels, including continuous venovenous hemofiltration (CVVH), hemodialysis (HD), continuous venovenous diafiltration (CVVHD),[6,7] continuous arteriovenous diafiltration (CAVHD)[8] or peritoneal dialysis (PD) (although this is much less effective). CVVHD is a mode of continual renal replacement therapy, which allows for the clearance of blood solutes both by diffusion across a semipermeable membrane (hemodialysis) and by convection of solutes across a membrane as they are separated from whole blood in response to hydrostatic pressure (hemofiltration). An additional technique involves the use of an extracorporeal membrane oxygenation (ECMO) pump system to drive a hemodialysis machine.[9]

Each method of dialysis has its own advantages and drawbacks. Although superior to previously used techniques such as exchange transfusion or pharmacological treatment alone, PD clears ammonia at a relatively slow rate of 3–5 ml min^{-1} and may take several days to reduce the level of blood ammonia. It should only be used where the other techniques are impossible (for example, in very small babies). CVVH clears ammonia at 10–30 ml min^{-1}, whilst ECMO/HD can achieve clearances of up to 200 ml min.$^{-1}$ CVVH has the advantage, however, of being better tolerated than HD in terms of cardiovascular stability, and it can be established more quickly in the majority of PICUs.

Dialysis techniques are less effective when the plasma ammonia levels fall below 200 μmol l^{-1} and dialysis can be discontinued at this point, although it is important to remain vigilant for any possible rebound in ammonia levels that may occur following this discontinuation. One should also consider discontinuation of dialysis if it is ineffective: if the ammonia level remains over 1000 μmol l^{-1} after 24 hours of effective treatment, then the outlook for the child is very poor.

The long-term management of patients with urea cycle disorders involves the use of a low-protein diet, supplementation with arginine (or citrulline) and administration of sodium benzoate and/or sodium phenylbutyrate to augment waste nitrogen excretion (see above). Most patients with branched-chain organic acidemias also require a low-protein diet. Carnitine supplements are usually prescribed and some patients with methylmalonic acidemia respond to treatment with vitamin B$_{12}$. In isovaleric acidemia, excretion of the organic acid is promoted by treatment with glycine. In methylmalonic and propionic acidemias, some of the organic acids are derived from gut bacteria and this can be reduced by giving metronidazole.

Plans need to be made for how to deal with periods of intercurrent illness and elective surgery because catabolism can precipitate episodes of metabolic decompensation. To minimize the risk of this, patients are given an emergency regimen, which involves stopping all dietary protein and administering drinks containing a glucose polymer every 2–3 hours. Drugs should be divided into small frequent doses to minimize the likelihood of vomiting. Vomiting or clinical deterioration necessitates hospital admission, for intravenous therapy and monitoring of the ammonia concentration.

Learning difficulties and neurological impairment are regrettably common. Other long-term complications include chronic renal failure in methylmalonic acidemia. Because of the poor outcome with conventional treatment, orthotopic liver transplantation is being performed in an increasing number of patients with severe urea cycle disorders and branched-chain organic acidemias. Management always requires a multidisciplinary approach, involving dietetics, genetic counseling, and often physical and occupational therapy, speech therapy, and educational services.

Initial assessment and management

Initial assessment and management of a child with hyperammonemia follows the ABC pattern:

A Airway

B Breathing

C Circulation

Neonates with symptomatic hyperammonemia should have their airways secured through endotracheal intubation and mechanical ventilation should be commenced. Frequently, such infants are dehydrated at presentation and may have circulatory compromise. Intravenous fluid resuscitation should be promptly administered if there are any signs of circulatory insufficiency.

Enteral feeds should be suspended and intravenous 10% dextrose should be commenced at a rate of at least 90 ml kg^{-1} per day in order to stop catabolism. Additional sodium can usually be excluded from maintenance fluids as the ammonia-lowering agents used in this condition contain large amounts. If hyperglycemia becomes a problem (consistently >13 mmol l^{-1} with glycosuria), do not reduce the dextrose infusion but infuse intravenous insulin, initially at 0.05 U kg^{-1} per h, whilst paying close attention to blood glucose levels.

Ammonia lowering agents should be administered at the referring hospital if they are available. Otherwise, they should be taken to the patient by the retrieving PICU team or commenced immediately on arrival at PICU if the patient is brought by the transport team of a referring hospital.

Drugs used in patients with undiagnosed hyperammonemia

Loading dose

> Sodium benzoate 250 mg kg^{-1}
> Sodium phenylbutyrate 250 mg kg^{-1}
> Arginine hydrochloride 600 mg kg^{-1}

All made up to a volume of 30 ml kg^{-1} with 10% dextrose and administered intravenously over 90 minutes.

Maintenance infusion

> Sodium benzoate 250 mg kg^{-1}
> Sodium phenylbutyrate 250 mg kg^{-1}
> Arginine hydrochloride 600 mg kg^{-1}
> L-carnitine 100 mg kg^{-1}

All are made up to a volume of 30 ml kg^{-1} with 10% dextrose and administered intravenously over 24 hours[10].

Dialysis techniques

Dialysis techniques should be undertaken if the plasma ammonia concentration is greater than 500 µmol l^{-1} or when the initial plasma ammonia is greater than 350 µmol l^{-1} and it is no lower after 3 hours of intravenous drug therapy with ammonia lowering agents.

CVVH or HD should be instigated in neonates weighing more than 2.5 kg but these techniques may not be possible in very small babies and in these circumstances PD may have to be considered.

Learning points

- Attention should initially focus on securing the airway and maintaining the breathing and circulation when approaching the child with hyperammonemia.
- Inborn errors of metabolism should always be considered as a differential diagnosis in the sick neonate as the initial features of hyperammonemia (poor feeding and drowsiness) may be present in many different diseases. The presence of a respiratory alkalosis due to direct stimulation of the respiratory center may be suggestive of hyperammonemia in a child otherwise thought to be suffering from sepsis.
- All feeds containing protein should be discontinued and intravenous glucose should be administered. Intravenous therapy with ammonia-scavenging drugs should be commenced whenever hyperammonemia is associated with central nervous system symptoms.
- All neonates with symptomatic hyperammonemia should be urgently transferred to an intensive care facility offering CVVH or hemodialysis.
- CVVH or hemodialysis should be commenced if the plasma ammonia concentration is greater than 500 µmol l^{-1} or when the initial plasma ammonia is greater than 350 µmol l^{-1} and is no lower after 3 hours of intravenous drugs.

References

1. Maestri NE, Clissold DB, Brusilow SW. Long-term survival of patients with argininosuccinate synthetase deficiency. *J Pediatr* 1995; **127**: 929–35.

2. Uchino T, Endo F, Matsuda I. Neurodevelopmental outcome of long-term therapy of urea cycle disorders in Japan. *J Inherit Metab Dis* 1998; 21 (Suppl 1): 151–9.

3. Hudak ML, Jones MD Jr, Brusilow SW. Differentiation of transient hyperammonemia of the newborn and urea cycle enzyme defects by clinical presentation. *J Pediatr* 1985; **107**: 712–19.

4. Chow SL, Gandhi V, Krywawych S *et al.* The significance of a high plasma ammonia value. *Arch Dis Child* 2004; **89**: 585–6.

5. Gebhardt B, Dittrich S, Parbel S *et al.* N-carbamylglutamate protects patients with decompensated propionic aciduria from hyperammonaemia. *J Inherit Metab Dis* 2005; **28**: 241–4.

6. Braun MC, Welch TR. Continuous venovenous hemodiafiltration in the treatment of acute hyperammonemia. *Am J Nephrol* 1998; **18**: 531–3.

7. Schaefer F, Straube E, Oh J *et al.* Dialysis in neonates with inborn errors of metabolism. *Nephrol Dial Transplant* 1999; **14**: 910–18.

8. Chen CY, Chen YC, Fang JT *et al.* Continuous arteriovenous hemodiafiltration in the acute treatment of hyperammonaemia due to ornithine transcarbamylase deficiency. *Ren Fail* 2000; **22**: 823–36.

9. Summar M, Pietsch J, Deshpande J *et al.* Effective hemodialysis and hemofiltration driven by an extracorporeal membrane oxygenation pump in infants with hyperammonemia. *J Pediatr* 1996; **128**: 379–82.

10. Summar M. Current strategies for the management of neonatal urea cycle disorders. *J Pediatr* 2001; **138**(Suppl 1): S30–9.

Further reading

Leonard JV Disorders of the urea cycle. In Fernandes J, Saudubray JM, van den Berghe G, eds. *Inborn Metabolic Diseases*, 3rd edn. Heidelberg, Springer-Verlag, 2000; 214–22.

Ogier de Baulny H, Saudubray J-M. Branched-chain organic acidurias. In Fernandes J, Saudubray JM, van den Berghe G, eds. *Inborn Metabolic Diseases*, 3rd edn. Heidelberg, Springer-Verlag, 2000; 196–212.

Management of acute heart failure in pediatric intensive care

Matthew Fenton and Michael Burch

Introduction

In this chapter we present a compilation of three short case reports, each representing a different age group. The reports illustrate aspects relating to the etiology, diagnosis, and management of acute heart failure in the pediatric intensive care unit.

Case history 1

A 6-month-old baby presented with severe cardiac failure to the local district general hospital. Delivery had been at term with no antenatal or neonatal problems. Parents were consanguineous and were from the Bangladeshi community in East London. Breastfeeding had gone well initially, although over the past week the baby's mother had noted that the child was more breathless whilst drinking and unable to complete a full bottle. On the evening of admission, the parents had noted the child to be severely breathless and unable to take any feeds during the day. On arrival at the local accident and emergency department the pediatric team were concerned that the infant was in acute heart failure. Despite intravenous furosemide, the baby was severely breathless, and initial blood gas showed a metabolic acidosis. There was poor peripheral perfusion. It was decided to electively ventilate and transfer was arranged via the regional retrieval team. On arrival at the cardiac intensive care unit, initial examination revealed very poor perfusion with capillary refill time of over 4 seconds. Peripheral pulses were all reduced. There was 5 cm of hepatomegaly. Saturations were normal in 50% oxygen. Chest X-ray showed gross cardiomegaly and severe pulmonary edema.

Echocardiography showed a structurally normal heart with no evidence of a congenital structural problem. The systolic function of the ventricle was very poor with a fractional shortening of less than 10%. There was significant mitral regurgitation. Both the left atrium and the left ventricle were grossly enlarged. Right ventricular function was better than the left. There was no evidence of an atrial septal defect.

Management

Intravenous central lines were sited and inotropic support was begun with adrenaline and milrinone. Initial dose of adrenaline was 0.01 mcg kg^{-1} per min and milrinone 0.7 mcg kg^{-1} per min. Initial U and Es showed a creatinine of 190 µmol l^{-1}. Urine output remained poor for the subsequent 6 hours and, despite inotropic support, the acidosis continued with a base deficit of −10. An elective decision was therefore made to provide mechanical support using extra-corporeal membrane oxygenation (ECMO). The cardiac surgical team was contacted and a cut-down via the neck vessels was performed. The child was then taken to the

Case Studies in Pediatric Critical Care, ed. Peter. J. Murphy, Stephen C. Marriage, and Peter J. Davis.
Published by Cambridge University Press. © Cambridge University Press 2009.

cardiac catheterization laboratory for a percutaneous atrial septostomy to be performed. Simultaneously with this procedure, a cardiac biopsy was performed to obtain myocardium for histology and PCR for viral analysis. Bloods were sent for metabolic and laboratory investigations including aclycarnitine, lactate, and pyruvate. A viral screen was taken from stool and respiratory secretions. PCR was performed on the blood for common viruses causing myocarditis.

After 6 days of ECMO support, no improvement in left ventricular function occurred. Viral PCR was positive in both myocardium and blood for enterovirus. ECMO support was continued for a further week and, at the end of the second 7 days, ventricular function improved enough for ECMO support to be withdrawn. Inotropic support was needed for a further week and then oral anti-failure therapy was begun with captopril, digoxin and diuretics. The infant was eventually discharged from hospital after a further 2 weeks of medical therapy. At follow-up 6 months from presentation, left ventricular function remained very poor, but at 1 year after presentation, left ventricular function improved substantially and anti-failure treatment was reduced.

Discussion

The differential diagnosis for the cause of cardiac failure in a child this age usually falls into one of the following categories:

1. Viral myocarditis cause by *Entero/Coxsackie virus*, *Adenovirus* and *Parvovirus*;
2. Familial cardiomyopathy/metabolic;
3. Cardiac structural abnormality (ALCAPA and coarctation of the aorta);
4. Idiopathic dilated cardiomyopathy.

The incidence of heart failure due to heart muscle disease is 0.87 per 100 000 for children under 16 in the UK and outcome is better for younger children. Overall, a third of children will die or require cardiac transplantation within the first year.[1]

The presentation of viral myocarditis in an infant can be very dramatic with severe heart failure, leading to a requirement for mechanical support early in the course of treatment. The most common viruses causing myocarditis in Europe are *Enterovirus/Coxsackie virus*, *Adenovirus* and *Parvovirus*. Prognosis of these infants is often poor and ECMO support may be required, ensuring adequate end-organ perfusion and preservation of function. From a recent publication of seven patients with *Enterovirus* positive myocarditis, three died and four required mechanical support, indicating that enteroviral myocarditis has a particularly poor outcome. In neonates it may be possible to ensure that the supply to the descending aorta is continued by providing support to the systemic circulation from the right ventricle through a patent arterial duct. If the right ventricular function is better than the left, this may provide adequate perfusion to allow time for the left ventricle to recover.[2] Some children do recover their left ventricular function to normal, although in many cases it can be over a year before this recovery occurs.[3]

Institutions differ in their approach to the use of immunoglobulin and subsequent steroid treatment when a viral myocarditis is suspected from the clinical history. Where the child has been previously well and the clinical course is short, immunoglobulin and steroid therapy is often considered. Current evidence on the effectiveness of both immunoglobulin and steroids remains uncertain. Initial studies in both adults and children showed promise, but randomized studies have failed to demonstrate a benefit.[4–6] This is most likely due to the high spontaneous recovery rate associated with acute myocarditis. A recent review on behalf of the Cochrane database did not find that administration of intravenous immuno-globulin was beneficial in improving outcome in adults with myocarditis and a prospective randomized trial in pediatric patients did not exist. It was their conclusion that immunoglo-bulin should not be included in the routine treatment of myocarditis.[7] However, it is still common practice to use high dose methylprednisolone and/or immunoglobulin to treat acute heart failure in children. The improvement in myocardial function may be related to a reduction in the cytokine response seen in heart failure and may not be related to the resolution of myocarditis.[8] The blanket use of immune suppression or immunoglobulin cannot be justified on current evidence, but it is important to consider that, for a number of rare causes of myocarditis, including giant cell myocarditis, systemic lupus erythematosus (SLE), and eosinophilic infiltration, immune suppression is the treatment of choice.[9]

Familial/metabolic causes are common, particularly in consanguineous parents, as recessive genes may be important in the etiology of a dilated cardiomyopathy. Often, a relative may be affected or another child may be symptomatic or have died in infancy.

An ECHO is required to exclude congenital heart disease and is particularly important in this age group. It is essential to ensure that the coronary artery origins are in the normal position, particularly that the left coronary artery is seen arising from the aorta and that diastolic flow is seen in the appropriate direction using colour Doppler. It is also prudent to ensure that there is no restriction to flow out of the left ventricle and that coarctation of the aorta is absent. In the early stages of treatment, before the result of viral PCR is obtained, echocardiography may help to differentiate the etiology of poor cardiac function though assessment of this is subjective. In myocarditis the left ventricular posterior wall diameter is relatively preserved when compared with the thin wall associated with a long-standing dilated cardiomyopathy.

In dark-skinned UK residents, there may be maternal hypocalcemia, which results in infant hypocalcemia if there is exclusive breastfeeding. This can cause a severe cardiomyo-pathy, which may recover during subsequent months with calcium replacement therapy. A recent review of cases of dilated cardiomyopathy in children in the south east of England highlighted 16 cases of severe cardiomyopathy in children with hypocalcemia and vitamin D deficiency. Three infants died in this series and cardiac function improved in the remain-ing patients with appropriate vitamin D replacement. All patients were from black or Indian ethnic groups.[10]

In the UK ECMO is used to bridge children with severe heart failure to recovery. Bridging infants under 10 kg to heart transplantation is a difficult problem to resolve. Using valuable and limited ECMO resources to provide support for these patients is questionable, given the limited availability of small hearts within the UK. While a lack of provision for ECMO support would put these children at a disadvantage in terms of their survival, it is important to understand that an exit strategy in the form of a suitable graft is unlikely to be forthcoming. Usually only three or four infant hearts will be offered over the course of a year with some of these being marginal donors. With the duration of an ECMO run currently limited to around 2 to 3 weeks, it is easy to understand the difficulty in applying finite resources to a scenario, which is likely to end in a donor organ not being available and the subsequent death of the patient. If more infant donors were available, as is currently the position in the USA, it would be possible to bridge these children to a successful cardiac transplantation.

In an attempt to widen the donor pool and increase the chances of a small infant receiving a cardiac graft, a number of institutions, including our own, have transplanted hearts that are not matched for blood group. This is known as an ABO mismatch transplant.[11,12] Under normal circumstances cardiac transplantation is performed with matching for blood group only, with further immunophenotyping identifying HLA mismatches between donor and recipients after the transplantation procedure. This mismatched transplant is possible because the infant's immune system is immature enough to accept unmatched blood groups. In order for an infant to receive an ABO mismatched heart, the plasma levels of anti-A and anti-B isohemagglutinins need to be sufficiently low so as not to cause hyperacute graft rejection. The plasma levels increase up to the age of 18 months after which performing an ABO mismatch transplant becomes impossible. Therefore, as part of a transplant assessment for a young infant, measurement of their isohemagglutinins is a valuable and important test that may increase the chance of receiving a donor organ.

Case history 2

A 4-year-old boy presented with familial dilated cardiomyopathy. No screening had been performed prior to admission, as it was felt that the presentation was unlikely to occur in early childhood, given that father and grandfather had remained asymptomatic until they were over 30 years of age. At presentation at the district hospital, the child was in severe heart failure and on examination jugular venous pressure was grossly elevated. Capillary refill time was over 4 seconds and peripheral pulses were all reduced. A central venous line was inserted and milrinone commenced intravenously. Transfer was organized to a tertiary cardiac center. Despite escalation in inotropic therapy, cardiac output continued to remain very poor and an elective decision was made to provide ECMO support. In view of the history of familial dilated cardiomyopathy, it was felt that the chance of recovery was small. After 2 weeks of ECMO support, no echocardiographic improvement of left ventricular function was seen, although renal and neurological function had been preserved. The decision was made that further long-term support would be required and a Berlin Heart would be used to bridge the child to cardiac transplantation. He made an excellent recovery after the insertion of this device. It was then possible to remove sedation, extubate, and feed enterally. After a number of days, the patient was able to play and interact with parents and staff. Support with the Berlin Heart was continued for 6 weeks until a suitable donor organ was found. An adult heart was used and post-operatively it was not possible to close the sternum until a week post-transplant. Initial post-operative renal failure was managed with calcineurin inhibitor-free immunosuppressive therapy using basiliximab and sirolimus.

Discussion

Familial dilated cardiomyopathy does not always present at the same age. It is common for children with severe heart failure to have parents that have not been symptomatic until adult life. Screening is advisable for children whose parents have dilated cardiomyopathy. ECMO support has drastically changed the results of end-stage pediatric heart failure.[13] A more aggressive approach to mechanical support has meant that fewer children die and more are successfully bridged to transplantation. The UK has an urgent transplant listing program, which was introduced in 1999. This has enabled children who are on ECMO support to be urgently listed and has increased their chances of a successful outcome with transplantation. We have now bridged a number of children with dilated cardiomyopathy to transplant with ECMO and all have survived the post-operative period, with subsequent successful discharge from hospital. The ECMO bridging to transplantation results have been collated and published for the UK.[14] In the UK the pediatric organ donation rate is less than that in North America and, as we have discussed, it is not possible realistically to bridge infants with chronic left ventricular failure to cardiac transplantation. It is crucial that pediatric intensivists consider and request a family's consent for organ donation when a child dies. Until now, the time frame available to bridge children to cardiac transplantation has been limited by the use of ECMO but it is hoped that, by using a left ventricular assist device, such as the Berlin heart, the duration of support will be extended and increase the chances of receiving a suitable donor organ increased.[15]

Although keeping a child alive and well enough to undertake heart transplantation has been the focus of the discussion so far, it is important to remember that the challenge to maximize the duration and function of the cardiac graft begins in the post-operative days on the intensive care unit early after transplantation. Current statistics for pediatric cardiac transplants demonstrate survival at 3 years across the pediatric age ranges to be between approximately 75% and 85%. (International Society for Heart and Lung Transplantation: quarterly reports (www.ishlt.org)). Mean survival for children followed up in the authors' institution since the start of the transplant program in 1988 is currently approximately 15 years. However, we would expect that, within the current era of improved immunosuppression and reduced 30-day mortality; current survival figures would be considerable better than this, maybe even as high as a mean of 20 years. These figures have improved dramatically over the previous decades but, for a child with dilated cardiomyopathy transplanted at age 4, the prospect of death or retransplantation as a young adult are currently a reality. The major causes for morbidity and mortality after cardiac transplantation are related to acute and chronic rejection, coronary allograft vasculopathy, renal failure, and malignancy secondary to immunosuppressive therapy, particularly Post-Transplant Lymphoproliferative Disease (PTLD). Current immunosuppressive regimes involve the use of steroids in the first 6 months after transplant in combination with calcineurin inhibitors (ciclosporin or tacrolimus) and purine synthesis inhibitors (azathioprine or mycophenolate mofetil). These agents are effective at providing protection from acute rejection but have many unwanted side effects, particularly renal toxicity in the case of ciclosporine and, to a lesser extent, tacrolimus. It is important that we limit post-operative acute renal failure, as early renal dysfunction not only increases 30-day mortality, but impacts on renal function in the long term after transplant.[16,17]

Post-transplant renal failure is a problem for children who have had mechanical support peri-operatively. Even when creatinine and urea have been virtually normal pre-operatively, we are still seeing significant renal failure in the early post-transplant period. The relative reduction in end-organ perfusion during mechanical support makes the kidneys particularly susceptible to the toxicity associated with the use of calcineurin inhibitors in the first few days after transplantation. Attempts to avoid the potential nephrotoxicity of these drugs are made by using a monoclonal antibody that helps prevent T cell activation (basiliximab) and hence prevents acute rejection. In combination with this strategy, it has been possible to provide adequate initial immunosuppression with a calcineurin inhibitor free regimen for a few days after pediatric cardiac transplantation.[18] In a number of other patients who have required renal dialysis post-operatively, a new anti-proliferative immunosuppressive agent called sirolimus has been used without the addition of calcineurin inhibitors. In adult recipients sirolimus has been effective at reducing the deterioration of renal function caused by ciclosporin when switched late after cardiac transplantation and its use as an adjunctive immunosuppressant may have a positive effect on the development of coronary vasculopathy seen years after transplantation.[19,20]

Case history 3

A 14-year-old boy had an idiopathic dilated cardiomyopathy, which was diagnosed when he was 6 years old. No underlying cause had been found. He had been under regular cardiac review since diagnosis and managed with anti-failure medication, including diuretics, angiotensin-converting enzyme (ACE) inhibitors and beta-blockers. He had remained stable with a fractional shortening of around 14%. However, 18 months ago he became more symptomatic and had reached New York Heart Association (NYHA) stage 3. Twelve months ago a biventricular pacing device was inserted in attempt to resynchronize his ventricular contraction but had not produced any lasting improvement. He had recently been admitted to hospital due to deteriorating symptoms. He was breathless in hospital with a raised JVP, hepatomegaly, and an S3 on cardiac auscultation. Blood pressure was 90/60. He was still producing urine and his blood gases were normal. Echocardiography revealed a dilated poorly functioning heart with minimal tricuspid regurgitation. He had severe mitral regurgitation.

Due to worsening symptoms and clinical signs of heart failure, he was admitted to PICU for intravenous diuretics and inotropes. He was started on 10 mcg kg^{-1} per min of dobutamine and showed some improvement with a reduction in weight, reducing hepatomegaly and an increase in urine output. Over the next 4 days there was no further improvement, and after a week of treatment he began to deteriorate despite escalating doses of dobutamine and the addition of milrinone. A formal transplant assessment was arranged and he was listed for cardiac transplantation. In order to increase his cardiac output, it was decided that levosimendan would be used for 24 hours to enhance his cardiac output. Inotropes were maintained for a further week and a successful cardiac transplant was performed from which he made a full recovery.

Discussion

This case reflects common clinical details of children presenting to a specialist pediatric heart failure clinic. The cause for their dilated cardiomyopathy is unknown, and deterioration occurs slowly during childhood with a more rapid deteriorating occurring around puberty. Standard anti-failure therapy involves the use of diuretics, including spironolactone, ACE inhibitors, low-dose digoxin and, when stable, the addition of beta-blockade usually carvedilol. These medications are titrated to weight and may be reduced if there is improvement in symptoms, fractional shortening, or left ventricular dimensions.

Clear benefit in all-cause mortality for all patients with heart failure has been demonstrated using ACE inhibitors for many years and beta-blockers over the last few. ACE inhibitors have been used as part of standard therapy for the failing heart and their effect on reducing mortality has been well documented.[21,22] Few large studies exist involving pediatric patients to date, but performing a randomized control trial in children when they have been used so effectively up until now would be ethically questionable.

For beta-blockers the mortality benefit is evident for patients with both mild and severe heart failure. A reduction in relative risk of death from 34% to 65% has been reported when used in combination with ACE and diuretics.[23–26] Within our specialist heart failure clinic beta-blockers are prescribed once the child is euvolemic (venous pressure not raised) and more than a month has passed since inotropic therapy. A small dose is given initially and titrated up to a therapeutic level over the first month. If the child becomes decompensated or requires inotropic support, the beta-blocker therapy is stopped for the duration of the episode and reinstated on recovery.

The use of loop diuretics such as furosemide in the management of cardiac failure is standard practice. More recently, large clinical trials in adults have demonstrated the benefit of potassium sparing diuretics for long-term treatment in heart failure. The RALES trial randomized patients to either the use of aldosterone plus standard therapy against standard therapy alone as control. This strategy produced a 30% reduction in all cause mortality and greatly reduced incidence of cardiac death in the aldosterone-treated group. It is thought that the direct benefits of aldosterone on mortality are not related to its diuretic effects but are due to prevention of myocardial fibrosis[27] and reduction of locally produced noradrenaline which may lead to arrhythmia. Patients enrolled in these trials did not experience a high incidence of dangerous hyperkalemia, but clearly careful monitoring of serum potassium levels is required.

The evidence for the use of low dose digoxin in patients with heart failure demonstrates benefits in patients with NYHA grade III and below, reducing hospital admission for worsening cardiac function. The use of digoxin in combination with standard therapy does not improve mortality rates. Digoxin levels should also be performed and maintained at less than $1.0 \, \text{nmol} \, l^{-1}$ to avoid the risk of sudden death.[28]

Cardiac Resynchronization Therapy (CRT) or biventricular pacing is a relatively new method of improving symptomatic cardiac failure. This technique has been extensively researched throughout the adult literature and derives from the observation that conduction delay is common in patients with heart failure, manifested by prolongation of the QRS complex. This indicates dyssynchrony associated with the contraction of the right and left ventricular mass, leading to a decrease in stroke volume, delayed relaxation, and increased mitral regurgitation. The procedure involves inserting pacing leads into the right atrium, right ventricle, and also laterally within the coronary sinus in order to activate the left ventricular free wall. Numerous investigators have shown that this technique has hemodynamic benefits when assessing both physiological and symptomatic aspects of patients with heart failure. The clinical evidence for using CRT exists for patients who have either ischemic or non-ischemic cardiomyopathy and heart failure with functional NYHA class III or IV on maximal medical therapy, left ventricular ejection fraction (LVEF) less than 35% and a wide QRS duration >120 ms.[29] To date, there is limited experience with this technique in children and evidence is restricted to a number of case reports. It is likely that, due to the small numbers of patients presenting with cardiomyopathy, a large randomized trial will take a number of years. However, this technique has been encouraging in adults and warrants further investigation, especially if any improvement in cardiac function delays the necessity for cardiac transplantation.

Deciding on a potential recipient's suitability for cardiac transplantation involves input from a number of specialties, including experienced nursing staff and clinical psychologists who ensure that the child and their family are informed about the benefits and pitfalls of life after cardiac transplantation. This process occurs over a number of days and involves medical assessment of the present cardiopulmonary hemodynamics. It is important that, during the course of the current illness, the pulmonary vascular pressures have remained low and are not likely to induce right ventricular failure in the post-operative period. For patients with a dilated cardiomyopathy, this can be assessed using echocardiography and an estimate of right ventricular or pulmonary artery pressure performed, using either the tricuspid or pulmonary valvular regurgitation velocity. For recipients with congenital heart disease or restrictive cardiomyopathy, a more accurate assessment is required with direct measurement within the cardiac catheterization laboratory.[30]

Patients are often admitted for inotropic support for worsening cardiac function either due to development of co-morbidity or because they are reaching a point when their cardiac output decreases sufficiently to make them symptomatic. This may occur unexpectedly and may indicate a suitable time at which cardiac transplantation should be considered. Once a patient has been listed for cardiac transplantation, there may be a significant period of time before an appropriate organ becomes available. During this period, it is often necessary to support cardiac output with inotropes. Initially, dobutamine is used and milrinone either substituted or added to maintain an inotropic effect over a number of weeks. However, the inotropic effect of dobutamine may decrease during the course of treatment. Recently, we have used the calcium sensitizing agent levosimendan to maintain cardiac output in a small number of patients. This novel agent does not increase myocardial oxygen consumption, preventing the downward spiral often seen when inotropic therapy is commenced. A recent review in adult patients described its potential superiority to dobutamine in improving cardiac output. However, some patients within the study continued with beta-blocker therapy, while receiving dobutamine, leading to antagonism between the two drugs.[31] However, the early use of levosimendan appears to be encouraging and may add to the arsenal available to treat pediatric cardiac failure in the future.

Learning points

- The differential diagnosis for the cause of cardiac failure in an infant usually falls into one of the following categories:

  1. Viral myocarditis cause by *Entero/Coxsackie virus*, *Adenovirus* and *Parvovirus*

  2. Familial cardiomyopathy/metabolic

  3. Cardiac structural abnormality (ALCAPA and coarctation of the aorta)

  4. Idiopathic dilated cardiomyopathy.

- Infants with cardiac failure require an ECHO to exclude congenital heart disease, ensure the coronary arteries are in the normal position and exclude obstructive lesions of the left ventricular outflow tract.

- The major causes for morbidity and mortality after cardiac transplantation are related to acute and chronic rejection, coronary allograft vasculopathy, renal failure and malignancy secondary to immunosuppressive therapy, particularly post-transplant lymphoproliferative disease (PTLD).

- In patients undergoing assessment for transplantation, it is important that pulmonary vascular pressures are low and stable, and are thus not likely to induce right ventricular failure in the post-operative period.

References

1. Andrews RE, Fenton MJ, Ridout DA, Burch M. New-onset heart failure due to heart muscle disease in childhood: a prospective study in the United kingdom and Ireland. *Circulation* 2008; 117(1): 79–84.

2. Inwald D, Franklin O, Cubitt D, Peters M, Goldman A, Burch M. Enterovirus myocarditis as a cause of neonatal collapse.

Arch Dis Child Fetal Neonatal Ed 2004; 89(5): F461–62.

3. English RF, Janosky JE, Ettedgui JA, Webber SA. Outcomes for children with acute myocarditis. *Cardiol Young* 2004; 14 (5): 488–93.

4. Drucker NA, Colan SD, Lewis AB *et al.* Gamma-globulin treatment of acute

myocarditis in the pediatric population. *Circulation* 1994; **89**(1): 252–7.

5. Mason JW, O'Connell JB, Herskowitz A *et al*. A clinical trial of immunosuppressive therapy for myocarditis. The Myocarditis Treatment Trial Investigators. *N Engl J Med* 1995; **333**(5): 269–75.

6. McNamara DM, Holubkov R, Starling RC *et al*. Controlled trial of intravenous immune globulin in recent-onset dilated cardiomyopathy. *Circulation* 2001; **103** (18): 2254–9.

7. Robinson J, Hartling L, Vandermeer B, Crumley E, Klassen TP. Intravenous immunoglobulin for presumed viral myocarditis in children and adults. *Cochrane Database Syst Rev* 2005; (1): CD004370.

8. Damas JK, Gullestad L, Aass H *et al*. Enhanced gene expression of chemokines and their corresponding receptors in mononuclear blood cells in chronic heart failure – modulatory effect of intravenous immunoglobulin. *J Am Coll Cardiol* 2001; **38**(1): 187–93.

9. Burch M. Heart failure in the young. *Heart* 2002; **88**(2): 198–202.

10. Maiya S, Sullivan I, Allgrove J *et al*. Hypocalcaemia and vitamin D deficiency: an important, but preventable, cause of life-threatening infant heart failure. *Heart* 2008; **94**(5): 581–4.

11. West LJ, Pollock-Barziv SM, Dipchand AI *et al*. ABO-incompatible heart transplantation in infants. *N Engl J Med* 2001; **344**(11): 793–800.

12. West LJ, Karamlou T, Dipchand AI, Pollock-BarZiv SM, Coles JG, McCrindle BW. Impact on outcomes after listing and transplantation, of a strategy to accept ABO blood group-incompatible donor hearts for neonates and infants. *J Thorac Cardiovasc Surg* 2006; **131**(2): 455–61.

13. McMahon AM, van Doorn C, Burch M *et al*. Improved early outcome for end-stage dilated cardiomyopathy in children. *J Thorac Cardiovasc Surg* 2003; **126**(6): 1781–7.

14. Goldman AP, Cassidy J, de Leval M *et al*. The waiting game: bridging to paediatric heart transplantation. *Lancet* 2003; **362** (9400): 1967–70.

15. Hetzer R, Potapov EV, Stiller B *et al*. Improvement in survival after mechanical circulatory support with pneumatic pulsatile ventricular assist devices in pediatric patients. *Ann Thorac Surg* 2006; **82** (3): 917–25.

16. Ostermann ME, Rogers CA, Saeed I, Nelson SR, Murday AJ. Pre-existing renal failure doubles 30-day mortality after heart transplantation. *J Heart Lung Transpl* 2004; **23**(11): 1231–7.

17. Ojo AO, Held PJ, Port FK *et al*. Chronic renal failure after transplantation of a nonrenal organ. *N Engl J Med* 2003; **349** (10): 931–40.

18. Ford KA, Cale CM, Rees PG, Elliott MJ, Burch M. Initial data on basiliximab in critically ill children undergoing heart transplantation. *J Heart Lung Transpl* 2005; **24**(9): 1284–8.

19. Groetzner J, Kaczmarek I, Landwehr P *et al*. Renal recovery after conversion to a calcineurin inhibitor-free immunosuppression in late cardiac transplant recipients. *Eur J Cardiothorac Surg* 2004; **25**(3): 333–41.

20. Keogh A, Richardson M, Ruygrok P *et al*. Sirolimus in de novo heart transplant recipients reduces acute rejection and prevents coronary artery disease at 2 years: a randomized clinical trial. *Circulation* 2004; **110**(17): 2694–700.

21. Effects of enalapril on mortality in severe congestive heart failure. Results of the Cooperative North Scandinavian Enalapril Survival Study (CONSENSUS). The CONSENSUS Trial Study Group. *N Engl J Med* 1987; **316**(23): 1429–35.

22. Effect of enalapril on survival in patients with reduced left ventricular ejection fractions and congestive heart failure. The SOLVD Investigators. *N Engl J Med* 1991; **325**(5): 293–302.

23. Effect of metoprolol CR/XL in chronic heart failure: metoprolol CR/XL randomised intervention trial in congestive heart failure (MERIT-HF). *Lancet* 1999; **353** (9169): 2001–7.

24. The Cardiac Insufficiency Bisoprolol Study II (CIBIS-II): a randomised trial. *Lancet* 1999; **353**(9146): 9–13.

25. Packer M, Bristow MR, Cohn JN *et al*. The effect of carvedilol on morbidity and mortality in patients with chronic heart failure. US Carvedilol Heart Failure Study Group. *N Engl J Med* 1996; **334**(21): 1349–55.

26. Packer M, Coats AJ, Fowler MB *et al.* Effect of carvedilol on survival in severe chronic heart failure. *N Engl J Med* 2001; **344** (22): 1651–8.

27. Weber KT. Aldosterone and spironolactone in heart failure. *N Engl J Med* 1999; **341** (10): 753–5.

28. The effect of digoxin on mortality and morbidity in patients with heart failure. The Digitalis Investigation Group. *N Engl J Med* 1997; **336**(8): 525–33.

29. Strickberger SA, Conti J, Daoud EG, Havranek E, Mehra MR, Pina IL *et al.* Patient selection for cardiac resynchronization therapy: from the Council on Clinical Cardiology Subcommittee on Electrocardiography and Arrhythmias and the Quality of Care and Outcomes Research Interdisciplinary Working Group, in collaboration with the Heart Rhythm Society. *Circulation* 2005; **111**(16): 2146–50.

30. Fenton MJ, Chubb H, McMahon AM, Rees P, Elliott MJ, Burch M. Heart and heart–lung transplantation for idiopathic restrictive cardiomyopathy in children. *Heart* 2006; **92** (1): 85–9.

31. Follath F, Cleland JG, Just H *et al.* Efficacy and safety of intravenous levosimendan compared with dobutamine in severe low-output heart failure (the LIDO study): a randomised double-blind trial. *Lancet* 2002; **360**(9328): 196–202.

Chapter 22

Tetralogy of Fallot

Roger Langford

Introduction

Tetralogy of Fallot (TOF) is the most frequently occurring congenital cyanotic heart lesion with an incidence of 1 in 3600. The tetralogy, as originally described, comprises a ventricular septal defect, overriding aorta, right ventricular outflow tract (RVOT) obstruction (valvular or infundibular) and right ventricular hypertrophy (Fig. 22.1). The obstructed right ventricular outflow results in inter-ventricular shunting of systemic venous blood from the right to left ventricle. The main implication of this, as well as right-to-left shunting of blood, is reduced pulmonary arterial blood flow. There are a variety of similar "Fallot's-type" cardiac lesions with similar flow characteristics that do not strictly conform to the original description, but may be managed in a similar manner.

The right-to-left shunt may be manipulated according to the balance between pulmonary and systemic blood pressure and vascular resistance. A further feature of TOF is the occurrence of an increase in tone of the muscular infundibular region of the right ventricle. This can lead to a further acute reduction in pulmonary flow and increased inter-ventricular shunt, often known as hypercyanotic "spelling."

Corrective surgery for TOF was traditionally undertaken after 18 months of age although this approach has been challenged in recent years and there has been a trend towards earlier full corrective surgery.[1] If symptomatic earlier in life, an initial palliative shunt procedure may be considered (such as a Blalock–Taussig or Central Shunt). Thus a child may present for corrective surgery at any age. Surgery for congenital cardiac disease carries a unique set of physiological problems and issues of significance in the post-operative period.

Case history

A 6-month-old boy with Trisomy 21 presented on a morning, elective operating list for correction of tetralogy of Fallot. He had previously undergone a modified Blalock–Taussig shunt at 2 weeks of age due to neonatal cyanosis and a single profound hypercyanotic spell. A recent cardiac catheter study indicated significant right ventricular outflow tract obstruction, reasonable sized branch pulmonary arteries (Fig. 22.2(a)). Coronary arteries were normal. The BT shunt (right subclavian artery to pulmonary artery) was patent (Fig. 22.2(b)) and provided adequate pulmonary blood flow such that arterial oxygen saturations were 75%. His chronic hypoxemic state had resulted in a polycythemia of hemoglobin 18g dl^{-1}. Other blood tests were unremarkable.

Developmentally, the child was just above the 25th centile for weight and height. No further hypercyanotic spells had been noted since the shunt procedure.

Case Studies in Pediatric Critical Care, ed. Peter. J. Murphy, Stephen C. Marriage, and Peter J. Davis.
Published by Cambridge University Press. © Cambridge University Press 2009.

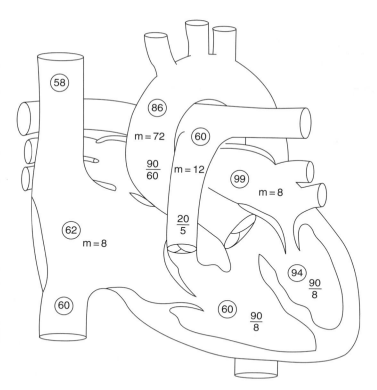

Fig. 22.1. Diagram of oxygen saturations (circled) and pressures in Tetralogy of Fallot. (From Nichols et al, 1995.)

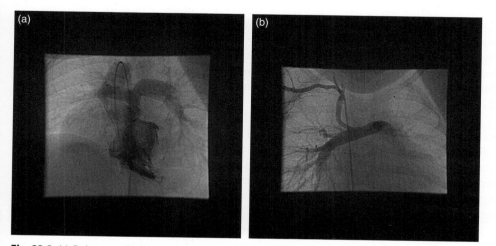

Fig. 22.2. (a) Catheter study showing right ventricular outflow tract obstruction and reasonably sized branch pulmonary arteries. (b) Catheter study showing patent right BT shunt.

Progress in the operating room

Following an inhalational induction with sevoflurane, nitrous oxide, and oxygen, vascular access was obtained and the trachea successfully intubated following the administration of pancuronium 0.2 mg kg^{-1} and fentanyl 2 mcg kg^{-1}. A right internal jugular central venous line, right radial arterial line, enterogastric tube, and urinary catheter were then sited. Throughout induction, cardiovascular observations were stable, oxygen saturations remaining between 70% and 85% and mean arterial pressure between 40 and 50 mmHg. Gentamicin 4 mg kg^{-1}, flucloxacillin 25 mg kg^{-1} and dexamethasone 0.5 mg kg^{-1} were administered shortly after induction and anaesthesia was maintained with isoflurane, nitrous oxide, and fentanyl to a total dose of 15 mcg kg^{-1}. Near-Infrared Spectroscopy (NIRS) monitors were applied to the scalp in order to monitor cerebral oxygenation throughout the procedure.

Surgical access was through a midline sternotomy and, following dissection, cannulae were placed in the superior and inferior vena cavae and in the aortic root. Heparin, 300 U kg^{-1} was given prior to bypass. The modified Blalock–Taussig shunt was closed by surgical tie prior to cardiac bypass. At the initiation of extra-corporal circulation, the mean blood pressure dropped significantly from 50 mmHg to 30 mmHg. Bypass flow rate was increased to 150% of the calculated cardiac output and 10 μg aliquots of phenylephrine were given until restoration of a mean blood pressure of 45 mmHg. Cardioplegia was achieved after application of the aortic cross-clamp and the patient cooled to 34 °C. Surgical repair was performed through right atriotomy and pulmonary arterotomy. A transannular patch was used and the right ventricular outflow tract was widened through resection of infundibular muscle. The ventricular septal defect was closed using a Dacron patch. The procedure went to plan, the aortic cross-clamp time was 60 minutes and the total bypass time was 95 minutes.

Towards the end of bypass, cardiovascular support was provided with a loading dose of milrinone, 75 mcg kg^{-1}, followed by infusions of dopamine, 5 mcg kg^{-1} per min and milrinone 0.25 mcg kg^{-1} per min. The patient was rewarmed to 37 °C. Removal of the aortic cross-clamp and reperfusion of the coronary circulation led to return of spontaneous electrocardiographical activity. An initial broad complex tachycardia was superseded by sinus tachycardia within a few minutes. Infusion of packed red blood cells and fresh frozen plasma demanded multiple boluses of calcium gluconate, titrated to arterial blood gas electrolyte measurement.

During the termination of cardiac bypass, there was a significant drop in mean arterial pressure from 40 to 32 mmHg. This responded to repeated boluses of fresh frozen plasma. Following termination of cardiac bypass, modified ultrafiltration was performed, removing a total of 50 ml kg^{-1} of filtrate. Epicardial pacing wires, intrapleural, and mediastinal drains were placed prior to closure and the remainder of the procedure was uneventful. He was transferred to the pediatric intensive care unit intubated, with infusions of milrinone and dopamine running.

Progress in pediatric intensive care

Day 1

On arrival to the intensive care unit, observations were as follows: pulse 145, blood pressure 55/35 mmHg, CVP 8 mmHg and temperature 36.8 °C. Arterial oxygen saturation was 97%

with an inspired oxygen fraction of 50%. Venous oxygen saturation, taken from the central line, was 76%. Intravenous sedation was instigated using morphine and midazolam infusions, and ventilation was achieved using intermittent positive pressure ventilation. Dopamine and milrinone infusions were continued at 5 and 0.25 mcg kg^{-1} per min, respectively. A standard 12-lead ECG was obtained as well as an atrial electrogram, taken by connection of the atrial pacing wire to the electrode in the V1 position; the initial ECG indicated sinus tachycardia and right bundle branch block with no discernable ischemic changes.

A post-operative chest X-ray indicated good central line and drain position, no pneumothorax, and no evidence of cardiac failure. Blood was taken for arterial blood gas measurement and analysis of FBC, U and E, LFT, magnesium, calcium, and phosphate. Clinical targets were set; mean arterial pressure 50–55 mmHg, oxygen saturation >90%, Urine output >0.5 ml kg^{-1} per h. Ventilation parameters were set to ensure normocapnea. Tidal volumes of 7 ml kg^{-1} were achieved using airway pressures of 18/5 cmH$_2$O with a FiO$_2$ 35%.

Over the next 6 hours, the child's condition remained stable. An initial blood gas revealed pH 7.39, PaO$_2$ 95 mmHg, PaCO$_2$ 35 mmHg, bicarbonate of 23 mmol l^{-1} and a lactate of 0.8 mmol l^{-1}. Other tests were unremarkable except for a serum potassium level of 3.4 mmol l^{-1} and magnesium level of 0.7 mmol l^{-1}. These were supplemented with appropriate electrolyte infusions. The post-operative hemoglobin was 12.4 g dl^{-1}.

Later that evening the child developed a pyrexia. His temperature rose from 37.4 to 38.5 °C. This was presumed due to an inflammatory response to surgery and was primarily managed using 15 mg kg^{-1} paracetamol. His pulse rate had also climbed steadily to 150 beats per minute. An arterial blood gas revealed pH 7.23, PaO$_2$ 65 mmHg, PaCO$_2$ 38 mmHg, bicarbonate 20 and a rising lactate of 2.9 mmol l^{-1}. Mean arterial pressure had fallen to 45 mmHg and the CVP had climbed to 12 mmHg. It was suspected that the child was developing a low cardiac output state. The FiO$_2$ was increased to 70% and a small fluid challenge of 5 ml kg^{-1} 4.5% human albumin solution was given. The CVP rose further to 15 mmHg but with no improvement in arterial pressure. The dopamine infusion was increased to 7.5 mcg kg^{-1} per min and the milrinone infusion increased to 0.5 mcg kg^{-1} per min.

At 23.00 h the pulse rate increased to 170 beats per minute, accompanied by a further drop in arterial blood pressure to a mean of 38 mmHg. On clinical examination, the child was peripherally shutdown, capillary refill was 4 cm centrally and a 3 cm liver edge could be palpated. A 12-lead electrocardiogram indicated a tachycardia with right bundle branch block. Immediate management included 100% oxygen and rapid administration of sequential doses of 100, 150 and 200 mcg kg^{-1} of adenosine. The cardiac rhythm remained unchanged. The PICU consultant was informed and the on-call cardiologist attended. The differential diagnosis comprised atrial tachycardia or junctional ectopic tachycardia (JET). An echocardiogram illustrated a lack of atrioventricular synchrony, an intact septal patch, and poor biventricular function with a dilated right ventricle. The maximum Doppler velocity across the right ventricular outflow tract was 2.8 m s^{-1} and there was prominent pulmonary regurgitation. A repeat atrial electrogram demonstrated atrioventricular dissociation with a ventricular rate of 170 and atrial rate of 100 beats per minute (Fig. 22.3), consistent with a diagnosis of JET.

Initial management was to correct any identifiable causes. Blood was taken for assessment of electrolytes, adequate sedation was ensured and a repeat chest X-ray was ordered. Electrolyte levels from the lab indicated mild hypomagnesemia, level 0.75 mmol l^{-1}. This was corrected using an infusion of 50 mg kg^{-1} magnesium sulphate over 20 minutes. Chest X-ray indicated extra-cardiac positioning of the central line tip and no pneumothorax. There was a

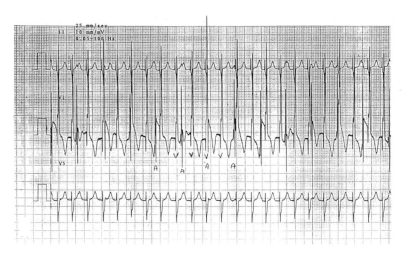

Fig. 22.3. ECG of JET.

significant increase in perihilar vascular markings consistent with cardiac failure. Active surface cooling was employed through use of a cooling air blanket to achieve a core temperature of 35 °C. A vecuronium infusion was initiated to prevent shivering and sedation increased to reduce any further endogenous catecholamine release. Regular blood gas analysis throughout the night allowed for aggressive correction of potassium, calcium, and magnesium levels with targets of greater than 4.5, 1.2 and 1.0 mmol l^{-1}, respectively. Cardiac overdrive pacing was attempted via the epicardial pacing wires in an attempt to increase atrioventricular synchrony; however, this resulted in a further drop in cardiac output and blood pressure. The issue of dopamine was considered carefully; although increased inotropy would be beneficial in the context of a failing ventricle, it was felt that the increased adrenergic stimulation would increase the heart rate further. The dopamine infusion rate was reduced to 5 mcg kg^{-1} per min.

Surface cooling and electrolyte supplementation resulted in a small clinical improvement. The heart rate dropped to 150 beats per minute and the mean arterial pressure rose to 53 mmHg. A blood gas analysis 2 hours after the onset of JET indicated pH 7.35, PaO$_2$ 80 mmHg, PaCO$_2$ 36 mmHg, bicarbonate 22 and a lactate of 4.5 mmol l^{-1}. Venous oxygen saturation at this point measured 64%.

Throughout the rest of the night, the clinical condition of the child remained unchanged. Pulse rate remained at 140 bpm and mean arterial blood pressure was between 50 and 55 mmHg. The lactate level ranged between 4.0 and 5.0 mmol l^{-1}.

Day 2

The following morning, a repeat echocardiogram indicated a slightly less dilated right ventricle; however, the atrioventricular asynchrony remained. A loading dose of 5 mg kg^{-1} amiodarone was administered over 1 hour. This was followed by an intravenous amiodarone infusion of 10 mcg kg^{-1} per h over the day. A chest X-ray indicated increased vascular markings and some right lower lobe sub-segmental collapse compared to the previous day.

Electrolyte levels were within the normal range, hemoglobin level was 11.1 g dl^{-1}, platelets were 342 and white cell count was 14 000. Furosemide 1 mg kg^{-1} b.d. was prescribed, the dopamine, milrinone, and sedation were left unchanged. Fluid drainage in the preceding

24 hours from the drains was 140 ml and 50 ml from the right and left intrapleural drains, respectively. A plan was formulated to leave the drains *in situ*. Three hours after the amiodarone loading, there was a change in cardiac rhythm to sinus tachycardia at a rate of 140 beats per minute, confirmed by ECG. There was an accompanying increase in arterial blood pressure of 10 mmHg. Serum lactate levels dropped over the next 2 hours to 2 mmol l^{-1}.

Despite a continuation of the amiodarone infusion, there was a recurrence of the arrhythmia later in the day. This episode was self-limiting and terminated within 45 minutes.

After a 6-hour period of sinus rhythm, the active surface cooling was stopped and the patient was allowed to warm to 37 °C. The vecuronium infusion was terminated. During rewarming, the CVP dropped from 11 to 5 mmHg, accompanied by a drop in the mean arterial pressure and an increased swing of the arterial waveform on the monitor. This responded to boluses of 5 ml kg^{-1} human albumin solution. Throughout the remainder of the day, the child's clinical condition improved. He was warm, well perfused with a capillary refill time of less than 2 seconds. The dopamine infusion was weaned over a period of 4 hours and the milrinone was reduced to 0.5 mcg kg^{-1} per min. The child developed a diuresis of 4 ml kg^{-1} per h, and staff were able to wean the ventilatory parameters to an inspired oxygen concentration of 35%, airway pressures of 15/5 and a respiratory rate of 18 b min^{-1}.

Day 3

Following a stable night, a plan was made to wean the ventilator settings in preparation for extubation early on day 3. Morphine and midazolam sedation was halted at 6 am. Standard blood tests were taken prior to the morning ward round. Current medications included potassium supplementation, furosemide b.d., milrinone, and amiodarone by infusion. Despite the persistence of sinus rhythm overnight, the amiodarone infusion was continued, with a plan to stop it the following day. A repeat echocardiogram indicated synchronized atrioventricular contraction and moderately good biventricular function. There was anterograde flow at the end of diastole noted in the pulmonary artery consistent with restrictive right ventricular physiology. Hemoglobin levels were 8.2 g dl^{-1} and a transfusion of packed red cells was provided to ensure a hemoglobin level above 10 g dl^{-1}. Electrolytes and renal function were stable. The child remained in good clinical condition and was triggering each ventilator breath by the end of the morning. Following appropriate movements and activity, he was successfully extubated onto 40% oxygen and nasal CPAP around midday. A post-extubation chest X-ray revealed clear lung fields with residual right lower lobe sub-segmental collapse. The chest drains were removed after minimal drainage overnight, but the epicardial wires were to remain until the fifth post-operative day. The child was moving all limbs, crying appropriately and appeared grossly neurologically intact. Oral fluids were commenced cautiously.

Day 4

The FiO$_2$ was reduced to 28% the next day and the non-invasive ventilation withdrawn. Amiodarone and milrinone infusions were discontinued and oral amiodarone commenced. The furosemide dose was increased to 1 mg kg^{-1} q.d.s. Plans were made to discharge the child to the cardiology ward later in the day.

Further developments

The epicardial pacing wires were removed on the fifth post-operative day. Resolution of the lobar collapse was noted on a subsequent chest X-ray. The child continued to make good progress and was discharged home on the tenth post-operative day. Amiodarone was stopped 1 week after discharge. Echocardiogram 3 months later confirmed persistence of right ventricular diastolic dysfunction; however, overall function was good. The child had a good exercise tolerance and was able to feed without excessive shortness of breath. There was no indication of ongoing cardiac failure.

Discussion

Pathology

Tetralogy of Fallot may occur in isolation or with co-existing cardiac malformations and genetic abnormalities, commonly Trisomy 21 and chromosome 22 q11 deletion. TOF incorporates a spectrum of pathological entities based on the anterior misalignment of the conoventricular septum. During fetal development, spiral separation of the truncus arteriosus fails to fully divide into the pulmonary artery and aorta, resulting in a smaller or even absent pulmonary artery and valve. The aorta and aortic valve tend to be larger than normal and, by overriding the intraventricular septum, result in formation of the VSD. Hypertrophy of the right ventricle occurs in response to increased right-sided pressures due to a narrow pulmonary outflow and VSD. The infundibular region of the right ventricle, below the pulmonary valve is also vulnerable to hypertrophy and can result in variable, dynamic obstruction of the right ventricular outflow tract, so-called infundibular spasm. The outflow tract obstruction may be at the level of the pulmonary valve, the right infundibulum or, more commonly, both. An absent pulmonary valve may exist in 3–6% of TOF.[2]

Physiology

It is the severity of RVOT obstruction that determines the degree of cyanosis. Hence the range of clinical presentations can vary from asymptomatic (the "pink variant") to severe persistent cyanosis from birth. If the VSD is of a reasonable size, the relative vascular resistance of the right and left outflow tracts determines the flow of blood shunting from the right ventricle to the left. The pulmonary resistance comprises the pulmonary vascular bed, the pulmonary valve and resistance to flow at the infundibular level. The left ventricular outflow resistance is predominantly a function of the systemic vascular resistance (SVR).

The SVR is affected by several physiological factors and may decrease following changes in posture, such as standing up or through dilation of vascular beds, notably after activity, food ingestion and after a warm bath. Vasodilating anesthetic agents can produce a similar effect. These situations can all lead to an increase in systemic blood flow and a reduced pulmonary flow.

Pulmonary vascular tone may be increased through hypoxia, hypercarbia, and increased pulmonary airway pressures, i.e. through mechanical ventilation. The balance of pulmonary and systemic flow will again be altered.

Increased infundibular tone may be spontaneous, due to increased sympathetic autonomic activity, due to positive inotropic drugs (including digoxin), or by direct stimulation during cardiac catheterization. It results in an increase in right-to-left shunting, increasing cyanosis and syncope (hypercyanotic spells). If not controlled, the hypoxia can lead to increased pulmonary vascular tone and further infundibular shutdown through increased sympathetic activity, aggravating the situation. Subsequent acidosis or even death may occur.

Treatment strategies

Tetralogy of Fallot is usually detected antenatally or shortly after birth in a clinically cyanotic neonate. Overall, survival in children with isolated tetralogy of Fallot has been placed at around 90% up to age 10.[3] Management of a child with TOF is dependent on the degree of cyanosis at presentation, usually as a neonate. The use of prostaglandins (PGE$_1$) to maintain ductal patency and to stabilize patients with severely diminished pulmonary blood flow, grants the surgical team time to arrive at the most appropriate surgical plan for each individual patient. If pulmonary blood flow is adequate, pharmacological options, prior to definitive repair, center on the management of consequent heart failure and the prevention of acute spells. Surgical options include a palliative shunt procedure to increase/maintain pulmonary blood flow or a full corrective procedure.

Pharmacological

Heart failure due to restricted pulmonary blood flow is uncommon, but may be managed using standard medications, such as diuretics and ACE inhibitors. These work predominantly by off-loading the ventricular preload and removing excess fluid. There is a risk of exacerbating any propensity to spelling if using an "off-loading" agent and this should be considered carefully. The use of beta-adrenergic blocking agents such as propranolol in TOF is widespread. The mechanism of action in TOF is to prevent infundibular obstruction through beta-mediated increased tone.

Hypercyanotic spelling

The management of spells aims to increase systemic vascular resistance and decrease pulmonary outflow tract resistance. Classically, squatting or, in an infant, flexion of the hips can reduce the shunt by compressing the aorta and iliac vessels, increasing systemic vascular resistance. Pharmacologic agents with alpha-agonist activity, such as metaraminol, phenylephrine or a noradrenaline infusion, can be used to increase the systemic vascular resistance. Expansion of the intravascular space with fluids will also help to increase the systemic vascular resistance, especially if the child is fluid deplete.

The pulmonary outflow obstruction can be reduced by terminating the infundibular spasm. Intravenous propranolol at a dose of 0.1 mg kg^{-1} is often successful, as is morphine (0.1 mg kg^{-1}). For morphine, the mechanism of action is not well understood in TOF, but it is thought that it may reduce the increased infundibular tone directly. Supplemental oxygen therapy may play a role in reducing pulmonary vascular tone, but is unlikely to have a major effect if used alone.

If unresponsive to pharmacological therapy and still deteriorating, it may be necessary to perform an emergency shunt procedure to increase pulmonary blood flow.

Surgical

Etienne Fallot first described the tetralogy in 1888 and the first surgical treatment for TOF was in 1945 by Alfred Blalock. The first successful intracardiac repair was completed in 1954 using human cross-circulation.[4]

Initial surgical management is largely dependent on the pulmonary arterial flow, which will vary according to the degree of right ventricular outflow tract obstruction. Surgical options in the neonate include construction of a palliative systemic-to-pulmonary shunt, such as a modified Blalock–Taussig (BT) or Central Shunt or a definitive corrective procedure.

In recent years there has been growing support for an early corrective procedure in the first few months of life.[4] There are several perceived benefits of early correction: reduced exposure to hypoxemia and polycythemia, due to a shorter interval of right-to-left shunting; reduced right ventricular hypertrophy; normal pulmonary flow and organ development; a single operation and reduced right ventricular muscle excision. Also, a decrease in shunt-induced left ventricular overload and a reduced incidence of late arrhythmias have been reported. However, there has been some concern over the effects of prolonged bypass at this age and increased overall mortality and morbidity including a prolonged ICU stay.[5] One of the key issues is that the right ventriculo-arterial junction may be more successfully repaired after it has been allowed to develop. Delayed repair (after the first 3 months of life) has been associated with a lower requirement for transjunctional patching and a better functioning native pulmonary valve. A number of studies have been published using early repair with excellent short- and medium-term results in the last 10 years.[4,6,7] Longer-term outcomes are still awaited.

The modified Blalock–Taussig shunt procedure carries a mortality of 0%–4%.[4] Complications are not insignificant and include differential blood flow to the lungs, shunt stenosis, thrombosis, and kinking of the shunt or involved vessels.[8] A central shunt from aorta to pulmonary trunk has been developed in an attempt to alleviate these complications with mixed results.

Definitive repair involves closure of the VSD and resection of the right ventricular outflow tract obstruction. It may occur through atriotomy or ventriculotomy. The later has been associated with immediate reduced right ventricular function, long-term arrhythmias and sudden cardiac death. A transpulmonary incision may damage the right ventriculo-arterial junction or the pulmonary valve itself, leading to regurgitation and right ventricular failure at a later stage. Use of a transjunctional patch leads to a higher incidence of pulmonary valve dysfunction and failure.[4] Atriotomy also has disadvantages, as surgical access may be impaired. Reduced access can result in inadequate resection of infundibular muscle and a residual right ventricular outflow tract gradient.[9]

Pre-operative concerns

A full cardiac work-up will include full blood count and electrolyte measurement, ECG and echocardiography. Polycythemia may be evident due to prolonged cyanosis and may be accompanied by iron deficiency (microcytosis).

A pre-operative cardiac catheterization procedure will allow for the determination of the degree of shunt, intracardiac pressure measurement, and provide an assessment of cardiac anatomy and function. Co-existing cardiac defects are associated with a higher mortality rate.[3] In some institutions pre-operative cardiac catheterization is not always deemed necessary. A catheter procedure is more likely if there are anatomical concerns or a previous BT shunt has been used.

The course of the coronary arteries is abnormal in 3%–8%. If there is a coronary artery crossing anterior to the RVOT, it may be compromised by a transannular incision and a right ventricle-pulmonary artery homograft may be preferred. This will require further replacement as the child grows.

The child may have had previous surgery in the form of a shunt procedure. These are usually performed via a thoracotomy; however, a midline sternotomy approach may have been used, especially if there have been concerns with severe spelling and the need for cardiopulmonary bypass or if a central shunt has been used. Scarring and abnormal anatomy results in a longer surgical time and a greater risk of hemorrhage. Additional intravenous access and use of the antifibrinolytic agent tranexamic acid may be considered.

Additional congenital abnormalities should be excluded. The 22 q11 chromosome abnormality, found in around 15% of patients with TOF,[2] is often related to immune dysfunction and hypocalcemia. If present, there is a risk of transfusion-related graft versus host disease. Γ-irradiation of transfused blood may be used to remove active T-cells and many centers will use this blood routinely without checking patient T-cell levels. Trisomy 21 carries with it additional anesthetic risks relating to the airway, sleep apnea, and cervical spine stability, to name but a few. Co-existing respiratory infection, such as respiratory syncytial virus, is associated with a high risk of post-operative complication.[10]

Signs and symptoms of cardiac failure include tachypnea, tachycardia, and hepatosplenomegaly. The child with TOF may exhibit clubbing, poor weight gain, and recurrent respiratory infection.

Beta-blocker medication doses should be adjusted in line with weight gain and should be continued up until surgery.

Peri-operative concerns

Attention must be given to the avoidance of tetrad spells and the maintenance of pulmonary blood flow. This may be accomplished by suitable premedication, using a benzodiazepine such as temazepam 0.5 mg kg^{-1} and a stable induction using ketamine or an inhalation agent. Inhalational induction using an agent such as sevoflurane can be used, but cautiously to avoid excessive vasodilation. Ablation of the sympathetic response to intubation is important to prevent spells. This may be achieved using fentanyl.

Consideration must be given to previous surgery, for example, arterial lines should not be placed in limbs affected by previous BT shunts.

Pre-operative cyanosis may be marked due to right-to-left shunting through the VSD or a prior surgical shunt. The goal is to maintain saturations at the pre-operative state or better until Cardiopulmonary Bypass (CPB) has been established. Any previously placed shunt will be closed surgically immediately prior to CPB to stop circulating blood from bypassing the extracorporeal circuit. Patients are often polycythemic prior to surgery and can tolerate a drop in hemoglobin at the commencement of bypass. It may still be necessary to prime the pump with blood however, especially in infants with a smaller circulating volume.

Surgery includes the resection of infundibular muscle within the right ventricle. Complications can arise if too much or too little is removed. If too much muscle is resected, the function of the right ventricle will be impaired, with resultant post-operative right ventricular failure. Resection may also encompass valvar tissue, leading to pulmonary valve dysfunction. Inadequate infundibular excision will leave residual right ventricular outflow tract obstruction, possibly requiring re-operation at a later date. Intra-operative ECHO has been used in an attempt to determine the RVOT obstruction post-resection, however, the values of acceptable parameters are controversial.[11] In addition, the measured intra-operative gradient can fall significantly in the post-operative period.

Modified Ultrafiltration (MUF) is a technique sometimes used after the termination of CPB. The bypass circuit is left in position and blood is circulated from the aortic cannula to the venous cannulae via a hemofilter. The main benefit of MUF is in reducing the total body water since CPB tends towards leaky vasculature and accumulation of fluid. It appears to be most effective in long bypass cases and in smaller children under 10 kg. Around 50 ml kg^{-1} of fluid is usually removed. Further perceived benefits are that inflammatory mediators, particularly interleukin 8 are removed from the circulation, attenuating the systemic inflammatory response to CPB and reducing post-operative capillary leak. There is evidence that MUF can increase systolic function, increase diastolic compliance, reduce post-operative ventilator days and reduce inotrope requirements in pediatric patients.[12,13] Post-bypass MUF needs to be instigated with caution as it is often accompanied by a significant drop in systemic blood pressure due to alterations in SVR combined with a relatively poor cardiac function post-bypass.

Post-operative concerns

In the immediate post-operative phase impaired right ventricular function is frequent.[14,15] This may manifest itself as ventricular diastolic dysfunction or an acute restrictive picture (so-called right ventricular restrictive physiology) and appears to increase the incidence of pleural effusions, low cardiac output and post-operative ICU stay.[14] It can be characterized on echocardiography by anterograde diastolic pulmonary flow during atrial systole, i.e. the stiff ventricle is acting as a conduit for blood flow from the right atrium to the pulmonary artery during atrial systole. The mechanism of right ventricular restrictive physiology is not clear, but contributing factors may be related to endomyocardial fibrosis, intra-operative myocardial injury and oxidative stress. It may be exacerbated by poor intra-operative cooling due to the anterior atrial position, inadequate cardioplegia of the hypertrophied muscle, or downregulated antioxidant properties of the chronically hypoxic myocardium.[15] There is also an association with the use of transannular patches.[14]

Prolonged cardiopulmonary bypass is associated with a systemic inflammatory response and capillary leakage syndrome and reduced myocardial function due to myocardial stunning.

Immediately following the repair of TOF, the pulmonary artery pressures will usually be higher. Pleural effusions, especially on the right side, are frequent and intrapleural drains are usually inserted peri-operatively. The drains may be removed in the post-operative period once output has decreased to a suitable level. In most units the drains will be removed before drainage has completely stopped, since residual pleural effusions may be treated medically with diuretics and the persistence of a drain increases the risk of empyema and reduces post-operative mobility.

Low cardiac output

Post-operative low cardiac output affects up to 25% of children following cardiopulmonary bypass. It results in reduced oxygen delivery to the tissues and may manifest as tachycardia, hypotension, poor urine output, reduced venous oxygen saturation and rising lactate.[16] Although the mechanism is usually due to reduced contractility of the myocardium, there are a number of potential contributing factors. There may be underlying pre-operative cardiac dysfunction due to structural abnormalities in TOF. Surgery involves resection of, and often dissection through, right ventricular muscle as well as placement of non-contractile artificial patches. Myocardial dysfunction may be exacerbated by long bypass and cross clamp times and an inadequate level of hypothermia. Patients are often intravascularly depleted due to interstitial fluid leak from the systemic inflammatory response and vasodilatation seen on warming post-CPB. Peri-operative fluid balance is difficult to assess and there is often a tendency to keep fluid therapy restricted in the immediate post-operative phase. There is usually an associated increase in systemic and pulmonary vascular resistance.

The assessment of oxygen delivery to the tissues is fundamental to the early recognition of a poor cardiac output state. As well as the basic cardiovascular parameters of pulse, blood pressure, and central venous pressure, other clinical observations can be useful in determining oxygen delivery and tissue perfusion. Core–periphery temperature gradient, urine output, and capillary refill are useful in determining organ and tissue perfusion. Serum lactate is a useful marker of anaerobic metabolism and is one of the best predictors of adverse outcome in this group. It has been shown that an elevated lactate on admission and at 4 hours is associated with significant adverse events.[16] The arterial–venous oxygen saturation differential is a global indicator of tissue oxygen extraction. A wide differential indicates a high oxygen extraction and can imply that the rate of oxygen delivery is low. These markers, when used together, can often provide a more accurate indication of cardiac output than invasive monitoring, which is difficult in this patient group.

There should be a low threshold for repeat echocardiography in the immediate postoperative phase if a low cardiac output state is suspected. Cardiac tamponade, patch failure, residual infundibular obstruction and an overloaded ventricle are just some of the potential causes that can be excluded by echocardiography.

The management of a low cardiac output state centers on both reducing tissue oxygen consumption and increasing oxygen delivery. Oxygen demand can be minimized by ensuring adequate sedation and analgesia to reduce endogenous catecholamine release and use of minimal amounts of exogenous catecholamines. The respiratory work can be reduced with the use of mechanical ventilation and body temperature should be maintained at normothermia. The metabolic rate of tissue increases by around 7% for each degree Celsius rise in body temperature.

Oxygen delivery can be improved by increasing the oxygen content or increasing the flow rate of circulating blood. The oxygen content of blood can be optimized by effective ventilation strategies, including use of positive end expiratory pressure (PEEP) and appropriate adjustment of arterial CO_2 and pH levels.

The mainstay of management of the low cardiac output state is the use of inotropic agents. Catecholamines are commonly used and act through the stimulation of myocardial β adrenergic receptors. Agents commonly used include dopamine, adrenaline, and dobutamine. Dopamine acts through some additional mechanisms. It appears to increase the release of noradrenaline from myocardial storage sites and reduce the degradation of noradrenaline. There is also some α-mediated pulmonary and systemic vasoconstriction although it appears that the renal and splanchnic vascular beds are dilated due to action on dopamine receptors. The balance of these effects is dependent, in part, on the dose of dopamine used with low doses (1–2 mcg kg^{-1} per min) acting on the renal and splanchnic beds and higher doses (2–10 mcg kg^{-1} per min) having a greater effect on the myocardium. Undesirable effects of catecholamines include an increase in arrhythmias, myocardial oxygen demand and an increase in the afterload of both the right and left ventricles. These can have a detrimental effect in the low cardiac output state and potentially make the situation worse.

Milrinone is a bipyridine derivative sometimes described as an inodilator. It is becoming increasingly popular in pediatric cardiac surgery.[12] The mechanism of action is through inhibition of the enzyme phosphodiesterase type III, responsible for the intracellular degradation of cyclic AMP. The effects on cardiac muscle are to increase stroke work index and there is also evidence of an increase in diastolic ventricular relaxation (lusitropy). There is little effect on myocardial oxygen consumption. A dose-related vasodilating effect results in a fall in systemic and pulmonary vascular resistance. These attributes make it a suitable drug to aid the termination of cardiopulmonary bypass in tetralogy of Fallot. Milrinone may be given as a loading dose during CPB and then weaned during the post-operative period once cardiovascular stability has been achieved. The combination of phosphodiesterase inhibitors with catecholamines, such as dopamine or dobutamine, has been shown to be effective following CPB[17] and a multicentre study has shown a decrease in the incidence of low cardiac output state in selected infants following cardiac surgery.[18]

Levosimendan has been shown to improve cardiac function in adult patients with cardiac failure,[19] although there is not much data available for pediatric usage yet. It is described as a calcium sensitizer and does not increase myocardial oxygen consumption. Further studies in pediatric patients are awaited.

Post-operative arrhythmia

The post-operative electrocardiogram will usually show right bundle branch block following repair of TOF, due to surgical access through the conducting tissue itself. The incidence of post-operative arrhythmia following TOF repair is around 35%.[20] Observed arrhythmias include sinoatrial block, bradycardias, accelerated junctional rhythm, supraventricular tachycardia (SVT), complete AV block, frequent ectopics and junctional ectopic tachycardia (JET).[20] Of these, JET is one of the most frequent, occurring in up to 22% of patients following TOF repair.[21]

Criteria for the diagnosis of JET include a narrow QRS tachycardia (unless pre-existing bundle branch block), rate 170–230 b min^{-1} and, crucially, atrioventricular dissociation. The ventricular rate is faster than the atrial rate or there is 1 to 1 retrograde AV conduction. Usual treatment modalities for SVT such as adenosine, DC cardioversion and overdrive pacing fail to terminate the rhythm.[21] Overdrive pacing may be used to increase cardiac output, however, by increasing atrioventricular synchrony.

JET is more frequently observed with greater muscle resection, higher bypass temperatures and relief of right ventricular outflow obstruction via a right atrial approach.[22] Other risk factors include a younger age, high post-operative troponin I levels and a longer aortic cross clamp time.[20]

JET carries a notable morbidity including increased mechanical ventilation time and ICU stay. The arrhythmia may continue for 2 to 8 days despite treatment[21] and, if left untreated, carries a significant mortality. JET may also be seen following other forms of cardiac surgery, but is most likely to occur subsequent to surgery around the conduction system, especially the atrioventricular node and bundle of His.

JET should be treated aggressively due to its malignancy. A number of steps have been shown to effectively reduce the duration of the arrhythmia.[21,23,24] Management should commence with active surface cooling and success has been reported using temperatures of 32–35 °C.[21,24] Mechanical ventilation and a deep level of sedation will minimize catecholamine release and use of a paralyzing agent will prevent shivering due to hypothermia. Biochemical abnormalities, especially pertaining to potassium, magnesium, and calcium levels, should be corrected. The use of inotropic agents is a difficult issue. On the one hand, catecholamines will tend to increase cardiac arrhythmogenicity; however, by the nature of the tachycardia, the heart is in a low output state. A rational approach would be to use minimal inotropic support, using as little beta-adrenoceptor agonist as is feasible.

Amiodarone is one of the few antiarrhythmic agents shown to have good efficacy in the treatment of JET.[21,24,25] An Australian group administered amiodarone as a bolus, followed by infusion, giving a median arrhythmia control time of 4.5 hours.[24] Complications of this therapy include hypotension and bradycardia, often effectively managed using IV fluids and cardiac pacing. In addition to the well-documented long-term side effects of amiodarone therapy, further life-threatening arrhythmias have also been reported, hence the need for adequate monitoring, pacing and resuscitation facilities.[24]

Other pharmacological agents shown to be useful in the treatment of JET include propofenone[26] and procainamide,[23] although the use of amiodarone has generally super-seded these in recent years.

(Narrow complex tachycardias are discussed in more detail elsewhere in this book.)

Long-term complications of tetralogy of Fallot repair

Preservation of the pulmonary valve is generally preferred during surgical repair of TOF, as it ensures that the valve will continue to grow with the child. Unfortunately, at present, homograft, xenograft, and prosthetic valves will all require periodic replacement due to the limited lifespan as the child grows, subjecting them to multiple operations, often with accompanying right ventricular dysfunction.[2] A trans-junctional incision and patch will increase the risk of pulmonary regurgitation in later life. These are avoided if possible[4] as pulmonary regurgitation is associated with right ventricular dilatation, reduced exercise tolerance, arrhythmias, cardiac failure and sudden death. Up to 50% of patients may develop severe pulmonary regurgitation following TOF repair.[27]

Right ventricular diastolic dysfunction has already been cited as a significant post-operative complication. Persistence of RV diastolic dysfunction may, paradoxically, be beneficial in the late post-operative period. It is thought that, due to the inability of the right ventricle to increase in size, the pulmonary outflow tract is relatively protected and there is less pulmonary insufficiency. It was seen in up to 50% of patients in one follow-up study.[28] Improved exercise tolerance and fewer ventricular arrhythmias are also reported.

Delayed ventricular dysfunction and arrhythmia (both tachy and bradyarrhythmia) can lead to unexpected premature death. A group of 162 patients were followed up for 32 years after TOF repair and 6% suffered sudden unexpected cardiac death in that time.[29] The etiology of the arrhythmia is unclear but may relate to the insult at the time of surgery, delayed right ventricular dilatation, residual VSD, residual RVOT obstruction or severe pulmonary regurgitation.[2,30] A prolonged QRS >180 ms late after repair is associated with inhomogeneous RV contraction and relaxation, an increased incidence of post-operative ventricular tachycardia and sudden death. Other recognized complications include continued obstruction of the right ventricular outflow tract and dilatation of the aortic root. Residual intracardiac abnormalities may increase the risk of early cerebrovascular events in young adults due to embolic phenomenon.[31]

New advances in the placement of percutaneous pulmonary valves may provide a non-surgical solution to the residual narrowing or regurgitation seen in these patients.[32] Current difficulties with this technique include size restrictions and, in pure pulmonary regurgitation with a dilated RVOT, a lack of stable tissue onto which the valved stent can be hinged.

Learning points

- There is growing support for full corrective repair of tetralogy of Fallot within the first 18 months of life.
- Oxygenation in TOF depends on a balance between systemic and pulmonary outflow resistance.

- The degree of cyanosis in TOF patients usually depends on the severity of the right ventricular outflow tract obstruction.

- Pre-operative concerns include exclusion of co-existing anomalies and syndromes, of which trisomy 21 and 22 q11 are more frequently observed.

- Modified ultrafiltration has been shown to reduce ICU stay. It can be used after cardiopulmonary bypass to remove excess body water and may have additional anti-inflammatory benefits.

- Phosphodiesterase inhibitors such as milrinone can provide increased ventricular diastolic relaxation and inotropy following TOF repair.

- Low cardiac output state is frequent and management principles center on reducing oxygen consumption and increasing oxygen delivery.

- Post-operative cardiac arrhythmia is common and should be monitored for. Junctional ectopic tachycardia is a malignant arrhythmia and should be managed aggressively.

- The management of JET centers on avoidance of catecholamine release and active cooling. Amiodarone appears to be an effective antiarrhythmic in this situation.

Acknowledgments

The author would like to thank Dr Damien Kenny and Dr Peter Murphy for assistance in editing, Elizabeth Jordan for assistance in obtaining source material and Dr Rob Martin for providing the catheter images.

References

1. Shrivastava S. Blue babies: when to intervene. *Ind J Paediatr*. 2005; **72**: 599–602.

2. Shinebourne EA, Babu-Narayan SV, Carvalho JS. Tetralogy of Fallot: from fetus to adult. *Heart* 2006; **92**: 1353–9.

3. Vobecky SJ, Williams WG, Trusler GA *et al.*, Survival analysis of infants under age 18 months presenting with tetralogy of Fallot. *Ann Thorac Surg* 1993; **56**: 944–50.

4. Dodge-Khatami A, Tulevski II, Hitchcock JF, de Mol BAJM, Bennick GBWE. Neonatal complete correction of tetralogy of Fallot versus shunting and deferred repair: is the future of the right ventriculo-arterial junction at stake, and what of it? *Cardiology in the Young* 2001; **11**: 484–90.

5. van Dongen EI, Glansdorp AG, Mildner RJ *et al.* The influence of perioperative factors on outcomes in children aged less than 18 months after repair of tetralogy of Fallot. *J Thorac Cardiovasc Surg* 2003; **126**(3): 703–10.

6. Hirsch JC, Mosca RS, Bove EL. Complete repair of tetralogy of Fallot in the neonate. *Ann Surg* 2000; **232**(4): 508–14.

7. Parry AJ, McElhinney DB, Kung GC, Reddy VM, Brook MM, Hanley FL. Elective primary repair of acyanotic tetralogy of Fallot in early infancy: overall outcome and impact on the pulmonary valve. *J Am Cardiol* 2000; **36**(7): 2279–83.

8. Gladman G, McCrindle BW, Williams WG, Freedom RM, Benson LN. The modified blalock-taussig shunt: clinical impact and morbidity in fallot's tetralogy in the current era. *J Thorac Cardiovas Surg* 1997; **114**(1): 25–30.

9. Malm T, Karl TR, Mee RB. Transatrial transpulmonary repair of atrioventricular septal defect with right ventricular outflow tract obstruction. *J Cardiac Surg* 1993; **8**(6): 622–7.

10. Khongphatthanayothin A, Wong PC, Samara Y *et al.* Impact of respiratory syncytial virus infection on surgery for congenital heart disease: postoperative

course and outcome. *Crit Care Med* 1999; 27(9): 1974–81.

11. Kaushal SK, Radhakrishanan S, Dagar KS, Iyer PU, Girotra S, Shrivastava S, Iyer KS. Significant intraoperative right ventricular outflow gradients after repair of tetralogy of Fallot: to revise or not to revise? *Ann Thorac Surg.* 1999; 68: 1705–13.

12. Stocker CF, Shekerdemian LS. Recent developments in the perioperative management of the paediatric cardiac patient. *Curr Opin Anaesthesiol* 2006; 19(4): 375–81

13. Chew MS. Does modified ultrafiltration reduce the systemic inflammatory response to cardiac surgery with cardiopulmonary bypass. *Perfusion* 2004; 19(suppl 1): S57–60.

14. Cardoso SM, Miyague NI. Right ventricular diastolic dysfunction in the post-operative period of tetralogy of Fallot. *Arq Bras Cardiol* 2003; 80(2): 198–201.

15. Chaturvedi RR, Shore DF, Lincoln C et al. Acute right ventricular restrictive physiology after repair of tetralogy of Fallot. *Circulation* 1999; 100: 1540–47.

16. Stocker CF, Shekerdemian LS. Recent developments in the perioperative management of the paediatric cardiac patient. *Curr Opin Anaesthesiol* 2006; 19: 375–81

17. Royster RL, Butterworth JF 4th, Prielipp RC et al. Combined inotropic effects of amrinone and epinephrine after cardiopulmonary bypass in humans. *Anesth Analg* 1993; 77: 662–72

18. Hoffman TM, Wernovsky G, Atz AM et al. Efficacy and safety of milrinone in preventing low cardiac output syndrome in infants and children after corrective surgery for congenital heart disease. *Circulation* 2003; 107(7): 996–1002

19. Follath F, Cleland J, Just H et al. Efficacy and safety of intravenous levosimendan compared with dobutamine in severe low-output heart failure (the LIDO study): a randomised double-blind trial. *Lancet* 2002; 360(9328): 196–202.

20. Pfammatter JP, Wagner B, Berdat P et al. Procedural factors associated with early postoperative arrhythmias after repair of congenital heart defects. *J Thora Cardiovasc Surg* 2002; 123(2): 258–62.

21. Dodge-Khatami A, Miller OI, Anderson RH, Gil-Jaurena JM, Goldman AP, de Leval MR. Impact of junctional ectopic tachycardia on postoperative morbidity following repair of congenital heart defects. *Europ J. Cardiothor Surg* 2002; 21: 255–9.

22. Dodge-Khatami A, Miller OI, Anderson RH et al. Surgical substrates of postoperative junctional ectopic tachycardia in congenital heart defects. *J Thorac Cardiovasc Surg* 2002; 123(4): 624–30.

23. Walsh EP, Saul JP, Sholler GF et al. Evaluation of a staged treatment protocol for rapid automatic junctional tachycardia after operation for congenital heart disease. *J Am Coll Cardiol.* 1997; 29(5): 1046–53.

24. Plumpton K, Justo R, Haas N. Amiodarone for post-operative junctional ectopic tachycardia. *Cardiol Young* 2005; 15: 13–18.

25. Raja P, Hawker RE, Chaikitpinyo A et al. Amiodarone management of junctional ectopic tachycardia after cardiac surgery in children. *Br Heart J.* 1994; 72: 261–5.

26. Reimer A, Paul T, Kallfelz HC. Efficacy and safety of intravenous andoral propafenone in paediatric cardiac dysrhythmias. *Am J Cardiol* 1991; 68(8): 741–4.

27. Frigiola A, Redington AN, Cullen S, Vogel M. Pulmonary regurgitation is an important determinant of right ventricular contractile dysfunction in patients with surgically repaired tetralogy of Fallot. *Circulation* 2004; 110(Suppl II): II153-7.

28. Gatzoulis MA, Clark AL, Cullen S, Newman CGH, Redington AN. Right ventricular diastolic dysfunction 15 to 35 years after repair of tetralogy of Fallot: restrictive physiology predicts superior exercise performance. *Circulation* 1995; 91(6): 1775–81.

29. Murphy JG, Gersh BJ, Mair DD et al. Long-term outcome in patients undergoing repair of tetralogy of Fallot. *N Engl J Med* 1993; 329: 593–9.

30. Gatzoulis MA, Till JA, Somerville J et al. Mechanoelectrical interaction in tetralogy of Fallot: QRS prolongation relates to right ventricular size and predicts malignant ventricular arrhythmias and sudden death. *Circulation* 1995; 92: 231–7.

31. Chow CK, Amos D, Celermajer DS. Cerebrovascular events in young adults after surgical repair of tetralogy of Fallot. *Cardiology Young* 2005; **15**: 130–2.

32. Khambadkone S, Coats L, Taylor A *et al.* Percutaneous pulmonary valve implantation in humans: results in 59 consecutive patients. *Circulation* 2005; **112**(8): 1189–97.

Further reading

- Critical Heart Disease in Infants and Children. Nichols DG *et al.* Mosby-Year Book Inc., 1995.

- Anesthesia for Congenital Heart Disease. Andropoulos DB *et al.* Blackwell Publishing, 2005.

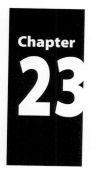

Chapter 23

The child with thermal injury and smoke inhalation

Sanjay M. Bhananker and Sam R. Sharar

Introduction

Burn-related injuries account for over 1 million emergency room visits, 50 000 acute admissions, and 4000 deaths in the USA annually. Children below 15 years of age account for approximately a third of burn admissions and burn deaths. Burns are second only to motor vehicle crashes as the leading cause of death in children older than 1 year. Flame burns account for about a third of pediatric burns and frequently involve inhalation injury. Although burns directly affect the skin, large burns alter the physiologic function of almost all other body organs and create increased risk of infection and death directly related in magnitude to burn size.

Case history

A 4-year-old boy and his 80-year-old grandmother were victims of an accidental house fire. While the grandmother succumbed to her injuries *en route* to hospital, the boy was brought to hospital by the paramedics. He had been responsive, but drowsy, at the scene of the accident. Upon arrival at the emergency department, he became unresponsive to commands, but moved all four extremities to pain. A Broselow length-based resuscitation tape was used to estimate his weight at 20 kg. His initial vital signs were: heart rate 174 b min^{-1}, BP 88/40 mm Hg, respiratory rate of 50 breaths min^{-1}, tympanic temperature 38.8 °C. His cervical spine was immobilized in an appropriately sized cervical collar. He was administered 100% oxygen via a non-rebreathing face mask and his transcutaneous oxygen saturation (SpO$_2$) was 99%. He had flame burns involving chest, abdomen, both his upper extremities, face, and parts of his lower extremities. He coughed up dark, carbonaceous sputum. In view of his unresponsiveness and possible inhalation injury, the on-call anesthesiologist was consulted to help with airway management. Intravenous access could not be obtained, so a right tibial intra-osseous needle was placed. Fluid therapy with Ringer's lactate solution was commenced. Following pre-oxygenation, a rapid sequence induction was performed by the anesthesiologist, using ketamine 40 mg (2 mg kg^{-1}) and succinylcholine 30 mg (1.5 mg kg^{-1}). He was intubated with a 4.5 mm uncuffed oral endotracheal tube and mechanically ventilated with 100% oxygen (O$_2$).

He was monitored with continuous ECG, NIBP at 5 min intervals, SpO$_2$, and end-tidal CO$_2$. A double lumen CVP line was placed in his right subclavian vein and an arterial line was placed in his left dorsalis pedis artery. Intra-osseous access was then discontinued. Blood was sent for complete blood count, electrolytes, urea, creatinine, arterial blood gases (ABG), carboxyhemoglobin levels, coagulation profile, and cross-matching. Continuous infusions of morphine and midazolam were started, and the rates adjusted as tolerated hemodynamically. A nasojejunal tube was placed and the position of the tube confirmed with abdominal X-ray.

Case Studies in Pediatric Critical Care, ed. Peter. J. Murphy, Stephen C. Marriage, and Peter J. Davis.
Published by Cambridge University Press. © Cambridge University Press 2009.

Table 23.1. *Findings on admission*

Examination	Airway clear but edematous, sats 99% on 100% Oxygen	
	Respiratory rate 50 min^{-1}	
	Chest clear, bilateral air entry, coughing up dark sputum	
	Heart rate 174 b min^{-1}, Capillary refill time = 3 seconds	
	Normal heart sounds, BP 88/40, peripheral pulses palpable	
	Temperature 38.8 °C	
	52% TBSA burns with smoke inhalation injury	
Investigations	Weight	20 kg (Estimated using Broselow tape)
	FBC	Hb 14.6 g dl^{-1}, Plat 410×10^9 l^{-1}
		WBC 13.4×10^9 l^{-1}
	U+Es	Na$^+$ 138 mmol l^{-1}, K$^+$ 4.2 mmol l^{-1}, Cl$^-$ 110 mmol l^{-1}
		Urea 15.9 mmol l^{-1}, Creatinine 100 μmol l^{-1}
		Ca^{2+} 2.1 mmol l^{-1}
	Glucose	12.5 mmol l^{-1}
	Albumin	25 g l^{-1}
	Arterial blood gas	pH 7.22, pCO$_2$ 50 mmHg, HCO$_3^-$ 16.2 mmol l^{-1}, BE −11.4, carboxyhemoglobin 30%

His bladder was catheterized with a Foley catheter. AP and lateral films of his cervical spine and a chest X-ray did not reveal any bony abnormalities.

Secondary survey revealed that he had suffered second- and third-degree burns to 52% of his total body surface area (TBSA) involving most of the anterior chest, abdomen, both arms, and parts of his face and lower extremities. An initial carboxyhemoglobin (COHb) level was 30%, and his ABG demonstrated a mixed respiratory and metabolic acidosis (Table 23.1).

Head and cervical spine CT was unremarkable. The pediatric intensivist and burn surgeon assumed his care and he was transferred to the PICU with full monitoring.

Presentation

Progress in the pediatric intensive care unit

Fluid resuscitation was continued with Ringer's lactate solution as per the Parkland (Baxter) formula (260 ml h^{-1} for the first 8 hours and then halved to 130 ml h^{-1} for the next 16 hours). Hourly urine output of >10 ml (0.5 ml kg^{-1} per h) was targeted. Intravenous infusions of morphine 0.1 mg kg^{-1} per h and midazolam 0.05 mg kg^{-1} per h were continued and additional boluses of these drugs ordered as necessary. He was ventilated with pressure-controlled ventilation (PCV) and the initial ventilator settings were a rate of 20 min^{-1}, pressure control of 20 cmH$_2$O, PEEP 5 cmH$_2$O, FiO$_2$ 1.0. The expired tidal volume was 180 ml (9 ml kg^{-1}). The initial PICU ABG showed pH 7.24, pCO$_2$ 58 mm Hg, pO$_2$ 392 mm Hg, HCO$_3$ 18, and BE −6, lactate 4.1 mmol l^{-1}. Ventilation rate was increased from 20 to

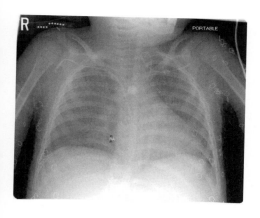

Fig. 23.1. Chest X-ray showing bilateral diffuse infiltrates in a child with smoke inhalation injury.

28 breaths min^{-1} to correct the respiratory component of acidosis. His parents and pediatrician were contacted. History obtained from these sources revealed that he was previously a healthy child, had no known drug allergies, and was not on any medication.

He was nursed in a warm room (temperature maintained at 30 °C). The burn areas were cleansed and dressed with silver sulfadiazine 1% cream, and covered with gauze. High caloric enteral feeds were commenced via the nasogastric tube. Arterial blood gases were monitored frequently to assess the adequacy of oxygenation and ventilation. Adequacy of fluid resuscitation was monitored by trending the HR, BP, urine output, capillary refill time, base deficit, and serum lactate levels.

Twenty-four hours later, the patient was opening eyes, and following simple commands. He was able to move all the extremities and, after a negative physical examination, the cervical collar was taken off to facilitate the care of burn areas in his upper chest and neck. He was judged to be in pain and the morphine infusion was adjusted upwards to 0.2 mg kg^{-1} per h. Additional pain relief was provided with nasogastric administration of acetaminophen (paracetamol) 300 mg (15 mg kg^{-1}) every 6 hours. His tympanic temperature was 39.5 °C and he had a sinus tachycardia at 190 b min^{-1}. Propranolol 10 mg every 6 hours was started via the NG tube. Target HR was set at 120–140 b min^{-1}. He was also started on Oxandrolone 10 mg every 6 hours to reduce the negative nitrogen balance.

Forty-eight hours later, his tidal volumes had dropped to 120 ml and the pressure control was gradually adjusted to 35 cm H$_2$O to maintain pCO$_2$ in the normal range. Despite the carboxyhemoglobin level dropping to <1%, 100% oxygen was now needed to maintain his oxygenation. Suctioning of his trachea revealed carbonaceous sputum. Fiberoptic bronchoscopy was performed and showed carbonaceous endobronchial debris and mucosal ulceration. Chest X-ray showed bilateral diffuse infiltrates (Fig. 23.1).

He was started on lung protective ventilation strategy and his ventilation parameters were set to SIMV, rate 30 min^{-1}, tidal volume 120 ml (6 ml kg^{-1}), PEEP 10 cmH$_2$O, FiO$_2$ 1.0. His peak inspiratory pressure was 40 cmH$_2$O and a leak around the tracheal tube resulted in inadequate minute ventilation. The tracheal tube was changed to 4.5 mm cuffed nasal endotracheal tube to allow adequate ventilation and proper fixation. High Frequency Percussive Ventilation (HFPV) was started at a frequency of 3 Hz (180 cycles min^{-1}) and the gas exchange gradually improved over the next 12 hours. HFPV was discontinued on day 5 and lung protective conventional ventilation was reinstituted using 6 ml kg^{-1} tidal volume,

Table 23.2. *Post-PICU course*

Day 9–14	Daily dressing changes in the "tank room" under deep sedation provided by an anesthesiologist. Daily range of motion exercises by physical therapist to try and prevent development of contractures.
Day 15	Taken to the OR for removal of the skin substitute, and autografting. Split thickness skin grafts harvested from his entire back and scalp and applied to the burn areas. He was brought to the PICU with endotracheal tube *in situ* as he was hypothermic (esophageal temperature of 34.6 °C). He was warmed gradually, weaned from the ventilator and extubated in the evening on the same day. He was started on supplemental oral transmucosal fentanyl (200 mcg) as required, and his 4-hourly oral morphine dose was escalated to 50 mg.
Day 16	Discharged back to the floor (pediatric ward)

PEEP of 12 cm H_2O and the rate adjusted to get acceptable pCO_2 (in the 50–70 range, pH >7.2, permissive hypercapnia, see below). Frequent tracheobronchial saline lavage and suctioning were performed to facilitate clearance of thick secretions.

By the seventh day, his lung injury was improving and his oxygen support was weaned down to FiO_2 0.5, PEEP 5 cm H_2O. His morphine infusion had been escalated in 0.025 mg increments to 0.4 mg kg^{-1} per h. He was scheduled for a primary excision and covering of his burn wounds with biosynthetic skin substitute (Integra). His tube feeds were continued through surgery. His burn wounds were excised and grafted with Integra. The surgical procedure lasted 4 hours and the estimated blood loss was 600 ml (30 ml kg^{-1}). The patient was transfused with 2 units (650 ml) of packed red cells, in addition to 2400 ml of crystalloid administration. He was returned to PICU with a temp 34.6 °C, HR 160 b min^{-1}, BP 90/44 mm Hg.

He was gradually warmed, using warm ambient room temperature, warm IV fluids, and a dry air convective heating blanket. On the ninth post-burn day, his trachea was extubated and he was able to maintain his airway and oxygenation. He was administered humidified oxygen via a face mask. Arterial line and subclavian line were removed, intravenous sedation was discontinued, and regular oral sedation/analgesia started. Oral morphine 40 mg every 4 hours and acetaminophen (paracetamol) 300 mg every 6 hours were supplemented with as-required doses of sublingual fentanyl and oral midazolam. He was transferred to a pediatric burn ward. His post-PICU hospital course is outlined in Table 23.2.

Discussion

A review of the management of a child with major thermal injury occurs elsewhere in this book; however, the following important points should be noted.

The primary determinants of severity of burn injury are the size and depth of burn area. Patient age, the body part burned, presence of pre-existing disease, and associated non-burn injuries also have an important impact on the outcome.

Children, especially those younger than 2 years of age, have a high surface area to body weight ratio, very thin skin, and minimal physiologic reserves causing higher morbidities and mortalities than in the older age groups. Severe burn injury results in vasoactive mediator release throughout the body to increase capillary permeability and third spacing of fluid in tissues both surrounding the burn, and distant from the burn (larger burn sizes > ~20% body

Table 23.3. *Classification of burn depth*

Classification	Burn Depth	Outcome
Superficial (first-degree)	Epidermis only	Heal spontaneously
Partial thickness (Second-degree)	Epidermis and dermis	
Full thickness		
Third-degree	Destruction of epidermis and dermis	Wound excision and grafting necessary
Fourth-degree	Fascia, muscle, bone burned	Complete excision required, functional limitation likely

surface area). Damaged skin is no longer able to retain heat and H_2O, consequently large evaporative losses ensue. Combination of these mechanisms results in hypovolemic shock acutely following burn injury.

Classification of burn depth
First-degree burns affect only the epidermis and are characterized by erythema and edema of the burned areas without blistering or desquamation. Second-degree or partial thickness burns involve the epidermis and a portion of the dermis. In most cases, these wounds can be expected to spontaneously heal in 7 to 28 days, although surgical treatment may be necessary for extensive or deep second-degree burns. Pain is characteristic of partial thickness burns. Third-degree or full-thickness burns extend entirely through both the epidermis and dermis and will not heal spontaneously (Table 23.3).

Metabolic complications
Metabolic complications are directly related to extent of burn. The core temperature in severe burn patients is reset to 38.5 °C. Thermal maintenance is critical in young children, especially those with burns of more than 10% TBSA. Body temperature is best maintained by a thermoneutral environment (room temperature of 28–32 °C), with the additional use of an overbed warming shield and warming of IV fluids. Dry-air warmers used directly over the burn wound can cause tissue desiccation.

Thermal injury leads to hypermetabolism and protein hypercatabolic state. Up to a ten-fold increase in circulating levels of catecholamines has been demonstrated following severe burn injury. These, along with wound-released mediators, hormones and bacterial products from the gut and wound, result in a systemic inflammatory response syndrome (SIRS), manifested as a hyperdynamic circulation and large increases in basal energy expenditure (*hypermetabolic response*). The secretion of glucagon and cortisol are increased and, together with post-injury insulin resistance, result in the use of amino acids to fuel production, with consequent muscle wasting and nitrogen imbalance. The supra-physiologic thermogenesis is associated with resetting of the core temperature to higher levels, proportional to the size of the burns. Damaged skin is no longer able to retain heat and water and the vasomotor thermoregulatory responses are impaired. Consequently large evaporative losses ensue. Concomitant sepsis can greatly exaggerate these metabolic demands (Fig. 23.2).

Adequate analgesia, anxiolysis, a thermoneutral environment, and control of infection are important steps in limiting catecholamine secretion and thus hypermetabolism.

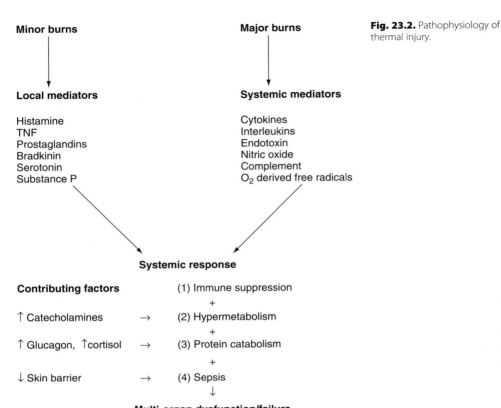

Fig. 23.2. Pathophysiology of thermal injury.

Infection prevention/control

Loss of barrier function of skin and blunting of immune response result in increased susceptibility to infection and bacterial overgrowth within the eschar. Sepsis is a leading cause of death in patients who survive the acute burn injury. Cutaneous burn toxin, a toxic lipid protein isolated from burned skin, is 1000 times more immunosuppressive than endotoxins.[1] Bowel permeability is increased in burn patients, leading to translocation of bacteria and absorption of endotoxins into the bloodstream. Burn wound infection, intravenous catheter associated septicemia, and ventilator-associated pneumonia are particularly common in burned children. Pyrexia, tachycardia, and leukocytosis are almost universal in burn patients and cannot be considered signs of sepsis. Blood cultures may be negative in up to half of septic patients. Hypotension, lactic acidosis, or intolerance of enteral feeds in the non-acute phase favor the diagnosis of infection. Quantitative cultures of wound biopsy help in identifying the offending pathogens and appropriately treating the infection. Systemic antibiotics should be reserved for treatment of proven infection and in the perioperative period.

Renal function

The incidence of acute renal failure in burn patients ranges from 0.5% to 38%, depending on the severity of burns. In the early post-burn period, the renal blood flow is reduced as a result of hypovolemia and decreased cardiac output. In addition, increased levels of catecholamines, angiotensin, vasopressin, and aldosterone contribute to renal vasoconstriction. Myoglobinuria and sepsis can also aggravate renal dysfunction. Despite an increase in the renal blood flow during the hypermetabolic phase of burn injury, tubular function and creatinine clearance may be reduced and renal function may be variable.

Pharmacologic changes

Burn injury also affects the pharmacodynamic and pharmacokinetic properties of many drugs. Decreased levels of serum albumin in these patients leads to increased free fraction of acidic drugs such as thiopentone or diazepam, while increased levels of α-acid glycoprotein result in decreased free fraction of basic drugs (with pKa>8) such as lidocaine or propranolol. Renal and hepatic functions may be impaired in patients with large burns and this may impair the elimination of some drugs, while increases in renal blood flow and glomerular filtration rate in the hyperdynamic phase of burns may enhance the renal excretion of drugs. It has been shown that some drugs, such as gentamicin, may be lost through the open wounds. The response to muscle relaxants is altered due to proliferation of acetylcholine receptors away from the synaptic cleft of the neuromuscular junction. Suxamethonium administration to patients >24 h after burn injury is unsafe, due to the risk of hyperkalemic ventricular dysrhythmias. The exact period of risk is unknown, but it appears that neuromuscular junction responses return to normal once the burn wound is healed. Pharmacokinetics of morphine are unchanged following burn injury. While lorazepam has an increased volume of distribution, increased clearance, and a reduced half-life, the elimination half-life of diazepam is significantly prolonged in burn patients.

Inhalation injury

Most injuries occur from inhalation of smoke, although rarely superheated air or steam produces direct thermal injury. Unless steam is involved, direct heat injury to airway is supraglottic. The pharyngeal mucosal lining acts as a heat reservoir and the vocal cords close, reflexly, in response to sudden exposure to hot air, thus limiting the physical effects of heat to the upper airway. The natural history of upper airway inhalation injury is edema that narrows the airway over the initial 12–24 h. Presence of stridor, wheeze, or voice changes is indicative of airway swelling and compromise. Circumferential burns to the neck can result in tight eschar formation which, combined with inhalation injury-induced pharyngeal edema, can exacerbate upper airway compromise.

Smoke inhalation is a combination of direct pulmonary injury and systemic and metabolic toxicity. The severity of smoke lung injury depends on fuels, intensity, duration, and confinement. Obvious concerns are obstructive edema, thermal tracheitis, hemorrhagic edema of bronchi. Gas phase constituents of smoke include carbon monoxide (CO), cyanide, acid and aldehyde gases, and oxidants. These can cause direct damage to mucociliary function, bronchial vessel permeability, alveolar destruction, and secondary edema. At the alveolar level, smoke exposure causes inactivation of surfactant and immediate atelectasis. Bronchial blood flow increases manifold and lung macrophages and neutrophils are activated in response to smoke exposure. The ensuing release of inflammatory mediators, oxygen derived free radicals, nitric oxide causes a large increase in the vascular permeability of the pulmonary circulation. The resultant airway edema, when combined with sloughing of necrotic epithelial mucosa and thick, viscid secretions, produces airway obstruction at various levels of the bronchial tree. Hypoxic Pulmonary Vasoconstriction (HPV) helps to

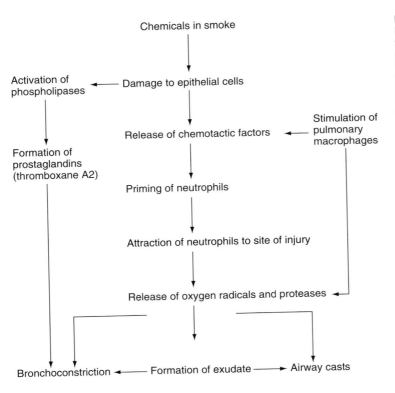

Fig. 23.3. Pathophysiology of tracheobronchial damage by smoke inhalation Adapted from Traber LD, Herndon DN: Pathophysiology of smoke inahalation. In Haponik EF, Munster AM, eds. Respiratory injury: Smoke inhalation and burns. New York, 1990, McGraw-Hill)

match lung ventilation to perfusion in normal lungs by causing pulmonary arterial smooth muscle constriction in response to localized alveolar hypoxia caused by airway obstruction. HPV is inhibited by nitric oxide. Concomitant cutaneous burn injury aggravates the lung damage by releasing pro-inflamatory mediators and causing hydrostatic pulmonary edema secondary to the lowered plasma oncotic pressure resulting from loss of plasma protein into the interstitial space. The end result is a mismatched V/Q ratio and hypoxemia. (Fig. 23.3).

There is strong evidence to suggest that mechanical ventilation can worsen lung damage (Ventilator Induced Lung Injury, VILI). Several factors such as shearing forces of large tidal volumes and excessive peak pressures (volutrauma, barotrauma), a high FiO_2 (oxygen toxicity), repeated opening and closing of alveoli due to insufficient PEEP contribute to the development of VILI. In addition, the non-homogeneous nature of ARDS leads to localized areas of over-inflation with conventional ventilatory modes. Over-distension of parts of lung has been shown to produce interstitial edema, hyaline membrane formation, and microatelectasis.[2]

Carbon monoxide (CO) poisoning is a leading cause of death in major burns with inhalation injury. CO has a 250-fold affinity for hemoglobin (Hb) as compared with O_2. CO displaces O_2 from Hb and also shifts the O_2–Hb dissociation curve to the left resulting in impairment of delivery of O_2 to tissues (Fig. 23.4).

CO also inhibits cytochrome oxidase a3 complex at the tissue level and thus interferes with aerobic cellular metabolism. Binding of CO to cardiac and skeletal muscles results in direct toxicity and impaired function, while central nervous demyelination can occur by a poorly understood mechanism. CO poisoning is diagnosed by co-oximetric estimations

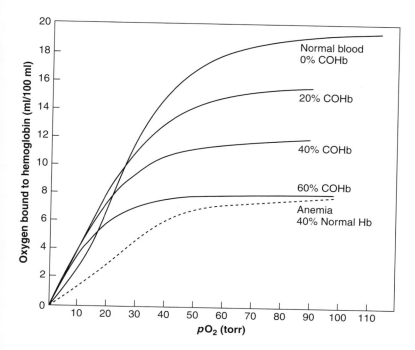

Fig. 23.4.
Carboxyhemoglobin-induced changes in the oxygen–hemoglobin dissociation curve (Fein, Leff, A, Hopewell PC. Crit Care Med 1980;8:94–8.)

of COHb and HbO_2. Pulse oximetry is unreliable in the presence of carbon monoxide poisoning, as it cannot detect COHb, and a falsely elevated oxygen saturation reading will be obtained. Treatment of CO poisoning relies on administration of oxygen. One-hundred percent oxygen administration results in fivefold reduction of half life of COHb from 2.5 h to approximately 40 min. Hyperbaric oxygen therapy is fraught with practical difficulties of transporting critically ill patients into hyperbaric chambers and, although useful in isolated cases of CO poisoning, is rarely used in the management of combined burn and inhalation injury victims.

Cyanide is released when natural and synthetic polymers such as wool, vinyl, and plastics are burned. Cyanide causes tissue hypoxia by uncoupling oxidative phosphorylation in mitochondria. Consider treating for cyanide poisoning in patients with unexplained severe metabolic acidosis associated with elevated central venous O_2 (therefore patients are clinically not cyanotic), normal arterial O_2 content and low carboxyhemoglobin.

Management of thermal injury and smoke inhalation

Initial assessment and management
Routine evaluation of the pediatric burn patient is the same as in any trauma patient. Wound care is of secondary importance until the ABCs of trauma care have been evaluated and treated.

A Airway
B Breathing
C Circulation

Oxygen is delivered by either mask or nasal cannula. Intravenous (IV) access is in a peripheral vessel. The access site is often a problem because of the distribution of the burn

Table 23.4. *Berkow chart for estimating percent of TBSA burned in various age groups*

Area	1 year	1–4 years	5–9 years	10–14 years	15 years	Adult
Head	19	17	13	11	9	7
Neck	2	2	2	2	2	2
Ant. trunk	13	13	13	13	13	13
Post. trunk	13	13	13	13	13	13
R buttock	2.5	2.5	2.5	2.5	2.5	2.5
L buttock	2.5	2.5	2.5	2.5	2.5	2.5
Genitalia	1	1	1	1	1	1
R U arm	4	4	4	4	4	4
L U arm	4	4	4	4	4	4
R L arm	3	3	3	3	3	3
L L arm	3	3	3	3	3	3
R hand	2.5	2.5	2.5	2.5	2.5	2.5
L hand	2.5	2.5	2.5	2.5	2.5	2.5
R thigh	5.5	6.5	8	8.5	9	9.5
L thigh	5.5	6.5	8	8.5	9	9.5
R leg	5	5	5.5	6	6.5	7
L leg	5	5	5.5	6	6.5	7
R foot	3.5	3.5	3.5	3.5	3.5	3.5
L foot	3.5	3.5	3.5	3.5	3.5	3.5
Total	100	100	100	100	100	100

wound, presence of subcutaneous edema, and reluctance to place a catheter through a burn. Access should be obtained percutaneously through unburned skin or through burned skin as a second choice. A venous cutdown may be performed through unburned or burned skin, if necessary. For large burns, two large bore peripheral IVs are recommended. A Foley catheter is inserted to evaluate hourly output of urine as a sign of adequate fluid resuscitation. A nasogastric tube is inserted to prevent gastric dilation. Periodic evaluations of the nose, pharynx, and lungs should be performed to determine adequacy of the upper and lower airways. Obstructive symptoms or evidence of airway involvement indicate the need for immediate endotracheal intubation.

The initial burn treatment algorithm determines whether the patient will be treated as an outpatient, be admitted, or will require transfer to a burn center. The extent of burn (% TBSA body parts involved and depth) should be estimated using age appropriate charts (Table 23.4).

The burned region is gently washed with dilute antiseptic soap and water. All loose tissue is removed. Partial thickness burns can be dressed in the emergency room with silver sulfadiazine, porcine heterograft, or Biobrane, applied as directed and covered with a simple snug gauze dressing. The wound is then inspected at 24 to 48 hours after application. If the dressing is adherent to the underlying burn, it is left intact. If non-adherent, the dressing is removed and replaced with silver sulfadiazine or neomycin. Wounds of indeterminate depth

Table 23.5. *American Burn Association (ABA) criteria for major burn injuries*

Partial thickness burns greater than 10% TBSA

Burns that involve the face, hands, feet, genitalia, perineum, or major joints

Third-degree burns in any age group

Electrical burns, including lightning injury

Chemical burns

Inhalation injury

Burn injury in patients with pre-existing medical disorders that could complicate management, prolong recovery, or affect mortality

Any patient with burns and concomitant trauma in which the burn injury poses the greatest risk

Burned children in hospitals without qualified personnel or equipment for their care

Burns in patients who require special social, emotional, or long-term rehabilitative intervention

are dressed with silver sulfadiazine, fine mesh gauze, and a simple gauze dressing. Wounds are washed daily to remove old topical agents and tissue debris. This is done in tap water with a washcloth and soap. New topical agent is then applied in a thin layer and dressed with gauze.

Optimal care of patients with major thermal injuries as outlined by the American Burn Association requires an organized approach best delivered by a specialized burn center facility (Table 23.5).

In addition to the general objectives of immediate care, special attention must be given to fluid resuscitation and maintenance of the airway and body temperature.

Fluid resuscitation

Children older than 2 years with more than 20% TBSA burns and all younger children regardless of burn size, require intravenous fluids for optimal management. The objective of resuscitation is to replace fluid losses and restore euvolemia with the minimal amount of fluid required to maintain organ function. The fluid requirements may be calculated using several different formulae, all of which achieve good results. There is no conclusive evidence re: *what* kind of fluid; *when* (how fast) to give; and *how* much to give. *Early* fluid resuscitation (within 2 hours of burn injury) helps in limiting the morbidity and mortality in pediatric burn victims.[3] The Parkland (Baxter) formula provides a simple, easily remembered basis for resuscitation (4 ml Ringer's lactate [RL]/kg per percent TBSA burned; one half to be given during the first 8 hours after injury and the rest in the next 16 hours).

The fluid volume determined by a burn formula is only the starting point of resuscitation. Exact volumes are individually adjusted, based on clinical response. It is widely believed that the Parkland formula tends to underestimate resuscitation volumes, especially in children. Studies using invasive monitoring in adults have reported use of significantly higher volumes (4.5–9.2 ml/kg per TBSA per 24 h) for adequate resuscitation, particularly in the presence of concomitant inhalation injury.[4] Goals of resuscitation include stable hemodynamics, urine output >1 ml kg^{-1} per h, and normal mentation. Serial lactate levels and base deficit can also be used to guide the adequacy of fluids. Isotonic fluids are currently preferred for resuscitation of burn victims. Dextrose-containing fluids and free water may be needed in infants less than 6 months of age. Cardiogenic failure, predominantly left-sided, is a major cause of a failing pediatric burn resuscitation. Information from pulmonary artery catheters can help direct therapy in such cases, by providing indications for vasopressors and modifying fluid resuscitation, but are rarely used in children.[5]

Inhalation injury and airway management
Inhalation injury is best divided into upper airway obstruction and lower airway injury.

Upper airway injury
Upper airway injury is usually an indirect heat injury causing swelling of the posterior pharynx and supraglottic regions, leading to upper airway obstruction. It is characteristically seen in patients with significant burns of the face and neck. The onset of acute obstruction may occur without any warning signs or symptoms, or may be preceded by increased respiratory rate or work of breathing, sudden increase in secretions, or progressive hoarseness over the first 12–24 hours after injury. Tracheal intubation serves both as prophylaxis and therapy and should be performed early when there is a suspicion of airway injury. Patients with marginal injuries should be monitored with elevation of the head of bed. Early tracheostomy is rarely required and when performed in children is safe, effective, and *not* associated with increased risk of infection.[6] Translaryngeal intubation for periods over 10 days may be associated with increased incidence of subglottic stenosis and a conversion to tracheostomy should be considered in children who require extended ventilatory support.[7] Steroids *do not* help in preventing the development of edema associated with burn injuries and may also increase the risk of infection too.

Lower airway or pulmonary parenchymal damage
This usually manifests 12 to 48 hours after the injury. Findings include dyspnea, rales, rhonchi, and wheezing. The clinical picture and radiographic findings (Fig. 23.1) are identical to that of acute respiratory distress syndrome and are caused by chemical irritation of the terminal bronchiolar tree. Meticulous pulmonary toilet is the cornerstone of early care. Tracheal secretions are often very viscous and may contain carbonaceous particles and pieces of mucous membrane. The small internal diameter of pediatric endotracheal tubes increases the risk of obstruction by secretions. Using as large an endotracheal tube as possible allows easy suctioning and fiberoptic bronchoscopy. Bronchoscopic findings include edema, ulceration, sloughing of the mucosa with thick, viscid secretions, and carbonaceous sputum (Fig. 23.5 and 23.6). Most large pediatric burn centers in North America frequently use cuffed endotracheal tubes in burned children.

Adequate fixation of the endotracheal tube is essential since facial burns can make fixation of the tube extremely difficult. Close proximity of topical burn wound agents, continual changes in size of the face and neck (because of burn edema), and fluid exuding through a facial burn often cause failure of the usual methods of fixation. Umbilical tape secured to the tube and passed around the head provides rapid fixation, as does wiring of the tube to firmly intact primary or secondary teeth.

Several strategies have been tried to minimize VILI, while allowing adequate oxygenation and promoting lung healing in patients with ARDS and smoke inhalation injury. These include use of Lung Protective Ventilation (LPV), permissive hypercapnia, inhaled nitric oxide, high frequency percussive ventilation (HFPV), high frequency oscillatory ventilation (HFOV) and

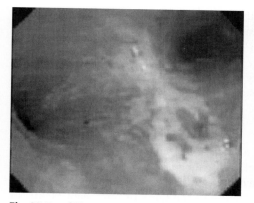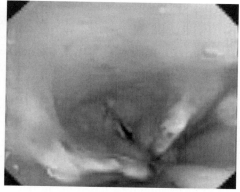

Fig. 23.5 and Fig. 23.6. Edema, ulceration, sloughing of airway mucosa at the level of carina and larynx as seen on fiberoptic bronchoscopy. (Images courtesy of Lee Woodson, MD, Ph.D.; University of Texas Medical Branch, Shriners' Burns Hospital; Galveston, TX.) (See color plate section.)

use of extracorporeal life support. The goal of ventilatory support is to provide adequate oxygentation and CO_2 removal at the lowest possible FiO_2 and peak (or mean) airway pressures

Permissive hypercapnia refers to the practice of accepting higher levels of $PaCO_2$ (in the 50–75 mm Hg range) and associated respiratory acidosis (generally pH >7.2). Despite the deleterious effects of acute hypercapnia (such as narcosis, cardiac depression, reduction of renal blood flow), chronic hypercapnia is generally well tolerated. Sheridan *et al.* have demonstrated lower rates of respiratory complications (pneumonia, barotraumas) and respiratory deaths in pediatric burn patients using permissive hypercapnia and conventional ventilation.[8]

HFPV is administered using a volumetric-diffusive respirator to deliver high frequency (0.6 to 15 Hz, 36 to 900 cycles min^{-1}), sub-dead space breaths. These pulsatile breaths are rapidly stacked to a selected peak airway pressure, followed by a phase of passive exhalation to the baseline continuous positive airway pressure (CPAP, generally 5–10 cm H_2O). Thus, the high frequency percussive waveform is superimposed on a sinusoidal, low frequency, cyclic waveform of increasing and decreasing airway pressures. In addition to reducing VILI, the percussive nature of the pulsatile breaths promotes mucokinesis and clearance of secretions. HFPV has been shown to allow lower peak airway pressures and achieve better PaO_2/FiO_2 ratios than conventional ventilation[9] and HFOV[10] in burned children and animals with smoke inhalation injuries.

HFOV has also been used successfully in burn patients with ARDS.[11] HFOV uses two principles:

1. Sustained inflation and recruitment of lung volume by the application of distending pressure (mean airway pressure, MAP) to achieve oxygenation and

2. Alveolar ventilation and CO_2 removal by superimposition of an oscillating pressure waveform on the MAP at a variable frequency (Hz) and an adjustable amplitude.

In a survey of North American Pediatric Burn Centers, a widespread but variable use of PCV, SIMV, HFOV, and mixed/other modes of ventilation was noted for the treatment of lung injury in burned children.[12]

Patients should be extubated as soon as the upper airway edema is resolved and the adequacy of gas exchange is confirmed. A leak around the endotracheal tube and direct laryngoscopic and/or fiberoptic visualization of the airway serve as clinical guides for resolution of airway edema. It is a common practice among North American pediatric burn centers to use steroids to diminish airway edema prior to extubation.[12]

Temperature homeostasis and nutritional support for pediatric burn victims are covered elsewhere in this book

Analgesia

Severe pain is an inevitable consequence of a major burn injury and analgesic requirements are frequently underestimated, especially in the peri-operative period. Anxiety and depression are common in a major burn and can reduce the pain threshold. Pain management should be based on an understanding of the types of burn pain (acute, or procedure-related pain versus background, or baseline pain), frequent patient assessment by an acute pain service team, and the development of protocols to address problems such as breakthrough pain. High-dose opioids are commonly used to manage pain associated with burn procedures, and morphine is currently the most widely used drug. There is an inter-individual variation in response to morphine, so "titration to effect" and frequent reassessment are important. Furthermore, most burned patients rapidly develop tolerance to opioids.

For background analgesia, analgesics such as acetaminophen (paracetamol) can be used for their opioid-sparing effect, and are combined with generous administration of oral opioids. Non-steroidal anti-inflammatory drugs have antiplatelet effects and may not be appropriate for patients who require extensive excision and grafting procedures. Burn patients can also manifest the nephrotoxic effects of non-steroidal anti-inflammatory drugs. Opioids and benzodiazepines can be used successfully together for both background and procedural sedation, as anxiety is a common component of burn pain associated with wound care procedures. Patient monitoring must be appropriate to the level of sedation. Breakthrough pain can be treated either with boluses of opiates using Patient Controlled Analgesia (PCA) or Nurse Controlled Analgesia (NCA) devices as dictated by the patient age or using rapidly acting transmucosal fentanyl lozenges.

Procedures such as dressing changes and wound care frequently require sedation and analgesia in pediatric burn patients. These procedures are often performed on a daily basis on the burn ward, making anesthesiologist involvement impractical. Nurse-administered opioid analgesics (IV, oral, or transmucosal) alone or in combination with benzodiazepine anxiolysis is the typical regimen. However, when wound care procedures are extensive, more potent anesthetic agents may be of benefit. Ketamine offers the advantage of stable hemodynamics and analgesia and has been used extensively as the primary agent for both general anesthesia and analgesia for burn dressing changes. Nitrous oxide with oxygen (Entonox) has been used effectively for analgesia during burn wound dressing changes. However, scavenging of the gas when administered outside of an operating room is problematic. Combination of nitrous oxide with opioids also carries a risk of inducing a state of general anesthesia with profound respiratory depression. The efficacy of general anesthesia administered by an anesthesiologist for procedures on a burn intensive care unit has been well documented. Music therapy, hypnotherapy, massage, a number of cognitive and behavioral techniques and, more recently, virtual reality techniques have been successfully used to reduce pain during debridement and wound care.[13]

Non-accidental trauma

Child abuse must always be considered when treating a burned child. Most of these burns occur in children younger than 4 years and in those with a history of tap water immersion. The pattern of burn injury should be carefully evaluated with special emphasis on the presence of multiple burns (recent or old), the presence or absence of splash marks, spared regions, bilateral symmetry (glove and stocking distribution), and well-demarcated water-lines. Cigarette burns should be looked for especially on the extremities. The soles of the feet should be always inspected for the presence of burn. Non-burn trauma, such as bruises, whip marks, fractures, and head trauma should be looked for, and old medical records reviewed for prior injuries. If abuse is suspected, skull, chest, and long bone radiologic series are obtained. Tell-tale signs of non-accidental burns include: the appearance, pattern, and depth of burn are not consistent with the history, history of events leading to the injury changes with repeated telling, and the pattern of burns is as described above. When suspicion is aroused, the social worker and child welfare department must be contacted. Due to the high incidence of further injury and death, it is vital that all persons caring for burned children maintain an appropriate index of suspicion for the possibility of non-accidental burn injury.

Drugs and materials used in patients with burns

Silver sulfadiazine cream 1%

Many topical antiseptics and antibiotics have been utilized as topical agents on burn wounds to prevent infection. Some antiseptics may be detrimental to wound healing, while some antibiotics have too many undesirable side effects. A 1% water soluble cream of silver sulfadiazine is most commonly used as it has a broad spectrum of activity against Gram-positive, Gram-negative bacilli and *Candida*. Precipitation of silver salts in the wounds imparts long-lasting bactericidal action, while the sulfadiazine has bacteriostatic properties. Some of the sulfadiazine may be absorbed systemically and give rise to transient leukopenia or skin rashes.

The two other common topical antimicrobials used are mafenide acetate (Sulfamylon) and silver nitrate.

Beta-blockers

Burn injury results in up to tenfold increase in the levels of circulating catecholamines. Beta-blockers are used in burned children to limit the detrimental effects of the increased levels of catecholamines in selected cases.

Oxandrolone

Is a synthetic testosterone analogue with potent anabolic effects. It has been shown to improve weight gain, increase muscle protein synthesis, and accelerate the healing of donor sites. Oxandrolone can be administered orally in contrast to testosterone or growth hormone, which have to be administered as injections.

Biosynthetic skin substitutes

Biosynthetic skin substitutes are made of animal or human cellular tissues and can be used as a temporary covering over full thickness and some partial-thickness burns until autografting is possible. They can be used also as a temporary covering for burn wounds that heal without autografting.

Biobrane and Integra were the first FDA-approved biologically based wound dressings. Biobrane uses an ultrathin silicone film into which is partially imbedded a nylon fabric. The nylon material contains a gelatin derived from pig tissue that interacts with clotting factors in the wound.

Integra is a two-layer membrane. The bottom layer, made of shark cartilage and collagen from cow tendons, acts as a matrix onto which a person's own cells migrate over two to three weeks. The cells gradually absorb the cartilage and collagen to create a new dermis, or "neo-dermis." This bottom layer is a permanent cover. The top layer is a protective silicone sheet that is peeled off after several weeks. A thin layer of the autologous skin is then grafted onto the neo-dermis.

The more recently approved cellular wound dressings are made with human tissue. OrCel is made of living human skin cells grown on a cow collagen matrix. TransCyte consists of human cells grown on nylon mesh, combined with a synthetic epidermal layer.

Learning points

- Attention should initially focus on securing the airway and on maintaining the breathing and circulation when approaching the child with burns.

- Direct pulmonary injury from hot gases, steam, smoke, and systemic and metabolic toxicity from the smoke constituents results in smoke inhalation injury

- Strategies to minimize ventilator induced lung injury should be employed early in children with smoke inhalation and ARDS.

- Adequate pain control, alleviation of anxiety, a thermoneutral environment, and treatment of infection are important steps in limiting catecholamine secretion and thus hypermetabolism.

- Early excision and grafting (covering the wounds) helps in reducing the morbidity and mortality associated with burn injuries.

References

1. Sparkes BG, Gyorkos JW, Gorczynski et al. Comparison of endotoxins and cutaneous burn toxin as immunosuppressants. *Burns* 1990; **16**: 123–7.

2. Dreyfuss D, Soler P, Basset G, et al. High inflation pressure pulmonary edema. Respective effects of high airway pressure, high tidal volume, and positive end-expiratory pressure. *Am Rev Respir Dis* 1988; **137**(5): 1159–64.

3. Barrow RE, Jeschke MG, Herndon DN. Early fluid resuscitation improves outcomes in severely burned children. *Resuscitation* 2000; **45**: 91–6.

4. Holm C, Melcer B, Horbranel F, et al. Haemodynamic and oxygen transport responses in survivors and non-survivors following thermal injury. *Burns* 2000; **26**: 25–33.

5. Reynolds EM, Ryan DP, Sheridan RL, et al. Left ventricular failure complicating severe pediatric burn injuries. *J Pediatr Surg* 1995; **30**: 264–9; discussion 9–70.

6. Palmieri TL, Jackson W, Greenhalgh DG. Benefits of early tracheostomy in severely burned children. *Crit Care Med* 2002; **30**: 922–4.

7. Barret JP, Desai MH, Herndon DN. Effects of tracheostomies on infection and airway complications in pediatric burn patients. *Burns* 2000; **26**(2): 190–3.

8. Sheridan RL, Kacmarek RM, McEttrick MM et al. Permissive hypercapnia as a ventilatory strategy in burned children: effect on barotrauma, pneumonia, and mortality. *J Trauma* 1995; **39**(5): 854–9.

9. Carman B, Cahill T, Warden G et al. A prospective, randomized comparison of the

Volume Diffusive Respirator vs conventional ventilation for ventilation of burned children. 2001 ABA paper. *J Burn Care Rehabil* 2002; **23**(6): 444–8.

10. Cioffi WG, deLemos RA, Coalson JJ *et al.* Decreased pulmonary damage in primates with inhalation injury treated with high-frequency ventilation. *Ann Surg* 1993; **218**(3): 328–37.

11. Cartotto R, Ellis S, Smith T. Use of high-frequency oscillatory ventilation in burn patients. *Crit Care Med* 2005; **33**(3 Suppl): S175–81.

12. Silver GM, Freiburg C, Halerz M *et al.* A survey of airway and ventilator management strategies in North American pediatric burn units. *J Burn Care Rehabil* 2004; **25**(5): 435–40.

13. Stoddard FJ, Sheridan RL, Saxe GN, *et al.* Treatment of pain in acutely burned children. *J Burn Care Rehabil* 2002; **23**: 135–56.

Further reading

Practice Guidelines for Burn Care. *J Burn Care Rehabil* 2001; **22**: S1-69.

Sheridan RL. Comprehensive treatment of burns. *Curr Probl Surg* 2001; **38**: 657–756.

A child with multiple trauma

Joshua C. Uffman and Monica S. Vavilala

Introduction

Trauma is the leading cause of mortality in children over 1 year of age and a significant cause of permanent disability in the United States.[1] Most injuries are the result of blunt trauma from Motor Vehicle Crashes (MVC), where the child is either an occupant or is struck by a vehicle. Traumatic Brain Injury (TBI) is the most common injury, but abdominal, chest, spine, pelvic, and long bone injuries also occur either alone, or in association with TBI. Other causes of injuries include falls, Non-Accidental Trauma (NAT), and sports.

Case history

A 7-year-old male was brought to the emergency department (ED) by the Emergency Medical Service (EMS) after being hit by a car while riding his bicycle. Witnesses reported that the car struck the un-helmeted child, forcing him off the bicycle then running him over. When EMS arrived, the child was crying and complaining of abdominal and left leg pain, with a Glasgow Coma Score (GCS) of 15. The child was able to give his name, phone number, and address. Initial vital signs were Heart Rate (HR) of 135 b min^{-1}, Blood Pressure (BP) 135/88 mmHg, Respiratory Rate (RR) of 36 breaths min^{-1} and SpO$_2$ 99%. Estimated weight was 25 kg. The child was placed on a rigid backboard and the neck was stabilized in a rigid cervical collar. Oxygen was administered via nasal cannula at 2 l min^{-1} and a 22G Peripheral Intravenous Catheter (PIV) was placed in his right antecubital fossa, through which a normal saline bolus of 20 ml kg^{-1} was administered. The child was transported to the region's level I pediatric trauma center without incident.

On arrival to the ED the patient was evaluated by the trauma service. Primary survey revealed a patent airway with bilateral breath sounds (45 breaths min^{-1}) and good air exchange. Pulse oximetry was 99% on 2 l O$_2$ via nasal cannula. He had strong peripheral pulses in four extremities, an HR of 135 b min^{-1} and BP of 95/50 mmHg. Neurological examination (disability) revealed intact cranial nerves II-XII. Pupils were equal and reactive. Pertinent positives on physical examination were: a line of ecchymosis from just under the right rib cage to the left pelvis, a tender distended abdomen, unstable pelvis and a left mid-shaft deformity femur fracture. The child could not cooperate with a motor or sensory exam of the lower extremities because of leg pain. He was log rolled, with the spine alignment maintained to examine the back. No obvious bone deformities or step-offs were noted.

As the primary survey was performed, an additional 20 G PIV was placed in the left forearm and blood obtained for Complete Blood Count (CBC) with platelets, liver profile, amylase, lipase, electrolytes, Blood Urea Nitrogen (BUN), creatinine, and coagulation profile. Blood was typed and crossed for 4 units of Packed Red Blood Cells (PRBCs). Anteroposterior (AP) and lateral cervical, AP chest, abdomen, and pelvic radiographs were obtained. Neck, chest, and abdominal radiographs were unremarkable. The pelvic radiograph revealed a right acetabular

Case Studies in Pediatric Critical Care, ed. Peter. J. Murphy, Stephen C. Marriage, and Peter J. Davis. Published by Cambridge University Press. © Cambridge University Press 2009.

fracture. Given the physical exam findings and mechanism of injury, computed tomography (CT) of the head, neck, abdomen and pelvis with oral and intravenous contrast was planned.

Thirty minutes after arrival at the ED, the patient became restless and confused. He vomited twice. His HR increased into the 150s and his BP decreased to 80/42 mmHg. A second 20 ml kg^{-1} bolus of normal saline was given with no effect. He became more somnolent and developed intermittent episodes of agitation. Laboratory evaluation revealed a hematocrit of 24%. Twenty ml kg^{-1} of un-cross-matched O negative blood was given. His BP improved to 90/50 mmHg but HR remained in the upper 140s with no improvement in mental status.

The trauma team decided to secure the airway by intubation. Preparations included arranging for: a ventilator, suction, styletted 5.0 and 5.5 cuffed tracheal tubes, Miller 2 and Macintosh 2 larygoscopes, drugs (etomidate and suxamethonium drawn up in syringes), and a No. 2.5 and No. 3 LMA at hand. The patient was pre-oxygenated with 100% oxygen by face mask. 0.1 mg kg^{-1} etomidate and 1 mg kg^{-1} suxamethonium were given intravenously. Cricoid pressure was applied, and the front of his collar was removed, while another assistant provided manual in-line stabilization. Direct laryngoscopy revealed a grade II airway. The tracheal tube was placed and confirmation of correct placement of the tracheal tube was made by inspection of chest rise, auscultation of bilateral breath sounds, and documentation of carbon dioxide via a disposable carbon dioxide detector for more than three breaths. The tracheal tube cuff was inflated, cricoid pressure released and the rigid cervical collar was replaced.

The patient was taken to the CT scanner where head, neck, abdomen and pelvic CTs were performed. The head and neck CT was remarkable for a right-sided Subdural Hematoma (SDH) with no midline shift (Fig. 24.1). The abdominal CT showed a grade IV liver laceration (Fig. 24.2). In addition, there were non-displaced transverse spine process fractures from T9–T12, a displaced right femur, and a right acetabular fracture (Fig. 24.3).

In the CT scanner, the child's BP decreased, requiring an additional 20 ml kg^{-1} PRBC. He was quickly taken from the CT scanner to the operating room (OR) because of the high-grade liver laceration and hemodynamic instability. In the OR, a 22 G right radial arterial line and an additional 18 G PIV were placed. Repeat hematocrit was 25%. General anesthesia was maintained using <1 MAC inhalational anesthesia in 50% oxygen, supplemented by

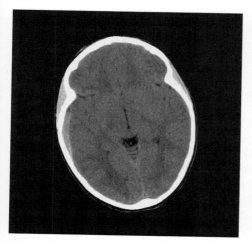

Fig. 24.1. Right-Sided Subdural Hematoma (SDH) with no mid-line shift.

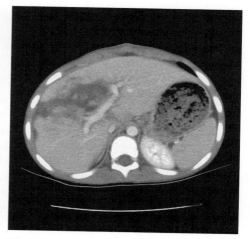

Fig. 24.2. Computed tomography of Grade IV liver laceration

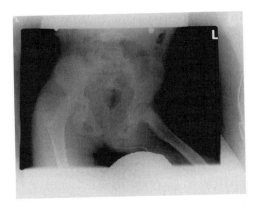

Fig. 24.3. Pelvic radiograph. Right acetabular fracture and dislocated right femur.

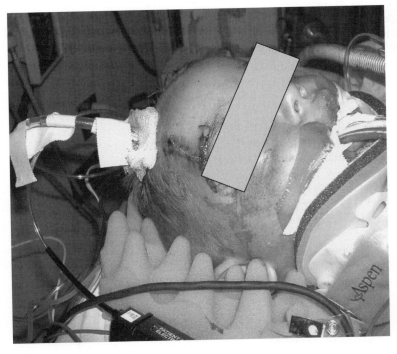

Fig. 24.4. Example of Camino fiberoptic intraparenchymal intracranial pressure monitor.

muscle relaxant and 5 mcg kg^{-1} intravenous fentanyl given incrementally. Because of the SDH, the need for general anesthesia, and likely prolonged sedation all making neurological assessment difficult, the neurosurgeon placed a Camino fiberoptic intraparenchymal intracranial pressure monitor (Fig. 24.4). Initial intracranial pressure (ICP) was 18 mmHg and cerebral perfusion pressure (CPP) 45 mmHg. After abdominal incision, a large amount of blood loss occurred and the BP dropped to 50/25 mmHg and the HR increased to 175 b min^{-1}. Four cross-matched units of PRBCs were given over the next 20 minutes, while the liver was packed and the patient was stabilized. BP increased to 80/45 mmHg and HR decreased to 145 b min^{-1}. Repeat hematocrit was 25% and an additional 6 units of PRBCs

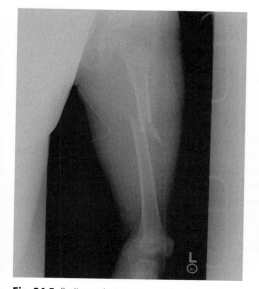

Fig. 24.5. Radiograph. Antero-posterior view right femur fracture.

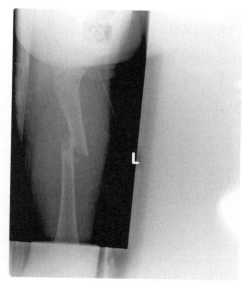

Fig. 24.6. Lateral view right femur fracture.

were ordered. There was no urine output over a 30-minute period and 40 ml kg^{-1} normal saline was administered incrementally to maintain a systolic BP >90 mmHg and CPP >40 mmHg. Coagulation studies revealed platelets of 90 000 × 10^9 l^{-1} and INR of 1.8; four units of platelets and four units Fresh Frozen plasma (FFP) were given. All fluids, with the exception of platelets, were given via a Level 1 fluid warmer. The skin was closed and the child was taken for repeat head CT prior to admission to the pediatric intensive care unit in critical condition.

On arrival to the ICU, the child had a temp of 35.5 °C, HR of 130 b min^{-1}, BP 90/ 50 mmHg, CPP 45 mmHg, and SpO$_2$ 99 % on volume controlled synchronized mechanical ventilation with pressure support (SIMV/VC/PS). The ventilator settings were: tidal volume (TV) 300 ml, rate 18 breaths min^{-1}, PS 8 cmH$_2$O, FiO$_2$ 40%, positive end-expiratory pressure (PEEP) 5 cmH$_2$O. On PICU admission, laboratory values were remarkable for a hematocrit of 27, platelet count of 155 000 × 10^9 l^{-1} and INR of 1.4. His urine output improved with continued fluid management to a goal of 0.5–1 ml kg^{-1} per h. Sedation was achieved with fentanyl and midazolam infusions ranging from 1–3 mcg kg^{-1} per h and 0.1– 0.3 mg kg^{-1} per h, respectively.

Additional radiographs of the lower extremities revealed a left femur fracture in addition to the right acetabulum fracture (Figs. 24.5 and 24.6). Both the femur and acetabulum were splinted. The child returned to the OR the next day for exploratory laparotomy and repair of the liver laceration. The operation and subsequent transport to the PICU were uncomplicated. On hospital day 2, he underwent an uneventful open repair of his acetabulum and placement of an intra-medullary rod in his femur. Over the next 5 days, he was weaned from his ventilator and his trachea was extubated. By hospital day 10, he was transferred to the general surgical floor for rehabilitation and was discharged home 4 weeks after his injury.

Discussion

Traumatic brain injury

Traumatic brain injury (TBI) is the most common injury in children following blunt trauma. This topic is discussed elsewhere in this book; however it is difficult to avoid a basic discussion of TBI when discussing pediatric trauma, since it is rare for a child to have significant injuries following trauma without associated TBI. The increased risk of TBI is largely due to their larger head-to-body ratio than adults, less central nervous system (CNS) myelination, and more compliant bones. Blunt trauma can result in an acceleration–deceleration injury, with cerebral contusion, intracranial hemorrhage, or Diffuse Axonal Injury (DAI). DAI is the result of tissue shearing, usually at the junction of two tissue types of differing densities, most commonly at the gray–white matter interface. DAI is a common cause of long-term disability in patients with TBI.

Diagnosis of TBI starts with the assumption of injury, even in the absence of neurological deficits, as children are more likely than adults to have neurological deficits present late in the course of injury. The modified GCS is helpful: more as a trend than an absolute number. The modified GCS takes into account the child's age in the derivation of the verbal and motor components (Table 24.1). In general, TBI is graded as follows: mild (GCS 13–15), moderate (GCS 9–12), and severe (GCS <9). Initial CT of the head may show intracranial bleeding and contusions, but patients with DAI may have a normal CT without evidence of injury until much later when cerebral edema becomes apparent.

Management of TBI is complex and current recommendations are the result of extrapolation from adult studies in most cases. In 2003, the Brain Trauma Foundation published "Guidelines for the acute medical management of severe traumatic brain injury in infants, children and adolescents" in *Pediatric Critical Care Medicine*[2], *Critical Care Medicine* and the *Journal of Trauma* as simultaneous supplements. They recommend preventing hypoxia, hypocarbia, and hypercarbia, maintaining SBP >fifth percentile for age and CPP >40 mmHg in children with severe TBI (Table 24.2). While the recommendations are for severe TBI, many providers also extrapolate the information to moderate head injury.

Spinal fractures and spinal cord injury

Overall, traumatic spine injuries are less common in pediatric than adult trauma patients, with an incidence of 1%–2%.[3,4] Most spine injuries are a result of MVCs, although falls and sports-related injuries are also common causes in younger children and adolescents respectively[4]. Of all Spinal Cord Injuries (SCI), 5% occur in children less than 16 years of age.[5] Despite this apparent low incidence, mortality is 15%–20% in C-spine injuries (CSI) because 50% of these children have associated TBI. In the presence of TBI, it should be assumed that the child has a CSI until proven otherwise.

The age of the child influences the level of spine injury. In patients younger than 11 years, the location of SCI is more likely to be C1–C4 whereas patients greater than 11 years are more likely to have injury to C5–C7, similar to adults.[4] Injury to the thoracolumbar spine is rare in children, accounting for only 10%–20% of spine injuries. Most thoracic spine injuries are from MVCs or falls resulting in compression injuries.

Table 24.1. *Modified Glasgow Coma Score for children*

Best eye response (modification for infants)	
4	Eyes open spontaneously (spontaneously)
3	Eyes open to speech (to speech)
2	Eyes open to pain (to pain)
1	Eyes don't open (don't open)
Best verbal response (modification for infants)	
5	Oriented and converses (coos, smiles, babbles, and interacts)
4	Confused (irritable and/or inappropriate interactions)
3	Inappropriate words (cries to pain and inconsistently consolable)
2	Incomprehensible sounds (moans to pain and inconsolable)
1	None (none)
Best motor response (modification for infants)	
6	Obeys verbal commands (normal spontaneous movements)
5	Localizes pain (withdraws to touch)
4	Withdraws to painful stimulus (withdraws to painful stimulus)
3	Abnormal flexion (abnormal flexion)
2	Extension posturing (extension posturing)
1	No motor activity (no motor activity)

GCS 13–15: Mild head injury.
GCS 9–12: Moderate head injury.
GCS <9: Severe head injury.
Modified from trauma.org website.

There are many postulates as to the different patterns of spine injury in children, but anatomic and social differences appear the most likely explanations. In younger children, the head represents a greater percentage of body weight resulting in the fulcrum of movement being C2–C3 compared to adolescents and adults where it is C5–C6. In addition, the cervical spine is less able to provide support because of greater muscle and ligament laxity and differences in spine body and facet orientation. Because of these differences, children are at risk of having SCI Without Radiographic Abnormality (SCIWORA). While this term was coined in the pre-magnetic resonance imaging (MRI) time, with its advent, most of these patients do have radiographic evidence of injury on MRI. SCIWORA injuries occur in 15%–25% of pediatric CSI[3,4] but are rare in adults. By 8–10 years of age, enough growth and development have occurred so that the anatomy, function, and pattern of injury approximate those of adults.

Diagnosis of spine injuries in children starts with spine immobilization while plain anterior posterior (AP) and lateral radiographs of the cervical and upper thoracic spine are obtained. Clearance of the cervical spine in children presents a unique dilemma since many children cannot reliably communicate if they have pain, let alone identify its location.

Table 24.2. *Recommendations for management of severe pediatric head injury*

Physiologic parameter	Recommendations
Blood glucose	• Avoid dextrose containing solutions • Maintain blood glucose <200–250 mg dl^{-1}
Temperature	• Avoid hyperthermia: cool patients to 36–37 °C • Hypothermia (32–34 °C) may be considered for refractory intracranial hypertension
Cerebral blood flow and pCO_2	• Mild or prophylactic hyperventilation (<35 mmHg) should be avoided • Mild hyperventilation may be considered if intracranial hypertension is refractory to sedation and analgesia, neuromuscular blockade, CSF drainage, and hyperosmolar therapy • Mild hyperventilation if evidence of acute brain stem herniation exist
Blood pressure	• Hypovolemia should be corrected to euvolemia as rapidly as possible • SBP should be maintained at least >fifth percentile for age • May be beneficial to maintain SBP in normal range (>50th percentile)
Cerebral perfusion Pressure (CPP)	• CPP >40 mmHg should be maintained • CPP 40–70 mmHg probably represents the age-related continuum for optimal treatment

CPP = cerebral perfusion pressure (mean arterial pressure – intracranial pressure).
CSF = cerebral spinal fluid.
SBP = systolic blood pressure.
Adapted from Adelson PD, Bratton SL, Carney NA *et al.* (2003).

The exact protocol for spine clearance varies by institution and practitioner but usually consists of the absence of radiological injury and absence of neurological deficit. If doubt exists about a neurological deficit, or if the patient is comatose, an MRI is performed looking for evidence of SCIWORA. Twenty-five percent of the time, SCIWORA presents well after the original injury[6]. Since thoracolumbar injuries are rare, routine screening for injury is not recommended.[7] The presence of thoracic or abdominal trauma should prompt a work up for SCI, beginning with plain radiographs.

The role of steroids in SCI is controversial. Several studies called the National Acute Spinal Cord Injury Study (NASCIS) I–III were undertaken to determine the value of steroids after spinal cord injuries.[8] The NASCIS III study of 1998 recommended the use of high-dose methylprednisolone with a loading dose of 30 mg kg^{-1} followed by 5.4 mg kg^{-1} per h for 24 hours if the loading dose is given within 3 hours of injury. If the loading dose is started 3–8 hours after injury, the hourly infusion of 5.4 mg kg^{-1} per h should be continued for 48 hours. While these recommendations are still followed in many institutions, others have abandoned them after other investigators re-examined the NASCIS data and found no benefit.[9] Further clouding the issue is the fact that these studies did not include any pediatric patients and there have not been any published reports looking at the value of steroids in children with SCI.

Cardiothoracic injury

Thoracic injury accounts for only 4%–10% of pediatric trauma,[10–12] yet isolated thoracic injuries carry a 5% mortality. When children present with thoracic and abdominal injury, mortality approaches 25% and if thoracic, abdominal, and head injuries are present, mortality increases to nearly 40%.[10] Between 60% and 80% of thoracic injuries are the result of blunt trauma, with the majority from MVCs.[7] However, NAT, bicycle, sports injuries, and personal violence are also causes with their incidence varying by age.

Unlike adults, rib fractures after thoracic trauma in young children are rare because of their pliable rib cage. As a result, children may have significant injury with no obvious external signs. If rib fractures are found, however, they indicate that a significant force was applied to the child's thorax and a thorough investigation should be undertaken. As the number of fractured ribs increases, so too does the risk of mortality.[13] In a child less than 3 years, the presence of fractured ribs should raise the concern for NAT.

Overall, the most common pediatric thoracic injury is pulmonary contusion[14] occurring in approximately 10% of pediatric trauma cases.[15] Chest radiography is nearly always diagnostic and contusion appears as areas of consolidation soon after injury. The timing of appearance may help to differentiate contusions from pulmonary infiltrates as a result of aspiration, which usually are located in the right lower lobe and may take several hours to appear. These patients may have alveolar hemorrhage and edema, resulting in increased ventilation–perfusion (V/Q) mismatch with hypoxia, hypercarbia, and decreased lung compliance. Pulmonary contusions themselves are rarely life threatening,[16] but they do present a nidus for infection.

Like pulmonary contusions, pneumothorax and hemothorax can occur without other physical evidence of injury. Unilateral breath sounds may indicate the presence of a pneumothorax but may be difficult to detect during resuscitation or in a crying child. A screening chest radiograph is particularly important. Definitive treatment is chest tube placement, although needle decompression is indicated in emergent situations until a formal chest tube can be placed.

Injury to the heart and mediastinal structures is less common than in adult trauma patients. The reported incidence of blunt cardiac trauma varies, depending on the particular study but ranges between 0% and 43%.[17] Many types of cardiac injuries have been described, but cardiac contusions are the most common, accounting for nearly 95% of cardiac injuries after blunt trauma.[18]

The diagnosis of cardiac contusions is difficult to make but is often associated with injury to at least one other anatomic site.[18] Chest pain, a classic symptom in adults, is present in less than 50% of alert and responsive pediatric patients with contusion.[18] Electrocardiogram can show a variety of changes including S–T changes, low voltage QRS complexes, conduction delays, as well as other arrythmias. However, these are present only 20% of the time.[18] Cardiac enzyme markers of injury, such as troponin I, may be elevated but are not as sensitive for cardiac contusion as they are of infarction. Echocardiography may help in significant injury, but has not been adequately studied in children with cardiac contusions.

Injury to the great vessels, esophagus, and diaphragm are exceedingly rare in the pediatric population. When they do occur, diagnosis can be delayed because of a low index of suspicion in children. The diagnosis of great vessel injuries is usually achieved with CT and esophageal injuries are often diagnosed with a water-soluble contrast upper gastrointestinal series. Mediastinal air observed on CXR with no other apparent cause prompts investigation of esophageal injuries.

Abdominal injury

Abdominal injuries are present in 8% of blunt pediatric trauma patients, with the spleen and liver being the most commonly injured intra-abdominal organs.[19] Compared with the adult, the child's organs are relatively larger and closer together, making them particularly susceptible to injury from blunt force. The compliant rib cage, with less abdominal fat and connective tissue, provides less of a protective barrier. Eighty-five to 90% of pediatric spleen and liver injuries can be managed non-operatively: a larger number than in adults.[20]

The diagnosis of abdominal injury begins with clinical suspicion based on physical findings. Abdominal abrasions and contusions, abdominal distension, and tenderness should prompt further investigation. Hemodynamically unstable patients with evidence of intra-abdominal injury are taken to the OR for exploratory laparotomy after the primary and secondary trauma surveys are completed. Hemodynamically stable patients should undergo routine X-ray examination of the abdomen and pelvis, followed by abdominal and pelvic CT with oral and intravenous (IV) contrast. Computed tomography is particularly important from diagnostic and management perspectives. Other diagnostic modalities are used variably amongst institutions. Diagnostic Peritoneal Lavage (DPL), bedside ultrasound, and routine laboratory studies have their place, but present significant limitations: especially early in the diagnostic phase. In a hemodynamically stable child, a positive DPL does not necessitate exploratory laparotomy because injuries like low-grade spleen lacerations that can be treated without surgery, result in a positive DPL.[19]

The liver is the most common intra-abdominal organ injured as a result of blunt trauma with the right lobe injured more commonly than the left lobe.[21] Patients with right upper quadrant (RUQ) pain and tenderness, RUQ abrasions, and contusions with right shoulder pain should be evaluated by CT. Liver injuries are graded from 1 to VI (Table 24.3) and in the absence of peritoneal signs, grades I–III are typically managed non-operatively.[20] The need for blood transfusion in the non-operative groups appears greater in patients with liver lacerations than splenic lacerations.[19]

Splenic injury is the second most common intra-abdominal organ injured after blunt trauma.[21] Physical findings suggestive of splenic injury are contusions or abrasions to the left upper quadrant (LUQ), LUQ pain and tenderness, and left shoulder pain known as Kehr's sign. CT examination in stable patients allows for grading the splenic injury (Table 24.4). For the most part, only grades IV and V require surgical intervention,[20] although this practice varies by institution. In one recent study, patients treated at pediatric trauma centers were significantly more likely to be treated non-operatively compared to similar patients treated at adult trauma centers or community hospitals.[22] If the splenic injury is isolated, only 5%–10% of children require transfusion of blood products: far less than non-operative liver lacerations.[21] With grade IV–V lesions requiring surgery, the current practice at the authors' institution is to avoid total splenectomy if at all possible, in an effort to minimize the risk of post-splenectomy infections.

The small bowel is injured less commonly than the spleen or liver but, when it occurs, is usually the result of *the seat belt syndrome*, a deceleration injury often the result of a poorly fitted seatbelt. In this syndrome, the torso folds over the lap belt with the lap belt exerting a force perpendicular to the spine. The bowel injury is usually the result of an abrupt increase in intraluminal pressure causing perforation of the bowel lumen. These injuries are often associated with horizontal fractures of the lumbar spinal bodies, called Chance fractures. Children with seat belt syndrome usually have contusions on the lower abdomen with

Table 24.3. *Liver injury scale*

Grade		Injury description
VI	Vascular	Hepatic avulsion
V	Laceration	Parenchymal disruption of >75% of hepatic lobe
	Vascular	Juxtahepatic venous injuries (major hepatic veins or retrohepatic inferior vena cava)
IV	Laceration	Parenchymal disruption of 25%–75% of a hepatic lobe
III	Hematoma	Ruptured subscapular or intraparenchymal >10 cm or expanding subcapsular >50% surface area or expanding
	Laceration	>3 cm parenchymal depth
II	Hematoma	Subcapsular comprising 10%–50% surface area or intraparenchymal <10 cm diameter
	Laceration	1–3 cm parenchymal depth and <10 cm length
I	Hematoma	Subscapular <10% surface area
	Laceration	Capsular tear <1 cm deep

Grades I–III more likely treated with non-operative medical management while Grade IV–VI more likely treated operatively. (GARCIA).
Adapted from American Association for the Surgery of Trauma presented on www.trauma.org/scores/ois-liver.html.

Table 24.4. *Spleen injury scale*

Grade		Injury description
V	Vascular	Hilar injury with devascularized spleen
	Lacertaion	Shattered spleen
IV	Laceration	Laceration of segmental or hilar vessels resulting in devascularization of >25% of spleen
III	Hematoma	Subcapsular involving >50% surface area or expanding. Ruptured subcapsular or parenchymal hematoma or intraparencymal hematoma >5 cm diameter.
	Laceration	Capsular tear >3 cm in depth or involving trabecular vessels
II	Hematoma	Subcapsular involving 10%–50% surface area or intraparenchymal <5 cm diameter
	Laceration	Capsular tear 1–3 cm in depth and not involving parenchymal vessels
I	Hematoma	Subcapsular involving <10% surface area
	Laceration	Capsular tear <1 cm depth

Grades 1–III more likely treated with non-operative medical management while Grade IV–V more likely treated operatively(GARCIA).
Adapted from American Association for the Surgery of Trauma presented on www.trauma.org/scores/ois-spleen.html.

associated abdominal and back pain (Fig. 24.7). Diagnosis is made with either serial physical examinations or free air on radiograph or CT. Additional finding on CT suggestive of bowel injury include free intraperitoneal fluid in the absence of solid organ injury and bowel wall thickening. Overall, CT is poor at identifying isolated bowel injury.

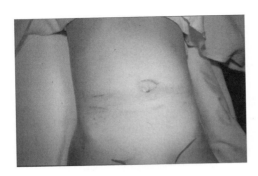

Fig. 24.7. Seat belt syndrome (see color plate section).

Orthopedic injuries

Orthopedic injuries other than spine injuries are very common, but are rarely the cause of death. However, interruption of ongoing bone growth from trauma can result in significant morbidity. Also ongoing growth and development can make radiologic diagnosis of bone injuries difficult for care providers not accustomed to normal changes of development.

Routine pelvic radiographs are appropriate for the pediatric trauma patient as they are for the adult patient. Pelvic injuries are associated with other injuries nearly 75% of the time. Their presence, therefore, is an indication of a significant blunt force and other injuries should be sought. Unlike adults, pelvic fractures in children are rarely the cause of hemodynamic instability.[23] Until definitive fixation, temporary pelvic stabilization can be achieved with bed rest, a pelvic sling, or external fixation as the medical condition allows.

Open fractures are urgent injuries that need to be repaired within 6 hours to minimize the risks of infection, further soft tissue, and muscle injury, and non-union or malunion of the bone. All fractures should be splinted as soon as medically possible after the secondary trauma survey. Irrigation and debridement should be performed as soon as possible and, if neurovascular injury is present, definitive repair should occur within 6 hours.

Closed fractures can appear less concerning than open fractures, but this can lead to a false sense of security if ongoing blood loss, neurovascular compromise, or compartment syndrome exist. Diagnosis begins with the physical exam during the secondary survey along with appropriate radiographs to confirm the diagnosis. Initial treatment is splinting while stabilization and treatment of more life-threatening injuries occurs followed by definitive repair and fixation when the patient has stabilized.

NAT

NAT, or child abuse, results in over 300 deaths each year in the USA. Head injuries, mainly subdural hematomas, as a result of blunt trauma or violent shaking (Shaken Baby syndrome) are the leading cause of death among children less than 1 year of age.[24] While it can sometimes be difficult to determine if a child was the victim of NAT, injuries out of proportion to the reported cause should alert the clinician to the possibility of NAT. For example, abdominal injuries as a result of a falling down stairs are rarely associated with bowel perforation.[25] Falls from table heights are rarely associated with fatal head injuries, and femur fractures in non-ambulatory children are almost non-existent in children not involved in significant accidents.[26] If the clinician suspects NAT, appropriate personnel who are trained to evaluate and navigate the public health system should be consulted. In addition, a careful examination for signs of other injuries should be undertaken including a full skeletal survey and ophthalmologic exam looking for evidence of retinal hemorrhages.

NAT is discussed further elsewhere in this book.

Fluid and transfusion management for the pediatric patient

Fluid and blood product management is a key part of trauma care and it is important to know the normal hemodynamic and blood volume values for various age groups (Tables 24.5 and 24.6). A few generalizations can be made. For example, the normal systolic blood pressure is twice the age in years plus 80 mmHg and the circulating blood volume for patients over 1 year of age is approximately 80 ml kg^{-1}.[27] Pediatric patients respond to hypovolemia with tachycardia like adults, but they are able to compensate for hypovolemia for a longer time. The pediatric patient can lose almost 25% of their blood volume before becoming hypotensive. The clinician needs to avoid the pitfall of underestimating the severity of the patient's condition, just because they appear "compensated."

According to the American College of Surgeons, initial fluid management for a pediatric trauma patient who is tachycardic (>130 b min^{-1}) is an isotonic fluid (normal saline, Ringer's

Table 24.5. *Normal hemodynamic values by age*

Age	Heart rate (beats/ minute)	90th percentile systolic blood pressure (mmHg)	5th percentile systolic blood pressure (mmHg)	90th percentile diastolic blood pressure (mmHg)	5th percentile diastolic blood pressure (mmHg)
1 year	120	105	72	69	48
3 years	110	105	78	62	48
5 years	100	108	78	67	48
8 years	90	112	82	73	52
10 years	91	117	89	75	54
13 years	85	124	95	79	59
16 years	85	131	103	81	60

Values are approximate and adapted from Update on the 1987 Task Force Report on High Blood pressure in Children and Adolescents. *Pediatrics*. 98(4) Oct 1996, Report of the task force on blood pressure control in children. *Pediatrics*. 59 (5) Suppl. May 1977, Adelson PD. Bratton SL, Carney NA *et al.* Chapter 4. Resuscitation of blood pressure and oxygen and prehospital brain-specific therapies for the severe pediatric traumatic brain injury patient. *Critical Care Med* 2003;4 (3 Suppl);S12–8 & Harriet Lane Handbook, 15th edn, 2000.

Table 24.6. *Estimated pediatric blood volumes by age*

Age	Estimated blood volume (EBV) (ml kg^{-1})
Premature infant	90–100
Full-term infant	80–90
3 months–1 year	70–80
>1 year	70

lactate or Plasma–Lyte R^{TM}) bolus of 20 ml kg^{-1}, representing roughly 25% of circulating volume. If this is unsuccessful in restoring normal blood pressure, a second 20 ml kg^{-1} bolus of the same solution should be given. If the patient either has ongoing blood loss or continues to be hemodynamically unstable, PRBC should be given. The overall goals of fluid resuscitation are to restore hemodynamic stability and ensure organ perfusion. End-points include normal heart rate and blood pressure for age, decreased skin mottling, increased warmth in extremities, improved sensorium, urine output >1 ml kg^{-1} per h, increased pulse pressure, and correction of sources of blood loss.

In virtually all hospitals, the administration of red blood cells is achieved with blood concentrates such as PRBC, as whole blood is rarely needed or available. Typical PRBC preparations have a hematocrit of around 50%–75%. For a 10 ml kg^{-1} bolus, the hematocrit should increase by approximately 10%.

Blood transfusion should be given to maintain oxygen-carrying capacity to the body. However, during the initial resuscitation, it can often be difficult to determine when transfusion is indicated. One helpful calculation is the maximum allowable blood loss (MABL), which gives a rough idea of how much blood the patient needs to lose to reach a targeted hematocrit.

$$\text{MABL} = (\text{Hct initial} - \text{Hct target})/\text{Hct Avg} \times \text{EBV}$$

It is unclear what the lowest allowable or target hematocrit should be in pediatric trauma. Guidelines for appropriate transfusion criteria in the pediatric population were published in 2002[28] (Tables 24.7 and 24.8). Many institutions, however, still target a hematocrit of 30%

Table 24.7. *Indications for transfusion of packed red blood cells (PRBCs) in children*

Clinical situation	Transfusion hematocrit goal (%)
Acute blood loss w/ hypovolemia not responsive to other treatment	>24
Emergency surgery with significant pre-operative anemia	>24
Intra-operative blood loss ≥15 % or more than maximal allowable by calculation	>24
Severe pulmonary disease	>40
Cyanotic heart disease	>40
ECHMO	>40

These end-points may be altered for different clinical situations. Adapted from Roseff SD, Naomi LC, Manno CS. (2002).

Table 24.8. *Guidelines for transfusion of platelets in children*

Age	Transfusion goals
Premature infant	$> 100\,000 \times 10^9\,l^{-1}$
Neonate	$> 30\,000 \times 10^9\,l^{-1}$
>1 month	$> 50–100\,00 \times 10^9\,l^{-1}$

Adapted from Roseff SD, Naomi LC & Manno CS (2002).

when deciding RBC transfusion, regardless of the clinical situation. Others attempt to take into consideration other factors like age, ongoing blood loss, evidence of cyanotic heart or sickle cell disease, and poor oxygen delivery, such as increasing serum lactate, when deciding to transfuse PRBCs. Previously healthy children can tolerate hematocrits well below 30% before adverse sequelae are seen.

PRBCs that have been cross-matched are the most desired form of red blood cell replacement. However, in acute, life-threatening situations, uncross-matched O blood should be used. There is no standard as to when to use O negative versus positive blood. In some hospitals, O negative blood is reserved for females to avoid alloimmunization to the Rh antibody, while boys get O positive blood. In other hospitals, all children receive O negative blood. If the blood type is known, type specific, un-cross-matched blood should be used rather than O blood. After massive transfusion, it is unclear when, or if, to switch to type-specific blood in type A, B, or AB pediatric patients when it becomes available.

After massive blood transfusion, dilutional thrombocytopenia, disseminated intravascular coagulation (DIC), hyperkalemia, hypocalcemia, hypothermia, and volume overload can occur. In actively bleeding patients during trauma resuscitation, platelet counts should be kept greater than $100\,000 \times 10^9\ l^{-1}$.[28] Administering $5–10\ ml\ kg^{-1}$ of random donor or apheresis platelets should raise the platelet count $50–100 \times 10^9\ l^{-1}$ in the absence of ongoing consumption as occurs with DIC.

FFP is indicated when there is bleeding associated with a coagulation factor deficiency, significantly prolonged prothrombin time, and/or partial thromboplastin time. While it is important to document a coagulopathy prior to administering FFP, it is often not clinically feasible. When resuscitation with massive transfusion is occurring, many clinicians administer FFP on the assumption that coagulation factors are critically low from dilution and/or consumption.

A relatively new adjunct to treating the bleeding trauma patient is recombinant activated factor VII (NovoSeven). While originally approved in the USA for hemophilia A and B patients with inhibitors to factor VIII or IX who were bleeding, it has been reported in limited case series to decrease transfusion requirements in adults[29] and children[30] following severe trauma. The future role of recombinant activated factor VII will depend on the results from larger studies but currently the high cost and limited supply have been a significant deterrent to more widespread use.

Management of the pediatric trauma patient

Initial management of the pediatric trauma patient is guided by the American College of Surgeon's Advanced Trauma Life Support (ATLS) protocols. The initial evaluation, called the primary survey, focuses on Airway, Breathing, Circulation, Disabilities, and Exposure/examination (ABCDEs) and spine immobilization. This is followed by the secondary survey where the remainder of the body is examined for evidence of injury. After stabilization has occurred, or in an effort to stabilize life-threatening injuries, definitive management occurs for the injuries sustained.

Evaluation and management of the airway is of paramount importance in the care of an injured child; there are several anatomic differences in children that need to be recognized. The size of the occiput of the child is significantly larger than the adult. This results in the child naturally resting in a flexed position. The tongue comprises a larger portion of the oral pharynx, and the epiglottis is more ovoid and less cartilaginous than the adult. The narrowest

Table 24.9. *Tracheal tube size by age*

Age	ETT Size (inner diameter in millimeters)
<30 weeks PCA	2.5–3.0
31–40 weeks PCA	3.0–3.5
Infant	3.5–4.0
1 year	4.0–4.5
3 year	4.5–5.0
5 year	5.0–5.5
8 year	6.0–6.5
10 year	6.5–7.0
12–18 years	6.5–7.5
>18 years	7.0–8.0

PCA: Post-conceptual age.
ETT: Endotracheal tube.
For cuffed ETT, use 0.5 mm smaller.
Adapted from Harriet Lane Handbook, 15th edn, 2000.

part of the airway is the subglottic region rather than the vocal cords and the distance from the vocal cords to the carina is relatively short compared to the adult.

Steps in evaluation include looking for signs of adequate respiratory effort followed by listening for air exchange in the chest and finally ensuring adequate oxygenation determined by pulse oximetry or arterial partial pressure of oxygen (PaO_2). If these are abnormal, an intervention is needed. Interventions include supplemental oxygen, suctioning the airway, oral or nasopharyngeal airway devices, jaw thrust, bag-mask ventilation, and tracheal intubation.

Until a complete evaluation can be undertaken, ensuring spine stabilization is important and can present some unique challenges to managing the airway. To minimize the natural flexion of the cervical spine from the large occiput, a rolled towel or sheet can be placed under the shoulders to align the spine. An appropriately sized rigid cervical collar is used in older patients and sandbags on either side of the head with tape across the forehead, can be used in younger children or if a rigid collar is not available.

If the patient is not adequately oxygenating or ventilating, despite non-invasive measures, or if the patient cannot protect their airway from the possibility of pulmonary aspiration, then tracheal intubation should be performed by an experienced laryngoscopist. Equipment that needs to be available prior to intubation includes suction, age appropriate tracheal tubes (Table 24.9), amnestic and paralytic drugs, back-up airway devices, a mechanism for delivering oxygen, and at least one person to assist with the procedure.

The patient should be considered to have a full stomach and, therefore, at risk of pulmonary aspiration. Induction should occur via a rapid sequence or modified rapid-sequence induction with cricoid pressure after pre-oxygenation with 100% oxygen. The spine needs to be stabilized during larygoscopy, which can easily be done with an assistant providing in-line stabilization while the anterior portion of the rigid collar is removed. Classic teaching has been to use un-cuffed tracheal tubes in children less than 8 years to minimize the risk of sub-glottic stenosis and cuffed tracheal tubes for children over 8 years.

However, some anesthesiologists use cuffed tracheal tubes in virtually all children. After tracheal intubation, the rigid collar should be replaced. Fiberoptic intubation can be considered for difficult intubations but is usually left to clinicians accustomed to performing pediatric fiberoptic intubations, and preferably not left as a rescue treatment to failed direct laryngoscopy. Lastly, nasotracheal intubation is rarely indicated in the trauma patient and is contra-indicated in the presence of basilar skull or nasal fractures.

Circulation is evaluated by feeling peripheral and central pulses and by assessing perfusion using capillary refill and blood pressure. While pediatric patients become progressively tachycardic as blood loss occurs, they are able to maintain their blood pressure until losses are greater than 25% of circulating blood volume.[31] After this time, decompensation can be rapid. Bradycardia is an ominous sign and may signify significant cardiac injury or raised intracranial pressure (ICP) as part of Cushing's triad (hypertension, irregular respirations, and bradycardia) in severe TBI. Regardless of the cause of bradycardia in young children, it results in decreased cardiac output (CO) as they have relatively fixed stroke volume (SV).

Venous access is an integral part of trauma care and adequate access depends on the size of the patient as well as the severity of injuries. For most children, a 22-gauge Peripheral Intravenous Catheter (PIV) is adequate to begin resuscitation. A larger second or third PIV should then be sought.[27] Typically, upper extremity veins are preferred. However, in the absence of significant abdominal trauma, saphenous veins provide a large vein in a predictable location that can be accessed either percutaneously or by cut-down. At the time venous access is obtained, baseline labs should be sent, including a complete blood count, coagulation studies, glucose, and blood for type and cross of PRBCs. In some centers, additional screening studies such as liver panel, amylase, lipase, and electrolytes are also obtained.

In the event that peripheral access cannot be obtained after two attempts or 90 seconds in an emergent situation, an intra-osseous (IO) line should be placed with either a packaged intra-osseous needle or any large bore (18–16 G) needle, such as a large spinal needle.[27] This technique has classically been recommended for children less than 6 years of age, but can be effective well beyond this age. The anteromedial surface of the proximal tibia is the most common site of insertion, but any non-traumatized long bone can be used. If the tibia is chosen, the needle is inserted 2 cm below and 1–2 cm medial to the tibial tuberosity, using a twisting motion until a loss of resistance is noticed indicating the tip of the needle is in the marrow cavity (Fig. 24.8). Often, bone marrow can be aspirated when the needle is in the

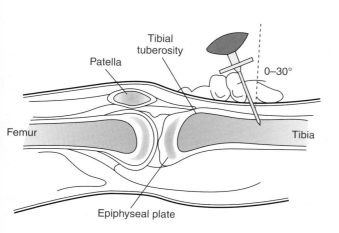

Fig. 24.8. Intra-osseous vascular access.

bone marrow. Inability to aspirate does not necessarily mean improper placement as long as there is not evidence of infused fluid in the soft tissue. The needle needs to be secured to the patient as well as possible recognizing the temporary nature of the IO line until more definitive access can be obtained. Substances that can be administered by the venous route can be given by the IO route; including crystalloid, medications, blood, and blood products.

Central venous access can be used as venous access as well as an indicator of volume status, but is best placed by experienced personnel to avoid iatrogenic injury. The femoral route is often the easiest to place but should be avoided when there is Inferior Vena Cava injury (IVC) or significant liver injury with ongoing bleeding.

Arterial line placement is often helpful and necessary and is most commonly performed in the radial artery with a 22G angiocatheter in all but neonates (24G) or a 20G angiocatheter in patients over 50 kg. Arterial cannulation is indicated when rapid changes in blood pressure or significant alterations in oxygenation and ventiliation are anticipated, or in cases where multiple blood tests are needed and no central venous access is present.

Both isotonic crystalloid (normal saline or Plasma-Lyte R^{TM}) and colloid solutions are acceptable choices for resuscitation. It appears best to avoid hypotonic solutions (Ringer's lactate) since they do not remain in the intravascular space for as long as isotonic solutions and potentially exacerbate fluid shifts to the interstitium, which can worsen an already increased ICP.

After the primary survey is complete, the secondary survey seeks out any disabilities by fully exposing and examining the patient from head to toe. A neurological assessment is made paying particular attention to any deficits as the clinical situation changes or as procedures need to be done. The GCS and modified GCS in infants are the most common neurological assessment tools used. Sedation or tracheal intubation may preclude a complete neurological evaluation either initially or as ongoing care is provided. The child needs to be serially evaluated to detect new or worsening neurological injury.

In most institutions, lateral cervical spine, chest, and pelvic radiographs are routinely obtained. After the secondary survey is concluded, additional studies can be performed to confirm or rule out injuries suspected by the exam. In some trauma centers, it is routine to do a screening ultrasound called Focused Assessment Sonography for Trauma (FAST) of the abdomen and chest cavity to look for free fluid, indicating the need for either additional studies or operative investigation. Currently, however, there is not a consensus on the utility of this in children.

The pediatric patient has a larger surface to body ratio compared to adults and therefore is more prone to heat loss. Those patients who arrive hyperthermic should be cooled to 36–37 °C. Normothermia should be sought in all patients except in those with refractory intracranial hypertension, in which case hypothermia (32–34 °C) may be considered (Table 24.2). Otherwise, patients should be warmed to 36–37 °C with warm blankets, lights, warmed IV fluids, and humidified oxygen.

Learning points

- Trauma is a leading cause of mortality and permanent disability in children over 1 year of age.
- Traumatic brain injury is the most common injury in children following blunt trauma.
- In the presence of traumatic brain injury it should be assumed that the child has a C-spine injury until proven otherwise.

- Rib fractures in young children imply that a significant force was applied to the child's thorax.

- Abdominal injuries are present in 8% of blunt pediatric trauma patients, with the liver and spleen most commonly injured.

- Pelvic fractures in children are rarely the cause of hemodynamic instability.

- Injuries out of proportion to the reported mode of injury should alert the clinician to the possibility of non-accidental trauma.

References

1. Fact Sheet 2. The National Pediatric Trauma Registry. October 1993. www.nemc.org/rehab/factsheet.html.

2. Adelson PD, Bratton SL, Carney NA et al. Guidelines for the acute medical management of severe traumatic brain injury in infants, children and adolescents. Pediatr Crit Care Med 2003; 4 (3) Suppl: S1–75.

3. Patel JC, Tepas JJ, Mollitt DL et al. Pediatric cervical spine injuries: defining the disease. J Pediatr Surg. 2001; 36 (2): 373–6.

4. Kokoska ER, Keller MS, Rallo MC et al. Characteristics of pediatric cervical spine injuries. J Pediatr Surg 2001; 36 (1): 100–5.

5. Hamilton MG, Myles ST. Pediatric spinal injury: review of 174 hospital admissions. J Neurosurg. 1992; 77(5): 700–04.

6. Proctor MR. Spinal cord injury. Crit Care Medi. 2002; 30(11): S489–99.

7. Bliss D, Silen M. Pediatric thoracic trauma. Crit Care Med. 2002; 30(11) Suppl: S409–15.

8. Bracken MB, Shepard MJ, Holdord TR et al. Methylprednisolone or tirilazad mesylate administration after acute spinal cord injury: 1-year follow up. Results of the third National Acute Spinal Cord Injury randomized controlled trial. J Neurosurg 1998; 89(5): 699–706.

9. Hulbert RJ. Methylprednisolone for acute spinal cord injury: an inappropriate standard of care. J Neurosurg Spine 2000; 93(1): 1–7.

10. Peclet MH, Newman KD, Eichelberger MR et al. Thoracic trauma in children: an indicator of increased mortality. J Pediatr Surg. 1990; 25(9): 961–5.

11. Peterson RJ, Tepas JJ, Edwards FH et al. Pediatric and adult thoracic trauma: age related impact on presentation and outcome. Ann Thorac Surg. 1994; 58(1): 14–18.

12. Stafford PW, Harmon CM. Thoracic trauma in children. Curr Opin Pediatr 1993; 5(3): 325–32.

13. Garcia VF, Gotschall CS, Eichelberger MR et al. Rib fractures in children: a marker of severe trauma. J Trauma 1990; 30(6): 695–700.

14. Smyth BT. Chest trauma in children. J Pediatr Surg. 1979; 14(1): 41–7.

15. Newman RJ, Jones IS. A prospective study of 413 consecutive car occupants with chest injuries. J Trauma 1984; 24(2): 129–35.

16. Cooper A. Thoracic injuries. Semin Pediatr Surg. 1995; 4(2): 109–15.

17. Baum VC. Cardiac trauma in children. Paediatr Anaesth 2002; 12: 110–17.

18. Dowd MD, Krug S. Pediatric blunt cardiac injury: epidemiology, clinical features and diagnosis. J Trauma 1996; 40(1): 61–7.

19. Gaines BA, Ford HR. Abdominal and pelvic trauma in children. Crit Care Med. 2002; 30 (Suppl): S416–23.

20. Garcia VF, Brown RL. Pediatric trauma beyond the brain. Crit Care Clin 2003; 19: 551–61.

21. Bond SJ, Eichelberger MR, Gotschall CS et al. Nonoperative management of blunt hepatic and splenic injury in children. Ann Surg 1996; 223(3): 286–9.

22. Davis DH, Localio AR, Stafford PW et al. Trends in operative management of pediatric splenic injury in a regional trauma system. Pediatrics 2005; 115(1): 89–94.

23. Silber JS, Flynn JM, Koffler KM et al. Analysis of the cause, classification and associated injuries of 166 consecutive pediatric pelvic fractures. J Pediatr Orthop. 2001; 21(4): 446–50.

24. Center for Disease Control: National Center for Injury Preventional and Control. Child

maltreatment: Fact sheet. 2005. www.cdc. gov/ncipc/factsheets/cmfacts.htm.

25. Huntimer CM, Muret-Wagstaff S, Leland, NL. Can falls on stairs result in small intestinal perforations? *Pediatrics* 2000; **106** (2): 301–5.

26. Feldman KW, Bethel R, Shugerman RP *et al.* The cause of infant and toddler subdural hemorrhage: a prospective study. *Pediatrics.* 2001; **108**(3): 636–46.

27. American College of Surgeons. *Advanced Trauma Life Support.* Chapter 10: *Pediatric Trauma.* Chicago, ACS, 1993.

28. Roseff SD, Luban NL, Manno CS. Guidelines for assessing appropriateness of pediatric

transfusion. *Transfusion* 2002; **42**(11): 1398–413.

29. Martinowitz U, Kenet G, Segal E *et al.* Recombinant activated factor VII for adjunctive hemorrhage control in trauma. *J Trauma* 2001; **51**(3): 431–9.

30. Kulkarni R, Daneshmand A, Guertin S *et al.* Successful use of activated recombinant factor VII in traumatic liver injuries in children. *J Trauma* 2004; **56**(6): 1348–52.

31. Wetzel RC, Burns RC. Multiple trauma in children: critical care overview. *Crit Care Med* 2002; **30**(11) Suppl: S468–77.

Further reading

1. www.Trauma.org.

2. Supplement to *Critical Care Medicine.* 2002; **30**(11): S383–523.

3. Adelson PD, Bratton SL, Carney NA *et al.* Guidelines for the acute medical management of severe traumatic brain injury in infants, children and adolescents. *Pediatr Crit Care Med* 2003; **4** (3): Suppl 572–5.

4. Baum VC. Cardiac trauma in children. *Paediatr Anaesth* 2002; **12**: 110–17.

5. Garcia VF, Brown RL. Pediatric trauma beyond the brain. *Crit Care Clin* 2003; **19**: 551–61.

6. Roseff SD, Luban NL, Manno CS. Guidelines for assessing appropriateness of pediatric transfusion. *Transfusion* 2002; **42**(11): 1398–413.

Chapter 25

Management of the patient with a failing fontan – morbidities of a palliative procedure

Heather A. Dickerson and Anthony C. Chang

Introduction

This case illustrates many of the post-operative complications encountered in the follow-up of the patient who has had a Fontan procedure. With decreases in mortality over the years, more patients are surviving to experience associated morbidities of this palliative procedure, even in those with a "perfect" Fontan circulation.[1] The procedure has also expanded to palliate patients with elevated pulmonary vascular resistance, borderline pulmonary artery anatomy, and those with complex single ventricle anatomy with other complicating factors such as anomalous systemic and pulmonary venous return, ventricular outflow tract obstruction, and atrioventricular valve abnormalities. Since the inception of the Fontan procedure, reported in 1971,[2] there have been many revisions in the way the surgery is performed. Current procedures involve staging with a bi-directional superior cavopulmonary anastomosis[3,4] and construction of a lateral tunnel[5] or an extracardiac conduit (20–24 mm)[6,7] to connect the inferior vena cava to the pulmonary arteries. These changes have been incorporated to attempt to relieve some of the morbidities associated with the atriopulmonary Fontan. These revisions have resulted in an earlier decrease in ventricular loading, improved flow dynamics and less atrial suture lines. The long-term results have yet to be elucidated though early- and mid-term follow-up has been encouraging. Current 10-year survival is 74%–91% after Fontan palliation.[3,8–9]

Case history

The patient is a 32-year-old female who was born with tricuspid atresia with normally related great arteries, a ventricular septal defect, and pulmonary stenosis. She underwent an atriopulmonary Fontan at 8 years of age. She initially did well with good exercise tolerance and no arrhythmias. She was maintained on no medications. At 28 years of age she presented with increased lower extremity edema, palpitations and poor exercise tolerance. Twenty-four-hour Holter monitoring revealed recurrent short runs of atrial tachycardia and a slow underlying sinus rate. An echocardiogram revealed a patent atriopulmonary Fontan connection without a discernable gradient into the pulmonary arteries, a severely dilated right atrium, mild to moderate left ventricular dysfunction, mild to moderate mitral regurgitation and a competent aortic valve. She was started on diuretics, an angiotensin-converting enzyme inhibitor and digoxin. She tolerated these medications well and had improvement in her symptoms of lower extremity edema and exercise intolerance.

She was able to return to work for several years but presented to the emergency room secondary to a prolonged episode of intra-atrial reentrant tachycardia (IART). A careful

Case Studies in Pediatric Critical Care, ed. Peter. J. Murphy, Stephen C. Marriage, and Peter J. Davis. Published by Cambridge University Press. © Cambridge University Press 2009.

history revealed that she was having recurrent palpitations that had been progressively increasing in frequency with some episodes lasting up to an hour. She had not had any symptoms of chest pain, shortness of breath, or neurologic deficits. An echocardiogram at this time documented the findings previously seen, but also showed a thrombus along the lateral right atrial wall and moderate left ventricular dysfunction. Pulse oximetry was 92% on room air and a CXR revealed small bilateral pleural effusions. Her coagulation studies were normal except a mildly elevated prothrombin time and a mild protein C deficiency. She required admission for heparinization and eventual DC cardioversion after resolution of her intracardiac thrombus. She was started on sotalol to control her atrial arrhythmias in addition to warfarin for anticoagulation. She had continued episodes of IART requiring cardioversion and her sotalol was transitioned to flecainide without significant effect. She had worsening exercise intolerance, was unable to work and had recurrence of her lower extremity edema. Her albumin and total protein levels were on the low end of the normal ranges and she did not have elevation in her stool α–1 antitrypsin. She did not have diarrhea.

She was taken to the cardiac catheterization laboratory for delineation of her hemodynamics and attempted ablation of foci involved in her atrial arrhythmias. Her right atrial pressure was 18 mmHg and there was a 2 mmHg gradient to her right pulmonary artery and no gradient to her left pulmonary artery. Her pulmonary vascular resistance was calculated to be 2.5 Wood units. She had a 2–3 mmHg gradient across her right pulmonary veins, which appeared compressed behind her enlarged right atrium and no gradient across her left pulmonary veins. Her coronary sinus was severely dilated. She had no mitral stenosis and her left ventricular end-diastolic pressure was 14 mmHg. She had no left ventricular outflow tract obstruction and no coarctation. Her left ventricular function was mildly to moderately depressed. She underwent mapping of multiple atrial foci. These sites were ablated with initial freedom from atrial arrhythmias, though they subsequently recurred. She was presented for Fontan conversion secondary to recurrent arrhythmias, left ventricular dysfunction, and progressive exercise intolerance. The findings at catheterization suggested several possibilities for surgical intervention, including relief of obstruction to the right pulmonary artery and right atrial debulking to decrease compression of the right pulmonary veins. It was also thought that her left ventricular dysfunction might improve if decreasing right atrial pressure would decrease coronary sinus pressure and improve coronary perfusion pressure.

She underwent conversion to an extracardiac, nonfenestrated Fontan with right atrial debulking, a right atrial Maze procedure, and placement of an epicardial atrial pacemaker. She was extubated less than 24 hours post-operatively and transferred to the floor on post-operative day 2. Her chest tubes were discontinued 3 days post-operatively. Her telemetry revealed AAI pacing at 80 b min^{-1} and no arrhythmias. She was restarted on warfarin and furosemide. She was discharged on post-operative day 10. At follow-up she has had improvement in her symptomatology. She has had no recurrence of arrhythmias, her exercise tolerance has improved, and she has had less edema. Her echocardiograms have shown some improvement in her left ventricular function, no intracardiac thrombi and no obstruction throughout her Fontan circuit or in her pulmonary veins. She has been able to return to work.

Discussion

The following sections discuss the morbidities associated with a Fontan circulation and possible management strategies.

Post-operative issues following a Fontan procedure

Fontan pathway obstruction

Factors which compromise flow through the Fontan circuit will diminish cardiac output and functional status and lead to many of the morbidities associated with this circulation. Associated morbidities often cannot be reversed or improved without addressing obstruction in the Fontan pathway. Hemodynamics indicative of obstruction in the Fontan pathway include an increased central venous pressure (CVP) with a low left atrial pressure (LAP) resulting in an increased transpulmonary gradient (CVP–LAP). After ruling out treatable pulmonary problems (pneumonia, poor ventilation, pleural effusions), circulatory causes must be investigated. Obstruction may occur within the systemic venous baffle, at the pulmonary arteries secondary to distortion or as a result of compression of the pulmonary veins. Bleeding around the Fontan circuit can cause external compression as well and present as obstruction. Obstruction can also be secondary to pulmonary thromboembolism. All of these abnormalities increase the resistance in the Fontan circuit leading to increases in the systemic venous pressure required to maintain flow. These obstructions are often hard to delineate by non-invasive means due to poor echocardiographic windows, low pressure gradients with non-pulsatile venous flow and the fact that many obstructions are in the distal pulmonary vasculature.

Patients frequently require cardiac catheterization for definitive diagnosis and possible concomitant transcatheter intervention.

Systemic venous baffle obstruction can occur at the proximal or distal anastomotic sites. Lateral tunnel baffles may obstruct due to kinking or may be relatively small if Fontan completion was performed at a young age with an extracardiac conduit. In patients with atriopulmonary connections there may be obstruction at the anastomosis between the atrium and pulmonary arteries (see Fig. 25.1). This obstruction is often exacerbated by progressive atrial dilation that can kink the connection. Pulmonary artery anastomoses can become stenotic at the suture lines or the pulmonary arteries can be distorted distally by

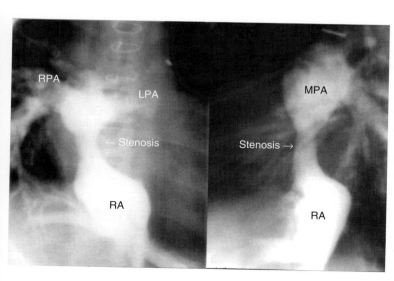

Fig. 25.1.
Atriopulmonary Fontan with stenosis in the atriopulmonary connection. RA = right atrium, RPA = right pulmonary artery, LPA = left pulmonary artery.

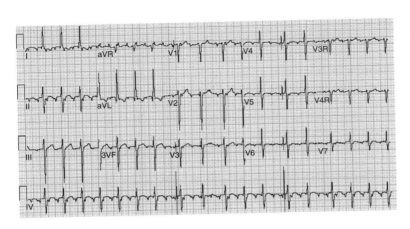

Fig. 25.2. Intra-atrial re-entrant tachycardia (IART) with 2:1 conduction (see color plate section).

previous surgeries or by congenital pulmonary artery anomalies or stenoses. Some of these stenoses are amenable to transcatheter intervention. The pulmonary veins on the right side may become narrowed behind an enlarged right atrium in atriopulmonary Fontans. This requires surgical intervention and responds well to right atrial debulking. If obstruction of the Fontan pathway is secondary to thromboembolism (see below), this can be treated with systemic heparinization or thrombolysis (either systemic or site-directed in the cardiac catheterization laboratory with tissue plasminogen activator (tPA)). Because of the compliance of the venous system, seemingly mild abnormalities or pressure gradients can have devastating effects in a circuit dependent upon passive flow to maintain cardiac output.

Atrial arrhythmias

The most frequent morbidities in patients with a Fontan circulation are atrial arrhythmias (10–40%).[3,9,10] These can be bradyarrhythmias or tachyarrhythmias and are poorly tolerated in patients with a functional single ventricle, where atrioventricular synchrony is of utmost importance.[11,12] Most patients with a Fontan circulation have sinus node dysfunction and chronotropic incompetence, which is exacerbated by exercise.[13] This is likely associated with damage to the sinus node during surgical interventions and right atrial dilation from elevated pulmonary/systemic venous pressure. Some patients with complex single ventricle anatomy can also have associated L-transposition of the great arteries with a high risk of complete heart block.

In the acute post-operative period there must be vigilance to document atrioventricular synchrony. Patients with Fontan physiology do not tolerate atrioventricular asynchrony, e.g. accelerated junctional rhythm. Patients should have temporary atrial pacing leads placed at the time of surgery and often require overdrive pacing if accelerated junctional rhythm occurs. The atrial or central venous pressure tracing can be helpful in determining atrioventricular synchrony. The tracing will show "cannon" atrial waves caused by the atria contracting against a closed atrioventricular valve, resulting in an acute rise in the atrial pressure. Another diagnostic maneuver is to connect the temporary atrial wires to an ECG machine to perform an atrial electrogram. This helps determine if atrial impulses correlate in a 1:1 relationship with the ventricular impulses and if the atrial impulses precede the ventricular impulses. Atrial arrhythmias should also be aggressively treated in the acute post-operative period and may require the institution of antiarrhythmic infusions.

In follow-up of these patients the most frequently encountered arrhythmia, other than sinus node dysfunction, is IART or "scar flutter" (see Fig. 25.2). This arrhythmia is often multifocal making it resistant to medical therapy and difficult to ablate in the catheterization laboratory.[1] IART impacts ventricular function from frequent atrial-ventricular asynchrony; it makes the patient more susceptible to intracardiac thrombi secondary to increased atrial stasis and often results in multiple hospitalizations for cardioversions.

Atrial pacing can be successful in certain patients to augment the underlying atrial rate diminishing episodes of atrial tachycardia. Many patients have residual intracardiac shunting limiting the placement of transvenous leads. In addition, there is often significant right atrial scarring, which limits effective right atrial pacing sites and increases the risk of circuit thrombosis. In patients with an extracardiac conduit there is no means of access to the atria from the systemic veins. As pacing leads must be placed epicardially,[11] associated hemodynamic abnormalities must be defined and addressed simultaneously.

Thromboembolism

The incidence of intracardiac thrombi ranges from 3%–20%[3,9,14,15] in patients with a Fontan circulation. The most frequent site for thrombus formation in this group of patients is in the right atrium or systemic venous baffle. This may occur secondary to venous stasis and is more frequently seen in those with poor hemodynamics (increased systemic venous pressure and poor venous flow) or arrhythmias. Thrombi have also been detected in pulmonary venous atria, hypoplastic ventricular cavities and ligated pulmonary artery stumps.[14] If clotting occurs, there must be investigation into possible etiologies – work-up should include investigation for arrhythmias requiring treatment or hemodynamically significant lesions such as systemic venous baffle obstruction or pulmonary artery distortion. Systemic venous baffle thrombi can lead to chronic pulmonary microemboli, which can increase pulmonary venous resistance and create a vicious cycle with worsening flow through the Fontan circuit and more impetus to form further thrombi.[16] These patients are also susceptible to right to left shunting through fenestrations or baffle leaks that can lead to intracerebral thromboembolism and neurologic complications. Transthoracic echocardiography is often not sensitive in delineating small thrombi or those in posterior systemic venous baffles. If there is clinical concern, transesophageal echocardiography should be considered.[17]

Studies have suggested associated coagulation deficits in this group of patients secondary to possible hepatic dysfunction resulting from chronic systemic venous hypertension. Researchers have found elevations in prothrombin times and factor VIII and deficiencies in protein C and S, factor VII and antithrombin III.[9,14,18] Diverse protocols exist for anticoagulation/platelet inhibition in patients with Fontan circulations, though there is little data supporting superiority of any of these protocols.[14] Some centers do not anticoagulate uncomplicated patients with Fontan physiology, while others use acetylsalicylic acid or warfarin on all patients. The risk of thrombus formation has to be weighed against the risk of bleeding secondary to anticoagulation. There is general agreement that patients require anticoagulation in the face of a previously documented thrombus or recurrent arrhythmias.

Cyanosis

Cyanosis can lead to exercise intolerance and may worsen myocardial and systemic oxygen delivery. Sources of cyanosis should be thoroughly investigated. This work-up frequently requires contrast echocardiography[19] or cardiac catheterization to delineate the presence of a fenestration or baffle leak, pulmonary arteriovenous malformations (AVMs) and venoatrial connections.[3] Shunting through a fenestration or baffle leak can increase if the hemodynamics worsen within a Fontan circuit as the difference between the systemic venous pressure and atrial pressure increases. Causes can include distal obstructions in the Fontan circuit as delineated above. Pulmonary AVMs may result in intrapulmonary shunting of venous blood directly from the systemic veins to the pulmonary veins. They are more likely if the patient has a history of a classic Glenn shunt, but can develop in its absence. Venoatrial connections can be absent initially, but develop in the face of worsening hemodynamics as these venous vessels recanalize or enlarge becoming clinically significant. In some patients with complex systemic venous connections the hepatic veins may return to the pulmonary venous atrium leading to desaturation and can be re-routed to the systemic venous side of the circulation. Some patients may have unrecognized defects in the wall of the coronary sinus and these can also lead to right to left shunting. Finally, cyanosis can be secondary to pulmonary venous desaturation from diffusion abnormalities as a result of chronic pulmonary microemboli leading to pulmonary infarctions, chronic lung disease, interstitial edema, or pneumonia. Other causes of pulmonary venous desaturation include pleural effusions or pneumothoraces.

Ventricular dysfunction/low cardiac output

Ventricular dysfunction and low cardiac output can be an ominous finding that responds poorly to medical interventions. Isolated ventricular dysfunction can be treated with afterload reduction and acutely with inotropes. Hemodynamics consistent with poor ventricular function includes an increased CVP in the face of an elevated LAP. The LAP reflects the end-diastolic ventricular pressure, which is elevated with decreased ventricular function. These hemodynamics contrast with those previously described (high transpulmonary gradient = increased CVP and low LAP) when there is a pulmonary problem or issue with obstruction in the Fontan circuit.

Treatment is complicated by the fact that cardiac output is dependant on venous return through the Fontan circuit. Conventional means of augmenting cardiac output such as inotropes may be ineffective in the absence of documented systolic dysfunction.[16] Mechanical ventilation, if required, can further compromise flow through the Fontan circuit as the bulk of flow through the Fontan circuit occurs during negative pressure spontaneous inspiration.[20] If cardiac output is compromised, the integrity of the Fontan circuit must be evaluated (see section on Fontan pathway obstruction). Patients with a Fontan circulation also do not tolerate atrioventricular asynchrony and this can lead to ventricular dysfunction as delineated above.

The right ventricle as a systemic ventricle has proven to have a higher incidence of failure than one of left ventricular morphology, possibly secondary to a higher incidence of valve failure.[21,22] Patients with single ventricle anatomy often have abnormal atrioventricular valves, which are more likely to become regurgitant, and this is poorly tolerated.[10] Mitral valves respond more favorably to attempts at repair than tricuspid valves but valve replacement is often required for promotion for orthotopic heart transplantation.[21]

Coronary sinus hypertension resulting in impaired coronary perfusion pressure may compromise myocardial perfusion and exacerbate ventricular dysfunction.[23,24] This can be seen in patients with a "failing" atriopulmonary Fontan or in those patients in which the coronary sinus was left to drain to the systemic venous side of the circulation. Late progression to a Fontan can be associated with worsened ventricular dysfunction (especially diastolic dysfunction) as the patient is left with prolonged pressure or volume overload lesions such as pulmonary stenosis, pulmonary artery banding or shunts.[3,16] This is one reason patients now undergo an interim bi-directional cavopulmonary anastomosis.[25] Some have also contributed ventricular dysfunction to ventricular volume overload from the presence of aortopulmonary collaterals; they are readily addressed in the catheterization laboratory. Diastolic ventricular dysfunction can be secondary to chronic underloading of the ventricle inherent in the dependence on passive venous return in this circulation.[12,16] There has been recent research into the fact that the Fontan circulation is associated with reduced mechanical efficiency that limits cardiac reserve, especially with exercise. The single ventricle must provide energy for both systemic and pulmonary flow and decreases in cardiac contractility (Ees) and increases in arterial elastance (Ea) worsen the ventriculoarterial coupling ratio and worsen the efficiency of the Fontan circuit.[25] Angiotensin-converting enzyme inhibitors have been used to attempt to improve or delay the development of ventricular dysfunction in these patients.

Protein Losing Enteropathy (PLE)

PLE can be an ominous finding in a patient with a Fontan circulation as there are few options for treatment (survival <50% at 5 years).[1,3] Fortunately, it is a less frequently diagnosed complication with incidences of 2.5%–13%.[3,9,10] PLE may present as edema or ascites from protein losses and chronic diarrhea. Patients can often have associated immunodeficiencies[8] and clotting disorders from loss of proteins in the stool. Diagnosis is made when a patient has low serum levels of albumin (<3 g dl^{-1}), a total protein (<5 g dl^{-1}), and elevated level of stool α–1 antitrypsin when compared with that found in the blood. Treatments include diet modification (low fat, high protein), diuretics, digitalis, and angiotensin-converting enzyme inhibitors. Some patients require intermittent albumin infusions and others are treated with steroids or high molecular weight heparin.[16]

All patients diagnosed with PLE require a cardiac catheterization to investigate possible causes of obstruction to flow through the venous pathway with the goal of intervening to improve obstructions if encountered. Fenestration of the systemic venous baffle has improved the symptomatology in certain patients with PLE, as it is thought that PLE is due to systemic venous hypertension which increases the pressure in the splanchnic circulation.[12,26] This can be accomplished in the catheterization laboratory in certain cases of atriopulmonary or lateral tunnel Fontans; however, it is often difficult to achieve fenestration in the catheterization laboratory in the presence of non-autologous tissue and may require surgical intervention. Patients with a fenestration that has diminished in size can have this defect balloon dilated to a goal systemic saturation of ~85%. There are also devices, currently in development, designed to maintain patency of the fenestration.[27] The patient should also be evaluated for the presence of arrhythmias, particularly sinus node dysfunction. Some patients have had resolution of symptoms of PLE with atrial pacing to improve cardiac output and maintain atrioventricular synchrony.[16,28] If there are surgically amenable abnormalities, some patients have benefited from Fontan conversion.[29,30] If all of these options fail, orthotopic heart transplantation is an option, though not uniformly successful.

Plastic bronchitis is thought to result from a similar mechanism with increased pressure in the pulmonary system leading to extravasation of chyle into the bronchi.[16] Patients with plastic bronchitis may be asymptomatic or may present with respiratory difficulties. Patients often expectorate tenacious casts from the bronchi. It is also very difficult to treat. In addition to the treatment listed above for PLE, long-term aerosolized tissue plasminogen activator and oral macrolides have been reported to improve symptoms of plastic bronchitis.[31]

Surgical strategies for failed Fontan circulations

Fontan conversion

There has been considerable success with Fontan conversions for patients with failing Fontan circulations leading to reduction in right atrial size, abatement or improvement in atrial arrhythmias, resolution of right pulmonary vein compression, resolution of pleural effusions, and clinical improvement (improvement in NYHA class and exercise tolerance).[17,23,24,29,30,32–38] Fontan conversions are most useful in patients with atriopulmonary Fontans with abnormalities amenable to surgical repair or in those with arrhythmias refractory to medical management or pacing (see Figs. 25.3 and 25.4). Lesions amenable to surgical intervention include systemic venous baffle obstruction, proximal pulmonary artery distortions, right pulmonary venous obstruction secondary to a dilated right atrium, atrioventricular valve regurgitation, and ventricular outflow tract obstruction. Series of conversions have included transitions to lateral tunnel baffles or extracardiac conduits, both aimed at streamlining flow through the Fontan circuit and diminishing atrial suture lines that predispose the patient to IART. These procedures are often scheduled in conjunction with right atrial debulking, cryoablation or radiofrequency ablation of foci generating atrial arrhythmias, right or biatrial maze procedures, and epicardial pacemaker placement.[17,24,30,34,35,37]

Orthotopic Heart Transplantation (OHT)

If there are no defects amenable to transcatheter or surgical therapy, OHT may be the only remaining option. Some centers promote this as a primary intervention for PLE[32,39] or significant ventricular dysfunction,[21,38] as other options often have less than satisfactory outcomes. OHT can be performed in these patients, though it often requires a surgeon with experience with congenital cardiac repairs as patients require pulmonary artery repairs and many patients have anomalies in their systemic and pulmonary venous return. Grafts are often harvested with extra venous and arterial connections to aid in anastomoses to the heart when placed *in situ*. Transplantation in these patients often

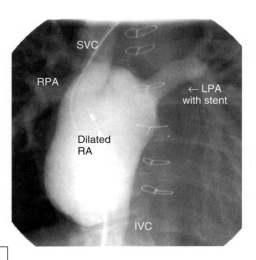

Fig. 25.3. Failing atriopulmonary Fontan with severe right atrial dilation and a previous stent in the left pulmonary artery. SVC = superior vena cava, RPA = right pulmonary artery, LPA = left pulmonary artery, RA = right atrium, IVC = inferior vena cava

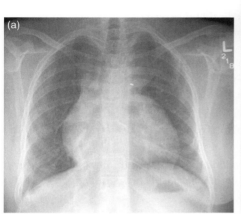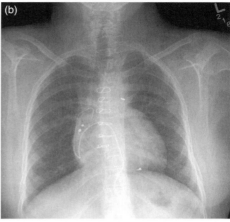

Fig. 25.4. Pre- and post-operative CXRs in a patient who underwent conversion from an atriopulmonary Fontan to a lateral tunnel Fontan with right atrial debulking and placement of an epicardial pacemaker showing a decrease in the cardiac size.

entails additional risk; these patients have had previous surgeries (often multiple), have multiple adhesions, and an increased risk of bleeding, have increased lymphocytotoxic antibodies secondary to blood transfusions, and may have elevated pulmonary vascular resistance which can cause difficulties with right ventricular failure post-operatively.[22,40] A case series of cardiac transplantation in patients with a Fontan circulation did not have an increased risk when compared with others with forms of congenital heart disease.[22] With these considerations, OHT may be the only viable option for some patients with a failing Fontan circulation.

Conclusions

Overall, the patient with a failing Fontan circulation presents a difficult clinical challenge requiring vigilance to diagnose repairable lesions as medical therapy is often unsatisfying. Medical therapy is aimed at improving symptomatology in a patient with a failing Fontan such as decreasing edema, preventing complications from thromboembolism, and diminishing the contribution of arrhythmias. Preservation of ventricular function is also of paramount importance as this can be an ominous finding with few therapeutic options. Blood work should be done to determine electrolytes, renal and liver function, coagulation studies, albumin, total protein, and α–1 antitrypsin determinations. Stool should also be collected for 24 hours to determine an α–1 antitrypsin level. Immunoglobulin testing can also be performed if there are signs of PLE. Signs of low cardiac output, edema, cyanosis, or PLE must be investigated to define lesions amenable to intervention (transcatheter or surgical). Testing includes determination of systemic saturations, Holter monitoring, echocardiography (transthoracic and transesophageal), and cardiac catheterization. Selective interventions to address hemodynamically significant lesions are often required. Other options include epicardial pacing, Fontan conversion, or OHT.

Patients with a Fontan circulation have become more frequent as a greater number of patients survive their initial operative interventions and as use of the Fontan procedure has been expanded to palliate more complex single ventricle lesions. The Fontan procedure remains palliative and even the "perfect Fontan" is likely to eventually fail. The focus on this group of patients is to continue to improve medical and surgical management in order to increase both the duration and quality of life for the patient with a Fontan circulation.

Learning points

- With recent decreases in early mortality, more patients are surviving to experience associated morbidities related to the Fontan circulation.

- Post-operative issues following a Fontan operation include: Fontan pathway obstruction, atrial arrhythmias, thromboembolism, progressive cyanosis, low cardiac output, and protein losing enteropathy.

- Fontan conversions are most useful in patients with atriopulmonary Fontans with abnormalities amenable to surgical repair or in those with arrhythmias refractory to medical management or pacing.

- If there are no defects amenable to transcatheter or surgical therapy, OHT may be the only remaining option for the failing Fontan.

- The Fontan procedure remains palliative and even the "perfect Fontan" is likely to eventually fail.

References

1. The Task Force on the Management of Grown Up Congenital Heart Disease of the European Society of Cardiology. Management of grown up congenital heart disease. *Eur Heart J* 2003; **24**: 1035–84.

2. Fontan F, Baudet E. Surgical repair of tricuspid atresia. *Thorax* 1971; **26**: 240–8.

3. Kaulitz R, Hofbeck M. Current treatment and prognosis in children with functionally univentricular hearts. *Arch Dis Child* 2005; **90**: 757–62.

4. Cochrane AD, Brizard CP, Penny DJ *et al.* Management of the univentricular connection: are we improving? *Eur J Cardiothor Surg* 1997; **12**: 107–15.

5. De Leval MR, Kilner P, Gewillig M, Bull C. Total cavopulmonary connection: a logical alternative to atriopulmonary connection for complex Fontan operations. Experimental studies and early clinical experience. *J Thorac Cardiovasc Surg* 1988; **96**: 682–95.

6. Humes RA, Feldt RH, Porter CJ, Julsrud PR, Puga FJ, Danielson GK. The modified Fontan operation for asplenia and polysplenia syndromes. *J Thorac Cardiovasc Surg* 1988; **96**: 212–18.

7. Nawa S, Teramoto S. New extension of the Fontan principle: inferior vena cavapulmonary artery bridge operation. *Thorax* 1988; **43**: 1022–3.

8. Stamm C, Friehs I, Mayer JE *et al.* Long-term results of the lateral tunnel Fontan operation. *J Thorac Cardiovasc Surg* 2001; **121**: 28–41.

9. Kaulitz R, Luhmer I, Bergmann F, Rodeck B, Hausdorf G. Sequelae after modified Fontan operation: postoperative haemodynamic data and organ function. *Heart* 1997; **78**: 154–9.

10. Driscoll DJ, Offord KP, Feldt RH, Schaff HV, Puga FJ, Danielson GK. Five- to fifteen-year follow-up after Fontan operation. *Circulation* 1992; **85**: 469–96.

11. Cohen MI, Vetter VL, Wernovsky G *et al.* Epicardial pacemaker implantation and follow-up in patients with a single ventricle after the Fontan operation. *J Thorac Cardiovasc Surg* 2001; **121**: 804–11.

12. De Leval MR. The Fontan circulation: what have we learned? What to expect? *Pediatr Cardiol* 1998; **19**: 316–20.

13. Harrison DA, Liu P, Walters JE *et al.* Cardiopulmonary function in adult patients late after Fontan repair. *JACC* 1995; **26**: 1016–21.

14. Coon PD, Rychik J, Novello RT, Ro PS, Gaynor JW, Spray TL. Thrombus formation after the Fontan operation. *Ann Thorac Surg* 2001; **71**: 1990–4.

15. Jacobs ML, Pourmoghadam KK, Geary EM *et al*. Fontan's operation: Is aspirin enough? Is Coumadin too much? *Ann Thorac Surg* 2002; **73**: 64–8.
16. Gewillig M. The Fontan circulation. *Heart* 2005; **91**: 839–46.
17. Setty SP, Finucane K, Skinner JR, Kerr AR. Extracardiac conduit with a limited maze procedure for the failing Fontan with atrial tachycardias. *Ann Thorac Surg* 2002; **74**: 1992–7.
18. Narkewicz MR, Sondheimer HM, Ziegler JW *et al*. Hepatic dysfunction following the Fontan procedure. *J Pediatr Gastroenterol Nutr* 2003; **36**: 352–7.
19. Podzolkov VP, Zaetz SB, Alekyan BG, Chiaureli MR, Yurlov IA, Chernikh IG. Surgical reinterventions after modified Fontan operations. *Ann Thorac Surg* 1995; **60**: S572–7.
20. Shekerdemian LS, Bush A, Shore DF, Lincoln C, Redington AN. Cardiopulmonary interactions after Fontan operations. *Circulation* 1997; **96**: 3934–42.
21. Mavroudis C, Stewart RD, Backer CL, Deal BJ, Young L, Franklin WH. Atrioventricular valve procedures with repeat Fontan operations: influence of valve pathology, ventricular function, and arrhythmias on outcome. *Ann Thorac Surg* 2005; **80**: 29–36.
22. Carey JA, Hamilton L, Hilton CJ *et al*. Orthotopic cardiac transplantation for the failing Fontan circulation. *Eur J Cardiothor Surg* 1998; **14**: 7–14.
23. McElhinney DB, Reddy VM, Moore P, Hanley FL. Revision of previous Fontan connections to extracardiac or intraatrial conduit cavopulmonary anastomosis. *Ann Thorac Surg* 1996; **62**: 1276–83.
24. Mott AR, Feltes TF, McKenzie ED *et al*. Improved early results with the Fontan operation in adults with functional single ventricle. *Ann Thorac Surg* 2004; **77**: 1334–40.
25. Szabo G, Buhmann V, Graf A *et al*. Ventricular energetics after the Fontan operation: contractility-afterload mismatch. *J Thorac Cardiovasc Surg* 2003; **125**: 1061–9.
26. Rychik J, Rome JJ, Jacobs ML. Late surgical fenestration for complications after the Fontan operation. *Circulation* 1997; **96**: 33–6.
27. Amin Z, Danford DA, Pedra CAC. A new Amplatzer device to maintain patency of Fontan fenestrations and atrial septal defects. *Cathet Cardiovasc Intervent* 2002; **57**: 246–51.
28. Cohen MI, Rhodes LA, Wernovsky G, Gaynor JW, Spray TL, Rychik J. Atrial pacing: an alternative treatment for protein-losing enteropathy after the Fontan operation. *J Thorac Cardiovasc Surg* 2001; **121**: 582–3.
29. Marcelletti CF, Hanley FL, Mavroudis C *et al*. Revision of previous Fontan connections to total extracardiac cavopulmonary anastomosis: a multicenter experience. *J Thorac Cardiovasc Surg* 2000; **119**: 340–6.
30. Kim WH, Lim HG, Lee JR *et al*. Fontan conversion with arrhythmia surgery. *Eur J Cardiothor Surg* 2005; **27**: 250–7.
31. Wakeham MK, Van Bergen AH, Torero LE, Akhter J. Long-term treatment of plastic bronchitis with aerosolized tissue Plasminogen activator in a Fontan patient. *Pediatr Crit Care Med* 2005; **6**: 76–8.
32. Van Son JAM, Mohr FW, Hambsch J, Schneider P, Hess H, Haas GS. Conversion of atriopulmonary or lateral tunnel cavopulmonary anastomosis to extracardiac conduit Fontan modification. *Eur J Cardiothor Surg* 1999; **15**: 150–8.
33. Vitullo DA, DeLeon SY, Berry TE *et al*. Clinical improvement after revision in Fontan patients. *Ann Thorac Surg* 1996; **61**: 1797–804.
34. Sheikh AM, Tang ATM, Roman K *et al*. The failing Fontan circulation: successful conversion of atriopulmonary connections. *J Thorac Cardiovasc Surg* 2004; **128**: 60–6.
35. Weinstein S, Cua C, Chan D, Davis JT. Outcome of symptomatic patients undergoing extracardiac Fontan conversion and cryoablation. *J Thor Cardiovasc Surg* 2003; **126**: 529–36.
36. Kreutzer J, Keane JF, Lock JE *et al*. Conversion of modified Fontan procedure to lateral atrial tunnel cavopulmonary anastomosis. *J Thorac Cardiovasc Surg* 1996; **111**: 1169–76.
37. Mavroudis C, Backer CL, Deal BJ, Johnsrude C, Strasburger J. Total cavopulmonary conversion and maze procedure for patients with failure of the

Fontan operation. *J Thorac Cardiovasc Surg* 2001; **122**: 863–71.

38. Conte S, Gewillig M, Eyskens B, Dumoulin M, Daenen W. Management of late complications after classic Fontan procedure by conversion to total cavopulmonary connection. *Cardiovasc Surg* 1999; **7**: 651–5.

39. Gamba A, Merlo M, Fiocchi R *et al.* Heart transplantation in patients with previous Fontan operations. *J Thorac Cardiovasc Surg* 2004; **127**: 555–62.

40. Michielon G, Parisi F, Di Carlo D *et al.* Orthotopic heart transplantation for failing single ventricle physiology. *Eur J Cardiothor Surg* 2003; **24**: 502–10.

Chapter 26

Sepsis in a BMT patient admitted to PICU

Farhan Bhanji and Sam D. Shemie

Introduction

Bone Marrow Transplant (BMT) recipients admitted to the pediatric intensive care unit (PICU) remain amongst the highest risk for mortality, particularly if they require intubation and mechanical ventilation. Negative perceptions exist amongst the healthcare team regarding their prognosis despite improving outcomes after ICU admission. Paradoxically, ICU outcomes are not principally linked to features of BMT itself, but rather related to the severity and temporal evolution of Multi-organ Failure (MOF), similar to any ICU patient.

Patients undergoing BMT are at particularly high risk for developing overwhelming sepsis and should be started on broad-spectrum antibiotics at the first signs of infection. Aggressive fluid resuscitation is frequently necessary and should be instituted rapidly. Inotropic support and invasive mechanical ventilation should be provided, as clinically indicated, but the family should be informed of the significant risk for mortality. Consideration should be given to withdrawal of support or non-escalation in therapy if the patient develops multiple system organ dysfunction.

Case history

A 3-year-old boy, on the oncology ward, was in second remission for Acute Lymphoblastic Leukemia (ALL). He underwent an allogeneic BMT 14 days ago and now presents with poor perfusion and a fever of 38.5 °C (axillary). The patient was evaluated 2 hours earlier by the junior resident because he did not "look well" according to the bedside nurse. There was no history of cough, runny nose, headache, vomiting, diarrhea, or urinary symptoms. The patient felt warm according to the parents but was afebrile (37.6 °C axillary) at that time. The young boy did not fully cooperate for the temperature measurement, as he was quite upset after being awoken. The remainder of his examination was unremarkable, aside from a heart rate of 160 min^{-1}, which persisted even when he stopped crying. The resident elected to wait and see the evolution of his condition, asking for vital sign assessment in 2 hours.

The patient received the bone marrow from his 5-year-old Human Leukocyte Antigen (HLA) matched sibling, following a preconditioning regimen of cyclophosphamide and Total Body Irradiation (TBI). Both the donor and recipient were CMV negative. A double-lumen subclavian broviac catheter was inserted into the superior vena cava (SVC) prior to transplantation and was functioning well. As expected, the patient had not yet demonstrated evidence of engraftment with the neutrophil count always remaining below 0.1×10^9 l^{-1}. He continued to require intermittent platelet transfusions, every 2–3 days. Fluconozole prophylaxis and Intravenous Immunoglobulin (IVIG) were given as per the local hospital protocol. Total parenteral nutrition (TPN) was started because of poor oral intake, worsened by significant mucositis.

Case Studies in Pediatric Critical Care, ed. Peter. J. Murphy, Stephen C. Marriage, and Peter J. Davis. Published by Cambridge University Press. © Cambridge University Press 2009.

Examination

The child looked generally unwell but was alert and protecting his airway. His respiratory rate was 35 breaths per minute with moderately increased work of breathing. Air entry was symmetric with no adventitious sounds appreciated. Oxygen saturation was difficult to record, but read 95% when the tracing was accurate. His heart rate was 180 beats per minute with a blood pressure of 80/50 mmHg by automated cuff. Capillary refill was prolonged at 5 seconds and the peripheries were cool to touch.

Initial resuscitation

The patient was immediately given oxygen via a face mask at $15 \, l \, min^{-1}$ and put on a cardiorespiratory monitor, which demonstrated a normal sinus rhythm. Additional intravenous access was obtained with a 20-gauge cannula in the right antecubital fossa. Blood was sent for FBC, coagulation profile (INR/PTT), U&E, glucose, venous blood gas, liver transaminases, bilirubin, C-reactive protein, and a blood culture. Bedside glucose measurement was mildly elevated at $9.1 \, mmol \, l^{-1}$. A fluid bolus of 300 ml of 0.9% saline ($20 \, ml \, kg^{-1}$) was given over 15 minutes with no change in perfusion. Blood pressure remained constant at 82/50 mmHg and heart rate did not change. The patient appeared agitated with a slight worsening of his respiratory status. A second fluid bolus of 300 ml was started, while the ICU fellow was called and intubation medications were being prepared.

Rapid sequence intubation was performed using atropine (0.15 mg), ketamine (30 mg), and suxamethonium (30 mg). A 4.5 uncuffed oral endotracheal tube was inserted using cricoid pressure to prevent aspiration of gastric contents. Good air entry was heard bilaterally and a disposable end-tidal CO_2 detector confirmed appropriate placement. The tube was secured with tape at 13 cm at the lips. The patient was placed on a portable ventilator with pressures of 18/5 and a respiratory rate of 20. The inspired oxygen concentration was left at 100%. A urinary catheter, placed for ongoing fluid management, drained only a small amount of concentrated urine. A sample was sent for urinalysis and culture. A nasogastric tube was also carefully inserted. Antibiotics were empirically started, given the high risk of sepsis; vancomycin, piperacillin/tazobactam and tobramycin as per the local protocol for febrile neutropenia.

Initial venous blood gas results (taken before mechanical ventilation) revealed a pH of 7.27 with a pCO_2 of 50 mmHg. Bicarbonate was low at $18 \, mmol \, l^{-1}$ and the base deficit was elevated at $7 \, mmol \, l^{-1}$. Electrolytes were normal, demonstrating a serum sodium of $143 \, mmol \, l^{-1}$, chloride of $105 \, mmol \, l^{-1}$, potassium of $4.2 \, mmol \, l^{-1}$, and blood glucose of $8.5 \, mmol \, l^{-1}$. Ionized calcium was normal at $1.15 \, mmol \, l^{-1}$. Urinalysis, by dipstick, showed mild ketones and a specific gravity >1.030 but no leukocytes, nitrites, or blood.

Vital signs were repeated and demonstrated ongoing tachycardia (sinus) at $190 \, min^{-1}$ with a blood pressure of 78/50 mmHg. Oxygen saturation recorded 100%, when it was reading appropriately. His peripheries remained cool to touch and capillary refill remained at 4 to 5 seconds. A third bolus of 300 ml of saline was started and a chest X-ray was undertaken to confirm endotracheal tube position. There was no evidence of pneumonia or interstitial disease noted (i.e. no ARDS). The ICU was prepared for urgent transfer.

Intensive care unit management

The patient was transferred into an isolation room of the ICU. Both lumens of the broviac were patent and functioned well for infusion. A blood gas was sent to measure mixed venous saturation and cultures were sent to assess for possible colonization. Ventilation was instituted using the Pressure Regulated Volume Control (PRVC) mode, at a rate of 20 and a delivered tidal volume of 10 ml kg^{-1}. The PaCO$_2$ was allowed to rise (permissive hypercapnia) so long as the pH remained greater than 7.25. The aim for PaO$_2$ was to remain between 80 and 100 mmHg. Inotropic support was started using dopamine at 5 mcg kg^{-1} per min via the broviac line. A 22-gauge left radial arterial line was also inserted for frequent bloodwork and accurate blood pressure monitoring. The initial readings correlated well with the blood pressure cuff, reading at 82/48 mmHg. The heart rate settled back to 180 min^{-1} as the atropine wore off. Central venous pressure monitoring, through the other lumen of the broviac, was instituted and demonstrated a reading of 10–11 mmHg. Sedation was accomplished with continuous infusions of fentanyl and midazolam. Vecuronium was given to maintain neuromuscular blockade.

Results from the original FBC became available, revealing a total white count of 1.0×10^9 l^{-1} and a manual neutrophil count of 0.1×10^9 l^{-1}. The hemoglobin was 10.5 g dl^{-1} and the platelet count was low at 54×10^9 l^{-1} but there was no active clinical bleeding. C-reactive protein was elevated at 20 mg dl^{-1}. The blood urea nitrogen was elevated at 9 mmol l^{-1} but the creatinine was normal, 50 mcmol l^{-1}. Liver transaminases (ALT and AST) and bilirubin were both within normal limits. The initial arterial blood gas demonstrated a pH of 7.30, pCO$_2$ of 44 mmHg and a pO$_2$ of 400 mmHg. The bicarbonate was low at 17 mmol l^{-1} and the lactate was 5.1 mmol l^{-1}. The measured venous saturation from the broviac was also low at 40%. The dopamine infusion was increased to 10 µg kg^{-1} per min in response to the clinical picture and the concern that the patient had not produced any urine in the past 45 minutes (i.e. since the catheter was placed).

An echocardiogram was requested and demonstrated moderately depressed biventricular function with no structural abnormalities or pericardial fluid. The heart appeared well filled and there was no evidence of pulmonary hypertension or valvar dysfunction. Clinically, there was minimal response to the increased dose of dopamine and the blood pressure remained 80/50 mmHg. Central venous pressure varied from 9–11 mmHg. The patient remained cool and clamped down peripherally with a capillary refill of 4 seconds. He started to produce a little urine (1.5 ml) over the previous half-hour. The lactate decreased slightly to 4.9 mmol l^{-1} and the mixed venous saturation improved mildly to 45%.

Given the clinical picture and current hemodynamics, it was decided to start adrenaline at 0.05 mcg kg^{-1} per min and titrate to effect. When the adrenaline was increased to 0.3 µg kg^{-1} per min the patient's heart rate increased up to 200 min^{-1} with the blood pressure remaining 82/50 mmHg. Urine output increased, slightly, to 0.3 ml kg^{-1} per h (4.5 ml h^{-1}) with a lactate of 4.7 mmol l^{-1} and venous saturation of 55%. After collaborative discussion amongst the ICU consultants and fellows, it was decided to try low dose sodium nitroprusside (SNP) to assess if a reduction in afterload might improve myocardial performance.

One hour after starting SNP and titrating up to 2 mcg kg^{-1} per min, the blood pressure remained stable and the heart rate decreased to 180 min^{-1}. Central venous pressure decreased to 6 mmHg, with a transient drop in blood pressure, but returned to 9 mmHg with a fluid bolus of 10 ml kg^{-1} of 5% albumin. Peripheral perfusion improved with capillary refill decreasing to 2 seconds and the extremities becoming noticeably warmer. The saturation probe began to read consistently, recording a saturation of 100%. Urine output improved to 0.75 ml kg^{-1} per h and lactate dropped to 4.0 mmol l^{-1} with mixed venous saturation increasing to 70%. The fraction of inspired oxygen was gradually decreased to 0.4 with no change in peripheral or mixed venous saturation. No further changes were made at this time and the patient's cardiovascular status remained stable.

Since it was possible that the patient would not be fed in the next day or two, he was started on ranitidine for protection against gastrointestinal bleeding. Intravenous antibiotics were continued with regular monitoring of levels. Daily laboratory monitoring included serum urea and creatinine, given the risk of nephrotoxicity. Other routine investigations included a daily FBC, electrolytes, and liver transaminases, along with bilirubin. Blood gases were performed as clinically indicated (i.e. change in patient status or ventilator) at least four times per day.

Over the course of his PICU stay, the patient's oxygenation gradually deteriorated despite escalation of PEEP to $14\,cmH_2O$. His PaO_2 remained near 70 mmHg with a FiO_2 of 0.8. The chest X-ray progressed to bilateral patchy infiltrates, consistent with ARDS. There was no air leak or effusion visible. A change in ventilator strategy to a lung protective mode (delivered tidal volumes of $6\,ml\,kg^{-1}$) was instituted to prevent barotrauma (volutrauma). Bronchoscopic guided bronchoalveolar lavage (BAL) did not grow any organism, nor did viral studies from the endotracheal tube and nasopharynx. The patient's cardiovascular status was essentially unchanged, requiring dopamine, adrenaline, and nitroprusside to maintain blood pressure and systemic oxygen delivery. Bacterial cultures, from both the broviac and peripherally, revealed the growth of a Gram-negative organism within 12 hours. Subsequent analyses allowed the identification of E. coli as the offending organism. Follow-up cultures, taken from the broviac and arterial line, remained negative, indicating clearance from the patient and the line. The patient became afebrile 48 hours after starting antibiotics and remained that way for the rest of the admission. Despite eradication of the identified organism and improvement in the hemodynamic status of the patient, he progressed to develop multi-organ dysfunction. As noted above, he developed worsening oxygenation with a PaO_2 to FiO_2 (or P/F) ratio of 87.5. The ALT and AST increased to $400\,U\,l^{-1}$ with a bilirubin of $80\,\mu mol\,l^{-1}$. The patient was noted to have significant fluid overload on the basis of oliguric renal failure with the creatinine rising to $250\,\mu mol\,l^{-1}$. Consideration was given to renal replacement therapy and high-frequency oscillation as a method of ventilation.

The primary nurse of the child verbalized his concerns of suffering and wondered if we (parents and healthcare team) should continue to be so aggressive in his management. He had accessed several web-based articles, as well as discussions debating the utility (futility) of mechanical ventilation in adult bone marrow transplant recipients. High frequency oscillatory ventilation was subsequently commenced. Ultimately, after much discussion over the next few days between the parents and both the oncology and intensive care teams, in view of the continued deterioration in his overall clinical condition with multi-organ failure despite increasing support, it was decided to withdraw treatment.

Discussion

Sepsis in a bone marrow transplant recipient, or any other immunocompromised patient, can be a life-threatening emergency. Depressed immunologic function and portals of entry, such as mucositis or indwelling central venous catheters, place these patients at high risk for infections. The initial assessment and management should focus on the ABCs of resuscitation: airway, breathing, and circulation. Broad-spectrum antibiotics are necessary to combat bacterial sources of infection (and the subsequent systemic inflammatory response) but should not delay active resuscitation. Patients are clearly at higher risk for mortality than the majority of PICU patients, but advances in care are improving outcomes. ICU admission and aggressive intervention should be initiated if clinically indicated. Outcome studies are limited by their retrospective nature, but collectively suggest that the severity and temporal evolution of MOF, rather than variables related to the BMT, are the principal determinants of survival.

Initial assessment and management

The majority of patients following bone marrow transplant are able to mount a febrile response to infection that brings about medical attention.[1] However, its absence should not exclude the possibility of infection. In the case scenario provided, the junior doctor did not adequately consider the possibility of infection when evaluating this child. Axillary temperatures may be misleading and under-recognize fever if there is inadequate positioning or poor skin perfusion. The thermometer may be influenced by ambient air, particularly with movement. In any situation of concern involving immunocompromised oncology hosts, it is most prudent to draw off cultures and commence broad-spectrum antibiotics pending the culture results. Perhaps the systemic inflammatory response in this case could have been attenuated with earlier initiation of antibiotics.

When the patient required more urgent evaluation, the focus was appropriately centred on the ABCs. The patient was protecting his airway appropriately but having significant difficulty with his breathing. Preparation was made early to take over his breathing with mechanical ventilation as it was anticipated that he would continue to deteriorate. Fluid resuscitation was likely to be very significant with subsequent development of pulmonary edema. Mechanical ventilation would have the added benefit of reducing his myocardial workload, if he is appropriately sedated. It must be recognized that bag–valve–mask ventilation and rapid sequence intubation may be quite difficult with severe mucositis and bleeding. Intubation should only be attempted by individuals with advanced airway skills. CPAP or BiPAP should be considered if the patient has isolated respiratory disease but not if there is significant hemodynamic compromise.

Atropine was used to prevent the vagally induced bradycardia that many young children experience with laryngoscopy. Use of the lower end of the dose range ($0.01 \, \text{mg kg}^{-1}$) limits tachycardia while providing vagolysis. An approach of drawing up atropine but not giving it unless the patient became bradycardic would be acceptable as this patient is out of the very high-risk group (under 1 year) and was quite tachycardic. Ketamine was used to ensure hemodynamic stability. Although ketamine is a direct myocardial depressant, it functions to increase blood pressure through the release of catecholamines. Caution should therefore be used in patients with chronic disease or end-stage heart failure who may be depleted of catecholamine stores.[2] The choice of neuromuscular blockade may also bring about discussion. Both suxamethonium and a rapid onset non-depolarizer such as rocuronium would be equally acceptable.

The patient clearly demonstrated signs of compensated shock (inadequate tissue perfusion with an acceptable blood pressure). Early and aggressive fluid resuscitation should be implemented as it has been shown to improve outcomes.[3] Patients in septic shock frequently require 40 to 60 ml kg^{-1} of crystalloid in the early resuscitative phase. The choice of crystalloid versus colloid remains a very active debate throughout critical care medicine. There is very little empirical literature on which to base fluid choice in this scenario, but the use of crystalloid is likely adequate.[4] In the case of ongoing fluid resuscitation, it may be more prudent to change to colloid as the additional fluid will ultimately need to be diuresed off. Initiation of the bolus should ideally occur prior to intubation and the patient should be followed closely post-intubation as there is a high risk of hemodynamic compromise.

Inotropic or vasopressor therapy should be considered in septic shock only after adequate initial fluid resuscitation. This can be based on an age-appropriate central venous pressure or often, in the absence of central pressure monitoring, on presumed adequate fluid resuscitation (40 to 60 ml kg^{-1} of crystalloid). Adults typically demonstrate a relative dysfunction in vasomotor tone in response to sepsis. They present with good cardiac output but low blood pressure with warm peripheries and bounding pulses, the so-called "warm shock." Children do not behave like adults and respond in a more variable manner to infection.[5] Most important to note is that children are often able to maintain blood pressure, despite falling cardiac output, through elevation of systemic vascular resistance. The child in this case demonstrated a classic example of "cold shock." The blood pressure was well maintained, despite significant myocardial depression and inadequate tissue oxygen delivery. The heart rate was markedly elevated in an attempt to maintain maximal cardiac output and there was significant vasoconstriction to maintain blood pressure. In fact, the drop in blood pressure of a child is a late and often worrisome finding. Age appropriate tables exist to estimate blood pressure but a simple clinical tool to estimate the fifth percentile for systolic blood pressure is 70 + (age × 2).

PICU management

Ventilation was implemented in the PRVC mode with delivered tidal volumes of 10 ml kg^{-1}. As the patient developed ARDS, ventilation was changed to reflect a more lung-protective strategy of 6 ml kg^{-1}.[5] Initial use of a fraction of inspired oxygen at 1.0 was to improve oxygen delivery to end organs. This was weaned as oxygen delivery improved. Transfusion of packed red blood cells could also be considered for the same purpose. It remains undetermined what the ideal transfusion threshold is and if the restrictive transfusion strategy (i.e. using a transfusion threshold of 7 g dl^{-1}) is safe or appropriate in the initial resuscitation of septic shock.[4]

The patient developed hypoxic respiratory failure after the initial resuscitation period, as demonstrated by the PaO$_2$/FiO$_2$ ratio. This clinical tool is applicable at the bedside, and easy to calculate, but is limited as it does not take ventilatory parameters into account (different from the oxygenation index). On a practical level, however, definitions of ARDS and acute lung injury are based on P/F ratios so physicians in PICU need to be comfortable with its calculation and use. ARDS is defined by the appearance of bilateral pulmonary infiltrates, a P/F ratio of less than 200 and no evidence of left atrial hypertension (however pulmonary artery wedge pressure is rarely done in pediatrics). In this case the patient deteriorated from a P/F ratio of 400 (pO_2 of 400 and FiO$_2$ of 1.0) to 87.5 demonstrating the evolution towards ARDS. Deterioration of the P/F ratio to less than 100, despite appropriate use of PEEP, is particularly concerning and reflects severe oxygenation impairment.

While pulmonary arterial catheterization and thermodilution cardiac output monitoring has frequently been performed in adults, the risk of complications in children limited its routine use. Indirect assessment of cardiac output relies on evaluation of end-organ perfusion, biochemical perfusion monitoring and non-invasive tests such as cardiac echocardiography and transesophageal Doppler. Urine output is a useful and easy bedside test to ensure adequate renal perfusion. Normal output should be at least 1 ml kg^{-1} per h in small children and 30 ml h in larger children and adolescents. Lactate and mixed venous saturation are other useful markers of perfusion, and hemodynamically unstable patients should have routine serial measurements. If oxygen delivery is inadequate to tissue vascular beds, they will change to anerobic metabolism and produce lactate as an end product. True mixed venous blood should come from the pulmonary artery, as this is the place where it can be assured that inferior vena cava (IVC) and superior vena cava (SVC) blood has adequately mixed. In children, central SVO_2 (SVC or IVC) blood may serve as a surrogate for mixed venous blood and is particularly useful for observing trends. It has been advocated to aim for a saturation of 70% in the SVC during sepsis to ensure adequate oxygen delivery.[6]

In this case, cardiovascular support was titrated to end-organ perfusion, aiming for good urine output, normal capillary refill (<2 seconds), warm limbs with no difference between central and peripheral pulses, decreasing lactate and a normal mixed venous saturation of greater than 70%.[4] Fluid resuscitation is frequently required beyond the initial resuscitation period. In this case, a central venous pressure of at least 8–9 mmHg was aimed for to ensure adequate preload to the heart.

In an improving patient, like the early post-resuscitative period of this case, the rising mixed venous saturation better reflects immediate changes in hemodynamic status. The initial use of dopamine is appropriate but may be inadequate. In patients with cold shock (normal blood pressure and poor cardiac output) the ideal choice is likely adrenaline (epinephrine), whereas warm shock (low blood pressure with low systemic vascular resistance) a vasocon-strictor such as noradrenaline (norepinephrine) or vasopressin may prove more efficacious. In cases of cold shock where inotropic support has not reversed the perfusion issues, but the blood pressure remains adequate, a vasodilator may be beneficial. Nitrovasodilators such as nitro-glycerin or SNP are ideal because of their short half-life. Care should be used to start at a low dose and increase slowly to prevent hypotension and worsening tachycardia (particularly with SNP). Milrinone may also be effective but is complicated by its long half-life.[7]

Corticosteroids may be considered in patients with catecholamine-resistant septic shock and those with known or suspected adrenal insufficiency.[4] The response to inotropes in this case was acceptable so the use of steroids was not pursued. Sedation was provided with fentanyl and midazolam to ensure patient comfort and reduce oxygen demand and total myocardial work. Neuromuscular blockade is appropriate to initiate in ventilated patients with profound shock or severe lung disease to further reduce oxygen consumption and lung injury. However, its use should be limited to the minimal time period necessary as there is increased risk of prolonged muscular weakness in bone marrow recipients.[8] Vecuronium was chosen as the patient was quite tachycardic. The longer-acting non-depolarizer pan-curonium would have otherwise been appropriate. The use of ranitidine, or other agents, for stress ulcer prophylaxis is commonly employed in pediatric sepsis. Its effect has not been adequately studied in pediatrics[4] but the potential benefit is large and the risk for harm is relatively low. It can be considered in all patients but would be highly recommended in those requiring mechanical ventilation, coagulation factors or corticosteroids for any reason.[9]

Although recombinant human activated protein C was successful in reducing mortality in a large adult study,[10] and it has been released for this indication, studies in sepsis following bone marrow transplant are lacking. It has been used successfully in an adult patient[11] but is use is now contra-indicated in all children due to the risk of bleeding.[4]

Issues related to bone marrow transplantation

Allogeneic transplants refer to the transplantation of stem cells between two, related or unrelated, individuals. In contrast, autologous transplants refer to blood or marrow that is removed from an individual and cryopreserved, to be returned after initial high-dose therapy. The source of stem cells can be either peripheral blood or bone marrow. Umbilical cord blood is useful for allogeneic transplants and may become a potential source for autologous trans-plants with the advent of umbilical cord blood banking.[12]

All patients are at risk of invasive infections following bone marrow transplantation, but the risk is higher amongst allogeneic patients as they receive a more aggressive initial myelosuppression. Other risk factors for infection include the development of Graft-Versus-Host Disease (GVHD) necessitating the use of ciclosporin and/or corticosteroids, use of bone marrow from unrelated donors,[13] the degree of mucosal disruption, bacterial colonization, and reactivation of latent viruses.[1]

Infectious pathogens following allogeneic transplant, vary according to the time elapsed following the procedure. In the early (pre-engraftment) time period, the risk for bacterial and fungal sepsis is highest for several reasons. Mucosal integrity is disturbed by toxic conditioning regimens, prolonged neutropenia results from myelosuppressive conditioning, and T and B-cells may be dysfunctional from induced immounosuppression to prevent GVHD.[14] Complicating the situation further is the routine use of indwelling intravenous catheters in pediatric patients. These conditions combine to create an ideal opportunity for invasive pathogens.

The organisms causing infection during the pre-engraftment time period are generally endogenous bacteria or fungi that colonize the intestinal tract.[15] Gram-positive organisms are isolated more frequently than Gram-negatives.[1] Organisms such as *Staphylococcus epidermis* tend to be associated with indwelling central lines, while others such as viridans *Streptococci* and *Stomatococcus mucilaginosus* are associated with chemotherapy-induced mucositis. Bacterial translocation of Gram-negative enteric organisms, such as *Pseudomonas aeroginosa*, *Escherichia coli* and *Klebsiella* spp., is a major issue as these organisms tend to be more aggressive, have higher associated mortality and are commonly resistant to antibiotics.[15] Fungal infections correlate with the degree and duration of neutropenia and generally tend to occur after a period of antibiotic therapy.[15] *Candida* spp. enter from the gastrointestinal tract and may be recoverable from blood cultures. *Aspergillus*, on the other hand, enters via the respiratory tract and is rarely isolated from blood cultures. Viral infections in this early period include the reactivation of *Herpes simplex virus* and respiratory viruses such as *Respiratory Synctial Virus* (RSV)[1] and *Parainfluenza type 3*. If respiratory viruses progress to involve the lower airways and cause an interstitial pneumonia, they are a high risk for mortality. In one retrospective pediatric study, none of the 11 patients intubated for viral pneumonitis survived.[16]

The second time period is that from engraftment until day 100 post-transplantation. CMV infection used to be quite common, but the prophylactic or early use of ganciclovir in at risk patients (i.e. patients with increasing viral load) has reduced its incidence. The major drawback of this medication is the induction of neutropenia[17] that may increase the risk of bacterial and fungal infections. For this reason many programs limit its use until the viral load is increasing. Bacterial infections, particularly Gram-negative organisms, decrease in this time period but Gram-positive infections, from indwelling catheters, do still tend to occur. Fungal infections can occur and may be aided by GVHD.

During the late post-transplant period (>100 days) there is usually a change in pathogen. Bacterial infections tend to be caused by encapsulated bacteria such as *S. pneumoniae*.[18] Catheter-related infections still occur if central lines are present. The presence of GVHD (and its associated therapy with steroids or ciclosporin) augment the risk. Varicella zoster is a common viral pathogen that tends to re-activate in this time period and is also associated with chronic GVHD.

Initial antibiotic coverage for febrile neutropenic patients following bone marrow transplant should be similar to the management of other chemotherapeutic-induced neutropenic patients with fever. Broad-spectrum antibiotics should be started based on the patient's colonization, the community antimicrobial resistance patterns and the hospital environment.[15] Our hospital standard antibiotics for febrile neutropenia include piperacillin/tazobactam and tobramycin. For patients with clinically suspected sepsis, vancomycin is added empirically to cover for viridans *Streptococci*, particularly if patients have significant mucositis, and *Staphylococcus epidermis*. Antifungals are not started at the onset of illness (particularly since fluconozole is used prophylactically) unless there is very high clinical suspicion. Patients who remain febrile despite antibiotic coverage should be started on an antifungal such as liposomal amphotericin B (less nephrotoxic than the non-liposomal preparation). Caspofungin, is equally effective with less toxicity [19] with 79% of courses in children with febrile neutropenia resulting in an overall favourable response in one retrospective study.[20]

Other methods to combat infection include G-CSF, which may be useful to promote neutrophil production and release. Its use may be particularly indicated some time after the BMT when the marrow may have at least partially engrafted. Granulocyte transfusions are also now feasible and should be considered as a possible adjunct in cases of severe infection.[17]

In this case, the patient presumably developed ARDS on the basis of overwhelming sepsis. The search for an etiology appropriately included a BAL. Although this procedure may be diagnostic, it is not the "gold-standard." In cases where the patient is not responding to empirical therapy, particularly if the BAL is not diagnostic (or if the patient is not responding to specific therapy after a diagnostic BAL), the procedure of choice is an open lung biopsy. A retrospective study demonstrated that the results of open lung biopsy led to a change in management for 76% (25 out of 33) of patients.[21] Complications, such as airleak, are common (45% of patients) but generally are easy to manage. More serious complications (such as the need for ventilation in non-intubated patients or prolonged ventilation) can occur therefore routine use prior to empirical therapy is not advocated.

Patient outcomes in PICU

Negative perceptions regarding bone marrow recipients still exist amongst intensivists despite research that demonstrates improving survival. This perception may be more pronounced amongst adult intensivists, whose patients have traditionally done quite poorly.[22] The literature in pediatrics, although not overwhelmingly positive, is significantly more encouraging. BMT preadmission characteristics, including underlying diagnosis, age, time of admission post-BMT, type of BMT, conditioning regimen, and GVHD, have no apparent influence on outcome.[23–25]

ICU measurements of disease severity, i.e. extent of multiorgan failure, are the dominant influences on short-term outcome. In comparison, the medium- and long-term outcomes are primarily influenced by underlying BMT or oncology-related conditions. The challenge remains to aggressively treat patients who may recover and identify those who cannot, in order to minimize suffering and apply limited resources appropriately.[26] Severity of illness scores, such as the Pediatric Risk of Mortality (PRISM) and Pediatric Index of Mortality (PIM), have not been helpful, tending to underestimate the true risk of mortality.[27]

Caution must be exercised when reviewing outcome data on bone marrow recipients in the PICU as most studies involve small numbers of patients reviewed in a retrospective manner. It is relatively clear that BMT patients have significantly worse outcomes if they require mechanical ventilation for any reason.[16,25] This should not, however, limit therapy as 44% of these patients may survive to PICU discharge and many were alive at 6-month follow-up (36%).[24] Similar outcomes were reported in patients requiring ventilation following sepsis-induced cardiovascular collapse (38% survival).[28] Although the survival is significantly lower than the vast majority of PICU patients, it is clearly not futile and therapy is indicated. Patients that develop multiple-organ failure are more concerning, with several studies demonstrating very poor outcomes.[23-25,27] The presence of three or more organ failures was associated with no survivors in one study (0/5)[27] and only 10% survival (1/10) in another.[23] A third study demonstrated 20% (4/20) survival in patients with failure of four or more organ systems.[24] Particularly poor outcomes were noted for patients who required renal replacement therapy for renal failure.

Attempts have been made to quantify risk for mortality in BMT patients requiring ICU admission.[27] The O-PRISM (oncological risk of mortality) score uses severity of GVHD, CRP level ($>10 \, \text{mg dl}^{-1}$) and presence of macroscopic bleeding combined with the standard score to identify patients at highest risk. Although quite helpful in that respect, the O-PRISM does not have enough of a positive predictive value for death to rely on it exclusively to make clinical decisions for withdrawal of support.

Continuous veno-venous hemofiltration (CVVH) has shown promise as a novel method to treat ARDS in BMT patients *without* renal failure.[29] The main mechanisms are considered to be improved lung function through removal of lung and body water, and removal of soluble proinflammatory mediators. If confirmed by further research, CVVH may have a great impact on the future outcome of these patients.

As a general rule, we would advocate that all bone marrow transplant patients requiring intensive care deserve a trial of conventional ICU therapy, so long as the family is well informed of the risk for mortality and agrees to intervention. More innovative therapy should be evaluated with the family on a case-by-case basis. Prognostic decisions and limitations to care should be based on the development and temporal evolution of multisystem organ failure and not on aspects on the BMT itself.

Withdrawal of support

The decision to limit or withdraw support on a pediatric patient is quite difficult. There is an inherent (and appropriate) bias towards giving the patient a chance for "life." At the same time parents and healthcare professionals do not want to prolong suffering if they can only delay the inevitable. The decision to limit or withdraw support should ideally be discussed with the family jointly by the oncology and PICU teams. The oncologist is likely to have a long-standing trusting relationship with the family, while the intensive care physician is best to provide current status and prognosis. Ultimately, the parents should guide when the right time is to withdraw support. Although difficult to be present at the time of withdrawal, most families appreciate being with their loved one at the time of death. Support services such as close family members, pastoral services, social workers, or other allied health professionals (based on the specifics of the PICU) may prove invaluable to the immediate family at the time of grieving.

Learning points

- The primary focus in a septic patient should be the ABCs:
  - Airway
  - Breathing
  - Circulation.

- Patients in septic shock need rapid fluid resuscitation with boluses of 20 ml kg^{-1} of crystalloid or colloid given over minutes.
- Inotropic support with dopamine (or dobutamine) should be started after 60 ml kg^{-1} of volume resuscitation.
- Pediatric patients are more likely to present with *cold shock* (vasoconstricted with inadequate cardiac output) than *warm shock* (vasodilated with good cardiac output).
- Second-line inotropic support should generally be adrenaline (epinephrine) for cold shock and noradrenaline (norepinephrine) or vasopressin for warm shock.
- Broad-spectrum antibiotics should be initiated early in the care of septic patients following bone marrow transplantation (or other immunodeficiency).
- The period of highest risk for sepsis is early after BMT, prior to engraftment.
- Although Gram-positive organisms are more common, Gram-negatives have a higher risk of significant morbidity and mortality.
- Patients requiring mechanical ventilation have significant risk of mortality. This risk is significantly lower for pediatric patients compared with adults.
- Pre-admission BMT characteristics have no apparent influence on ICU outcomes.
- Limitation or withdrawal of support should be considered in cases with advancing multi-system organ failure, as this is the primary determinant of ICU outcome.

References

1. Einsele H, Bertz H, Beyer J *et al.* Infectious complications after allogeneic stem cell transplantation: epidemiology and interventional therapy strategies. Guidelines of the Infectious Disease Working Party (AGIHO) of the German Society of Hematology and Oncology (DGHO). *Ann Hematol* 2003; **82** Suppl 2: S175–85.

2. Gerardi MJ, Sacchetti AD, Cantor RM *et al.* Rapid-sequence intubation of the pediatric patient. *Ann Emerg Med* 1996; **28**: 55–74.

3. Carcillo JA, Davis AL, Zaritsky A. Role of early fluid resuscitation in pediatric septic shock. *J Am Med Assoc* 1991; **266**: 1242–5.

4. Dellinger RP, Levy MM, Carlet JM *et al.* Surviving Sepsis Campaign: International guidelines for management of severe sepsis and septic shock: 2008. *Crit Care Med* 2008; **36**: 294–327.

5. Carcillo JA. Pediatric septic shock and multiple organ failure. *Crit Care Clin* 2003; **19**: 413–40.

6. Carcillo JA, Fields AI. Clinical practice parameters for hemodynamic support of pediatric and neonatal patients in septic shock. *Crit Care Med.* 2002; **30**: 1365–74.

7. Barton P, Garcia J, Kouatli A *et al.* Hemodynamic effects of i.v. milrinone lactate in pediatric patients with septic shock. A prospective, double-blinded, randomized, placebo-controlled interventional study. *Chest* 1996; **109**: 1302–12.

8. Banwell BL, Mildner RJ, Hassall AC *et al.* Muscle weakness in critically ill children. *Neurology* 2003; **61**: 1779–82.

9. Trzeciak S, Dellinger P. Other supportive therapies in sepsis: an evidence-based review. *Crit Care Med* 2004; **32** (11 Suppl): S571–7.

10. Bernard GR, Vincent JL, Laterre PF *et al.* Efficacy and safety of recombinant human activated protein C for severe sepsis. *New Engl J Med* 2001; **344**: 699–709.

11. Pastores SM, Papadopoulos E, van den Brink M *et al.* Septic shock and multiple organ failure after hematopoietic stem cell transplantation: treatment with recombinant human activated protein C. *Bone Marrow Transpl* 2002; **30**: 131–4.

12. Pizzo PA, Poplack DG. *Principles and Practice of Pediatric Oncology.* Philadelphia, Lippincott Williams & Wilkins, 2002; 429–51.

13. Matsui H, Karasuno T, Santo T *et al.* Analysis of sepsis in allogeneic bone marrow transplant recipients: A single-center study. *J Infect Chemother* 2003; **9**: 238–42.

14. Devine SM, Adkins DR, Khoury H *et al.* Recent advances in allogeneic hematopoietic stem-cell transplantation. *J Lab Clin Med* 2003; **141**: 7–32.

15. Long SS, Pickering LK, Prober CG. *Principles and Practice of Pediatric Infectious Diseases.* Philadelphia, Churchill Livingstone, 2003; 561–7.

16. Hayes CH, Lush RJ, Cornish JM *et al.* The outcome of children requiring admission to an intensive care unit following bone marrow transplantation. *Br J Hematol* 1998; **102**: 666–70.

17. De Bock R, Middelheim AZ. Febrile neutropenia in allogeneic transplantation. *Int J Antimicrobial Agents* 2000; **16**: 177–80.

18. Pizzo PA. Fever in imuunocompromised patients. *New Engl J Med* 1999; **341**: 893–900.

19. Walsh TJ, Teppler H, Donowitz GR *et al.* Caspofungin versus liposomal amphotericin B for empirical antifungal therapy in patients with persistent fever and neutropenia. *N Engl J Med* 2004; **351**: 1391–402.

20. Koo A, Sung L, Allen U *et al.* Efficacy and safety of caspofungin for the empiric management of fever in neutropenic children. *Pediatr Infect Dis J* 2007; **26**: 854–6.

21. Kornecki A, Shemie SD. Open lung biopsy in children with respiratory failure. *Crit Care Med* 2001; **29**: 1247–50.

22. Barnes RA, Stallard N. Severe infections after bone marrow transplantation. *Curr Opin Crit Care* 2001; 7(3): 62–6.

23. Jacobe SJ, Hassan A, Veys P, Mok Q. Outcome of children requiring admission to an intensive care unit after bone marrow transplantation. *Crit Care Med* 2003; **31**: 1299–305.

24. Rossi R, Shemie SD, Calderwood S. Prognosis of pediatric bone marrow transplant recipients requiring mechanical ventilation. *Crit Care Med* 1999; **27**: 1181–6.

25. Diaz MA, Vicent MG, Prudencio M. Predicting factors for admission to an intensive care unit and clinical outcomes in pediatric patients receiving hematopoietic stem cell transplantation. *Haematologics* 2002; **87**: 292–8.

26. Shemie SD. Bone marrow transplantation and intensive care unit admission: what really matters? *Crit Care Med* 2003; **31**: 1579.

27. Schneider DT, Lemburg P, Sprock I *et al.* Introduction of the oncological pediatric risk of mortality score (O-PRISM) for ICU support following stem cell transplantation in children. *Bone Marrow Transplant* 2000; **25**: 1079–86.

28. Warwick AB, Mertens AC, Ou Shu X *et al.* Outcome following mechanical ventilation in children undergoing bone marrow transplantation. *Bone Marrow Transplant* 1998; **22**: 787–94.

29. DiCarlo JV, Alexander SR, Agarwal R, Schiffman JD. Continuous veno-venous hemofiltration may improve survival from acute respiratory distress syndrome after bone marrow transplantation or chemotherapy. *J Pediatr Hematol Oncol* 2003; **25**: 801–5.

Further reading

Kache S, Weiss IK, Moore TB. Changing outcomes for children requiring intensive care following hematopoietic stem cell transplantation. *Pediatr Transpl* 2006; **10**: 299–303.

Martin PL. To stop or not to stop: how much support should be provided to mechanically ventilated pediatric bone marrow and stem cell transplant patients? *Resp Care Clin North Am* 2006; **12**: 403–19.

Raman T, Marik PE. Fungal infections in bone marrow transplant recipients. *Expert Opin Pharmacotherapy* 2006; **7**: 307–15.

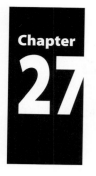

Chapter 27

Management of sagittal sinus thrombosis in a child

David J. Grant

Introduction

Cerebral Venous Sinus Thrombosis (CVST) is a clinically diverse disease in its causation, extent, and clinical presentation. Its outcome is unpredictable and can vary greatly among patients.

Thrombosis of the cerebral veins and sinuses are cerebrovascular disorders that occur most commonly in young adults and children. In children the estimated annual incidence is 7 per 1 million children.[10,22]

A prothrombotic risk factor or a direct cause is identified in almost all cases of CVST in children and up to 85% of adults.[10,21,22]

The management priorities, in the acute phase, are to stabilize the patient, by optimal resuscitation, and prevention/reversal of cerebral herniation. Following stabilization, attention should turn to preventing progression of the thrombus and/or thrombolysis. Treatment should be started as soon as the diagnosis is established and should aim to reverse the underlying cause (if known), control seizures, control intracranial hypertension, and commence antithrombotics. Heparin should be the first-line antithrombotic agent used.[7]

Case history

An 18-month-old girl presented to her primary care physician with a 1-day history of vomiting and lethargy.

She had been diagnosed with nephrotic syndrome 3 weeks ago and 1 week later she presented to her local hospital with diarrhea and vomiting. Her illness was severe enough to warrant hospitalization for intravenous fluid administration. Rota-virus was isolated in her stool and she seemed to recover from the gastroenteritis without any sequelae.

She had been well since discharge and had taken no medication other than the prednisolone (2 mg kg^{-1} per day) for treatment of her nephrotic syndrome. The nephrotic syndrome seemed to be steroid sensitive as she had her first "protein-negative" urinary dipstick 2 days prior to her current presentation.

Examination

On examination she was lethargic with sunken eyes and dry mucous membranes. In view of these findings and her history, the general practitioner administered some oral rehydration solution and referred her to the local hospital.

In hospital the history and clinical findings were as documented by the primary care physician, but the senior house officer (SHO) felt that her lethargia seemed out of keeping with her illness. She was reassured by her registrar who felt that she was dehydrated and lethargic secondary to a viral gastroenteritis.

Case Studies in Pediatric Critical Care, ed. Peter. J. Murphy, Stephen C. Marriage, and Peter J. Davis. Published by Cambridge University Press. © Cambridge University Press 2009.

Table 27.1. *Results of investigations*

	Admission 14:00	Day 2 09:30	15:00	20:15	Day3 01:30
Full blood count:					
Hb g dl^{-1}	12.4	9.8			
WCC (x10^9 l^{-1})	14.4	6.5			
PLT (x10^9 l^{-1})	280	229			
Coagulation:					
INR	1.2	1.0			
APTT ratio	1.1	1.2			
Fibrinogen	4.2	3.6			
Serum U&Es:					
Na^{2+}mmol l^{-1}	148	114	113	113	136
K$^+$ mmol l^{-1}	4.5	4.3	4.4	4.1	3.2
Ur mmol l^{-1}	8.2	2.6	2.6	2.0	1.6
Cr mmol l^{-1}	80	30	30	26	22
Osmolality	305	264	262	260	290
Albumin	23	21			
CRP (N<5)	7	<5			
Urine U&Es:					
Na$^+$ mmol l^{-1}		211			
K$^+$ mmol l^{-1}					
Osmolality	568	542	521	503	
Dipsticks	No protein/blood				
CT brain with contrast: DGH	No evidence of cerebral edema or hydrocephalus. ? Thrombus in superior sagittal sinus				
PICU	Thrombus superior sagittal sinus with extension into both lateral sinuses and extensive venous infarcts				

After obtaining IV access and taking bloods for blood cultures, C-reactive protein (CRP), biochemistry, full blood count, and clotting she was resuscitated by giving a 20 ml kg^{-1} normal (0.9%) saline fluid bolus. Her perfusion improved and she was commenced on 0.45% saline plus 5% dextrose as intravenous maintenance fluid. Full maintenance requirements plus 100 ml kg^{-1} was prescribed at a rate to rehydrate her over a 24-hour period.

The results of her initial CRP, biochemistry, full blood count, and coagulation screen are depicted in Table 27.1. She was admitted to the pediatric ward at 16:00 that afternoon and seemed to respond well to the fluid therapy. During the night the doctors were asked to review her because she was quite difficult to rouse. The same registrar whom saw her in the emergency department reviewed her and felt that she was merely tired after the events of the last couple of days and that she was sleeping as it was late at night. He commented that if she was at home she would be sleeping now. He felt no need to discuss her case with the consultant on call.

By the following morning she still had a reduced level of consciousness, but was now also having episodes of bradycardia. In view of these findings and the fact that she continued to vomit despite her diarrhea having been resolved and her clinical hydration status improved, there was concern that she may have meningitis. It was therefore decided to perform a full septic screen including a lumbar puncture.

The fluid obtained from the lumbar puncture was clear and colorless, but flowed at a rate suggesting that it was under increased pressure leading to concerns that she may have raised intracranial pressure.

After the lumbar puncture, she required intubation due to further deterioration in her level of consciousness. An urgent CT head with contrast was arranged. As they were waiting to move to the CT scanner, the results depicted in Table 27.1 were phoned through. Her serum sodium was $114 \, \text{mmol} \, l^{-1}$, with a serum osmolality of 264, and no obvious laboratory indicators of infection. She had been started on IV cefotaxime after the septic screen had been completed and it was continued.

The local pediatric intensive care unit was contacted about the patient and retrieval and advice was requested. They were advised to change her maintenance fluid to 0.9% saline and 5% dextrose and to restrict the fluid rate of infusion to 60% of her normal daily fluid requirements. They were also told to recheck the serum electrolytes regularly and adjust the fluids so as not to exceed a rise of more than $0.5 \, \text{mmol} \, l^{-1}$ per h of sodium. They added that, if she started seizing or deteriorated further, consideration should be given to affecting a more rapid rise in the serum sodium by the administration of hypertonic saline. The PICU team undertook to leave as soon as possible, and requested to be contacted with the CT result to discuss further management. The expected travel time by road was 4 hours.

The CT scan was reported by the local radiologist. In summary the report read that there was no evidence of cerebral edema or hydrocephalus, but there was some suggestion of a thrombus in the superior sagittal sinus. However, it was felt that this was most likely to be an artifact.

On arrival of the retrieval team at the referring hospital, the patient was intubated and ventilated. Her ventilation parameters and O_2 requirement suggested that she was easy to ventilate and oxygenate. The main concern was that she was poorly perfused with cool peripheries. She was given $20 \, \text{ml} \, kg^{-1}$ 0.9% saline, which improved her perfusion and blood pressure significantly. The results of the serum electrolytes, sent just before the arrival of the retrieval team, are shown in Table 27.1 (15:00).

Prior to their departure, the retrieval team placed a 4.5Fr triple lumen central line in her right femoral vein and a 24G right radial arterial line. During the transfer she was managed under the assumption that she had raised intracranial pressure. She was nursed in a 10° head up position with her head in a neutral midline position. She was sedated with morphine and midazolam and paralyzed for the journey. Her SaO_2 were maintained >95% and her end-tidal CO_2 was maintained at $35\text{-}40 \, \text{mmHg}$ (intermittently calibrated with a blood gas done on an iStat machine). They assumed her intracranial pressure to be $+/-20 \, \text{mmHg}$ and thus her mean BP was maintained >65 mmHg in order to approximate a cerebral perfusion pressure of 45 mmHg.

During transfer she was hemodynamically labile with episodes of hypotension. These episodes were treated with fluid boluses, but inotropic support was not started. She was given a total of $60 \, \text{ml} \, kg^{-1}$ of 0.9% saline during the transfer.

Progress in the pediatric intensive care unit

The results of her biochemistry on arrival at PICU are depicted in Table 27.1 (20:15). She now started developing episodes of bradycardia with associated hypertension. On examination, there was no evidence of pupillary asymmetry and both pupils were reactive to light. Owing to concern regarding raised intracranial pressure and the presence of two of the components of the Cushing's triad, she was treated as if she was coning. This was done by hyperventilation and a dose of $0.5 \, g \, kg^{-1}$ mannitol. Whilst she was being treated, an urgent repeat CT with contrast was arranged.

The repeat CT showed extensive thrombosis of the superior sagittal sinus with extension of the thrombus into both lateral sinuses. There was also evidence of extensive bilateral venous infarcts with surrounding cerebral edema (Fig. 27.1).

Immediately upon her return to PICU, she was commenced on a heparin infusion. In order to allow the evaluation of her neurological status, it was decided to discontinue her paralysis in the first instance and, after a normal train of four nerve stimulation tests, all her sedation was also discontinued.

The following morning she was stable with all the treatment measures for raised intracranial pressure in place, but she remained comatose. Review of the patient and comparison of the two CTs done, respectively, at the referral hospital and the tertiary center by the pediatric intensivist, neurologist, and neuroradiologist led them to believe that performing local thrombolytic therapy was indicated. This view was based upon a combination of the extent of the thrombus and venous infarcts and the speed at which they progressed as well as her comatose state.

Local thrombolysis using recombinant tissue type Plasminogen Activator (rt-PA) was performed. There were no complications and after a period of 24 hours she had recovered sufficiently to be extubated. She was fully alert, but remained on PICU for a further 24-hour period of observation before being discharged to the ward on warfarin. A subsequent MRI venography confirmed complete resolution of the thrombus.

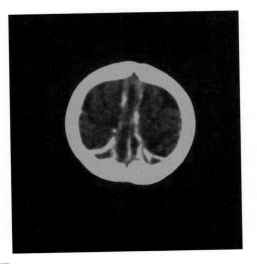

Fig. 27.1. Filling defects in lateral and sagittal sinuses.

Discussion

Cerebral venous sinus thrombosis (CVST) is a poorly understood, unpredictable condition presenting with a wide range of symptoms and etiologies making the standardization of a treatment protocol more difficult. Although relatively rare, it is diagnosed with increasing frequency due to greater clinical awareness and improved neuro-imaging.

Thrombosis of the cerebral veins and sinuses is a cerebrovascular disorder which, unlike arterial stroke, occurs most commonly in young adults and children. This is reflected in the fact that it only accounts for 1%–2% of all strokes in the adult population.[4] The estimated annual incidence is 3–4 per 1 million total population and 7 per 1 million among children.[10,21,22]

The dural sinuses that are most commonly affected are the transverse sinuses (86%), superior sagittal sinus (62%) and less commonly the straight sinus (18%). Figure 27.2 shows the structures that are most frequently involved. Studies have shown that between 33% and 49% of all cases have more than one sinus involved plus or minus cortical or cerebellar vein thrombosis.[10,20,22]

Causes and risk factors

In adult patients a direct cause or prothrombotic risk factor is identified in approximately 85% of all cases of sinus thrombosis. A recent prospective study of children presenting with

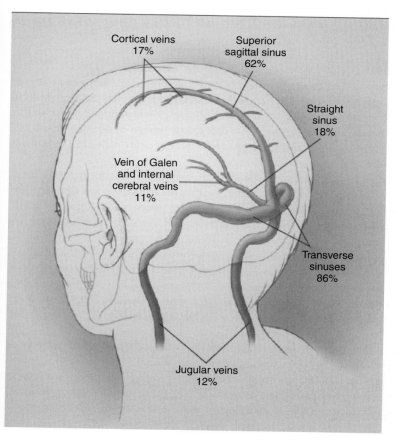

Fig. 27.2. Structures most frequently involved in CVST.

CVST in five European centers found clinical risk factors in all their patients.[21,22] Among children presenting with CVST, approximately 40% have known previous illnesses while ± 60% are previously well children.[10,21]

In children with pre-existing illnesses the most common etiologies are prothrombotic disorders and anemia ± microcytosis. The prothrombotic disorders account for between 33 and 62% of this group.[5,10,20,21] In the group of children studied by Sebire *et al.* the most common prothrombotic conditions were found to be high levels of Factor VIII and homozygosity for thermolabile methylene tetrahydrofolate reductase polymorphism.[21]

In previously well children infection and microcytosis (suggestive of iron deficiency) appears to be particularly common triggers. Studies have found that anemia and/or microcytosis were as common (62%) an etiological factor as prothrombotic conditions. Although anemia as an association with CSVT has received little attention in the adult literature, iron deficiency anemia (± thrombocytosis) has been well described in children with CVST, and should thus be sought and treated.[3,15,17,18] It is thought that high erythropoietin levels with an accompanying increase in adhesive reticulocytes might predispose to CVST in recovering iron deficiency, hemolytic/aplastic anemias and nocturnal hemoglobinuria. This theory is further supported by a report of CVST in a patient treated with poetin alpha.[14]

In children and the elderly there are no significant sex preponderances, but there is a significantly higher incidence of CVST in young adult females of child-bearing age.[10,21]

In up to 33% of cases presenting with CVST the etiology remains unknown, while others have not one but a combination of multiple risk factors.[5,10,20,21] (see Table 27.2 for list of risk factors).

Clinical manifestations

The clinical manifestations can be life threatening and may cause long-term neurological deficits. Unfortunately, as with so many other diseases in children, the presenting symptoms can be very non-specific and thus, unless a high index of suspicion is maintained in children with predisposing illnesses, the diagnosis can be delayed or missed altogether. There is a broad spectrum of presenting symptoms and signs and it may be acute, subacute, or chronic depending on the extent of venous collateralization.

The median duration of symptoms at presentation is around 5 days in the majority of patients presenting with acute symptoms (seizures, focal signs, and symptoms of raised ICP such as headache and reduced level of consciousness), while patients with subacute symptoms (chronic headaches, vomiting, lethargy, anorexia, and drowsiness) present with a history of 3 weeks or more.[10]

In practice, 28% of patients present with acute symptoms, 41% with subacute, and 31% with chronic symptoms. The etiology to some extent determines the nature of the symptoms. Acute symptoms are most commonly associated with an infective etiology, whereas subacute and chronic symptoms are more frequently associated with patients with inflammatory disease. Other factors determining the presentation are the location and rate of progression of the thrombus.[1,6,20]

There is evidence that the neurological manifestations at presentation differ between neonates and children outside of the neonatal period. Non-neonates present with manifestations similar to those reported in adult studies: headaches, focal neurological signs such as hemiparesis, and cranial nerve palsies and decreased level of consciousness and, in contrast, neonates present with seizures and diffuse neurological signs such as abnormal movements.[10] The most common presenting symptoms and signs in children are lethargy, anorexia,

Table 27.2. *Etiologies and risk factors associated with cerebral venous sinus thrombosis*

Prothrombotic conditions		
Genetic:	Antithrombin deficiency
	Protein C and S deficiency
	Factor V Leiden mutation
	Prothrombin mutation
	Homocysteinemia
Acquired:	Nephrotic syndrome
	Antiphospholipid antibodies
	Homocysteinemia
	Pregnancy and puerperium
Infections		
Otitis media, mastoiditis, and sinusitis		
Meningitis		
Systemic infectious diseases		
Inflammatory diseases		
Systemic lupus erythematosus		
Wegener's granulomatosis		
Sarcoidosis		
Inflammatory bowel disease		
Behçet's syndrome		
Hematological conditions		
Anemia		
Thrombocythemia		
Leukemia		
Polycythemia		
Drugs		
Oral contraceptives		
Asparaginase		
Trauma		
Head injury		
Jugular vein or sinus injury secondary to jugular catheterization		
Neurosurgical procedures		
Lumbar puncture		
Miscellaneous		
Dehydration		
Oncological process		

headache, vomiting, diffuse neurological signs (76%), seizures (58%), focal neurological signs (42%), and coma.[10,21]

Focal neurological signs that develop secondary to venous thrombosis may often localize to a unilateral hemisphere only to be followed within days by bilateral signs. These manifestations may take the form of seizures, behavioural symptoms, or coma.

Seizures occur in approximately 40%–60% of patients and are usually focal, but may generalize. Behavioral symptoms are most commonly found secondary to thalamic lesions, which may lead to coma if they occur bilaterally. Coma can also be caused by unilateral infarcts or hemorrhages that compress the diencephalon and brainstem. If left untreated, these patients die due to cerebral herniation.[10,22]

Involvement of the deep venous system (straight sinus and its branches) may result in the infarction of basal ganglia, thalamus, hypothalamus, ventral corpus callosum, medial occipital lobe, and upper cerebellum. These patients may deteriorate rapidly into a coma with long tract signs in the absence of signs of raised ICP or seizures.[20]

Patients with isolated intracranial hypertension have headaches, but in general do not have other neurologic signs unless they have already developed papilledema. Such patients will present with symptoms and signs of diplopia.

All of the above symptoms and signs of CVST is better understood when we consider the two different mechanisms contributing to it. Thrombosis of the cerebral veins causes local effects due to venous obstruction, whilst thrombosis of the major sinuses leads to the development of intracranial hypertension.

Venous occlusion of the cerebral veins can lead to localized swelling and venous infarction. Pathological examination show enlarged swollen veins, edema, ischemic neuronal damage, and petechial hemorrhages. These hemorrhages can merge to become large hematomas causing midline shift of the brain. Cerebral edema may develop secondary to the ischemic damage of energy-dependent cellular membrane pumps (cytotoxic edema), or secondary to disruption of the vascular integrity leading to leakage of plasma into the interstitium (vasogenic edema). The vasogenic edema is a reversible component that will resolve once the underlying cause is treated.

The normal absorption of cerebrospinal fluid (CSF) occurs in the arachnoid villi from where it is drained to the superior sagittal sinus. Occlusion of the sinuses leads to increased venous pressure and thus impaired absorption of CSF. The reduction in CSF absorption, in turn, leads to a rise in intracranial pressure and thus intracranial hypertension. Owing to the fact that the obstruction to the CSF absorption occurs at the end of the transport pathway there is no development of a pressure gradient between the ventricles and the subarachnoid spaces. This explains why hydrocephalus is not a common complicating factor of sinus thrombosis. Approximately 20% of patients have signs of intracranial hypertension in the absence of signs of venous thrombosis.[13]

Diagnosis

In most first-world hospitals, a CT scan of the head is almost routinely available in emergencies. A CT scan is useful to exclude other pathologies, but may be normal in up to 20%–40% of patients with CVST.[20,21] CT venography is diagnostically superior to normal CT. The pathognomonic signs are the cord sign (hyperdense thrombosed vein on unenhanced CT) and the delta sign (intraluminal thrombus within enhancing dural sinus walls of the superior sagittal sinus). Unfortunately, there are difficulties with interpreting these signs as the delta sign may be mimicked by a high split of the SSS, an epidural abscess, subdural hematoma, subarachnoid hemorrhage, or septations within the sinus. Other CT findings may include edema of the brain (focal or generalized), venous infarction, parenchymal hemorrhage, and subdural hematoma.[20] The spectrum of venous infarcts includes unilateral or bilateral infarcts or hemorrhages of the deep gray structures (secondary to thrombosis of the deep cerebral veins and straight sinus) or the cortex and underlying white matter (secondary to thrombosis of the sagittal, transverse, and sigmoid sinuses).[21]

The superior method of diagnostic imaging for CVST is thought to be a combination of magnetic resonance imaging and magnetic resonance angiography.[7,21] The most sensitive examination technique is a MRI combined with magnetic resonance venography. A T1$^-$ and T2$^-$ weighted MRI will show a hyper-intense signal from the thrombosed sinuses, although it may vary depending on the age of the thrombus. During the acute phase, the thrombus may be isosignal on T1$^-$ weighted and low signal on T2$^-$ weighted imaging. However, the combination of an abnormal signal in a sinus with the absence of flow on magnetic resonance venography confirms the diagnosis of a thrombus. MRI is not only better diagnostically, but will also allow parenchymal lesions to be more readily seen.[21,22]

Treatment

Supportive therapy

Historically, the treatment of CVST has generally been supportive. This usually takes the form of rehydration, seizure control, treatment of infectious etiologies, and implementation of measures to reduce ICP.

The combination of acutely raised intracranial pressure (ICP) and large venous infarcts can lead to cerebral herniation and be fatal within hours. The priority in the acute phase is to stabilize the patients condition (ABC) and then to prevent or reverse the cerebral herniation. This may require medical management by administration of intravenous mannitol or surgical management to remove the hemorrhagic infarct or perform a decompressive hemi-craniectomy. Of equal importance are the investigation and diagnosis of an underlying etiology (i.e. infection, etc.) in order to treat it as early and effectively as possible.

Once the emergency management and stabilization of the patient has taken place, attention should turn to specific treatment measures.

Specific treatment

Anticoagulation

In the past the evidence for safety and efficacy of antithrombotic therapy in children was extrapolated from adult research, but there have since been several pediatric studies that have confirmed the adult findings in children.[2,9–12,16,21]

Sebire et al. found that children treated with heparin were more likely to have a good cognitive outcome, but found no evidence of a statistically significant reduction in mortality. The study was, however, not powered to detect a difference in mortality.[21]

In a recent Cochrane review of anticoagulation in cerebral sinus thrombosis only two trials met the inclusion criteria. The fact that they were small trials meant that the review was based on data obtained from only 79 patients. It is therefore not surprising that no statistically significant results were found. They found that anticoagulant therapy had a pooled relative risk (RR) of death of 0.33 (95% CI 0.08–1.21) and of death or dependency of 0.46 (95% CI 0.16–1.31). What is, however, important to note is that no new symptomatic intracerebral hemorrhages were observed in any of the patients receiving anticoagulation therapy and, despite the fact that the RR 95% CI includes 1, there is a potentially important reduction in the risk of death or dependency.[23]

Heparin is the most commonly used first line of treatment to prevent local extension of the thrombus and pulmonary embolism. Sebire *et al.* demonstrated, in the group of children they studied, that 78% of patients who demonstrated complete recanalization received heparin, while in the group with persistent thrombosis only 33% were treated with heparin.[21]

Venous infarcts occur in approximately 40% of all patients with CVST and due to the tendency of venous infarcts to become hemorrhagic, heparin therapy is not without controversy. Several studies have investigated the effect of anticoagulant therapy in patients with CVST, but they have unfortunately all had major methodological flaws or were not powered to detect a significant difference in outcome. Despite these shortcomings, none of the trials showed an increase in the incidence of new cerebral hemorrhages or the extension of existing cerebral hemorrhages after treatment with heparin was commenced.[2,9–12,16,21] Thus most neurologists will now start heparin therapy as soon as the diagnosis is confirmed, even in the presence of a hemorrhagic infarct.

There have been no prospective studies to compare the effect of fractioned versus non-fractioned heparin in patients with CVST. However, in patients with thrombosis of leg veins, it has been shown that treatment with a fixed high dose of subcutaneous, low molecular weight heparin caused less major bleeding episodes than treatment with unfractionated heparin having similar antithrombotic efficacy.[24]

The optimal duration of anticoagulant therapy after the acute phase is unknown, but usually vitamin K antagonists are given for 6 months after a first episode of sinus thrombosis, or longer if the patient has predisposing factors. Therapy should be aimed at achieving an international normalized ratio of 2.5.

Thrombolysis

There have been no randomized controlled trials and thus no good evidence to support or advise against the use of thrombolysis. Systemic thrombolysis has been tried with varied success and is not recommended. Local thrombolysis is, however, indicated in very rare patients who deteriorate despite adequate anticoagulation or present with coma from the outset.[7,20]

Thrombolytic agents are plasminogen activators that convert plasminogen to plasmin, which then dissolves the fibrin to soluble Fibrin Degradation Products (FDP). The most commonly used products are recombinant tissue type plasminogen activator (rt-PA) and urokinase. Most centers prefer rt-PA because it has a greater affinity for plasminogen bound to thrombus than circulating plasminogen and thus restricts the systemic effects. Other advantages are that it has a short half-life of 4–5 min, is not antigenic, produces fewer FDPs and recanalization occurs faster than with other fibrinolytic agents.

Local thrombolysis can be performed via selective local delivery of the thrombolytic enzyme directly into the thrombosed sinus. This is usually performed via a transvenous femoral route. A guide catheter is advanced into the jugular bulb, and a micro-catheter and guide wire is then retrogradely manipulated through the guide catheter to the site of the thrombus where the rt-PA is delivered directly into the clot. Either hand-delivered boluses or infusions of the thrombolytics can be used.

These methods appear to restore flow more frequently and more rapidly than heparin alone, but there are currently no data to confirm better clinical outcome. This method should, however, only be attempted in centers with staff experienced in interventional radiology and should be restricted to patients with poor prognosis.[20]

Treatment of isolated intracranial hypertension

In patients whom only have symptoms of chronic intracranial hypertension, the first priority is to rule out any space-occupying lesions and to confirm sinus thrombosis as the etiology.

In the absence of contraindications such as large infarcts or hemorrhages, a lumbar puncture should be performed to measure the CSF pressure and to drain CSF. This should be combined with oral acetazolamide treatment (to reduce CSF production), which should be continued for weeks to months. The aims of these therapies are to reduce the ICP, relieve headaches and reduce papilledema.

If the combination of repeated LPs and acetazolamide proves to be ineffective in controlling the ICP within 2 weeks, surgical drainage via a lumbo-peritoneal shunt should be considered.

In the event of visual field deterioration, fenestration of the optic nerve sheet has been advocated.[7]

Prognosis

The prognosis of CVST is variable and can be very poor. In adults the mortality ranges from 5.5%–30%, while a further 15%–25% will incur permanent neurological deficits.[1,19,25] An international multicentre prospective observational study assessed patients for primary outcome measures of death or dependence as assessed by a modified Rankin scale score > 2. At the end of follow-up, they found 57% of patients were asymptomatic, 22% had minor residual symptoms, 7.5% had mild impairments, 3% were moderately impaired, and 2.2% were severely handicapped, while 8.3% died.[13]

De Brujn et al. showed in their study of adult patients that 44% of patients had cognitive impairment 1 year after the cerebral thrombotic event. There was no significant difference between the incidences of cognitive impairment in the heparin versus the placebo group.[8] This number is very high and does not correlate with other adult long-term follow-up studies where the incidence of neurological impairment, including blindness, cognitive impairment, and focal neurological deficits were found to be 14.3%.[19]

In follow-up studies of children with CVST 30%–50% of patients survived without neurologic deficit, 54%–62% survived with persisting neurological deficit and 8%–12% died. The nature of the neurological deficit can be diverse. Predictors of adverse neurological outcome are seizures at presentation and venous infarcts.[10] In a Canadian study the neurological deficits were motor impairment in 80%, cognitive impairment in 10%, developmental delay in 9%, speech impairment in 6%, and visual impairment in 6% of cases, respectively.[10] Sebire et al. studied a group of 42 children with CSVT in five European centers. Five of them (11.9%) died, three during the acute presentation and two at a later stage. The remaining 37 patients were followed up over a 10-year period. Of the 37 patients, 11 (29.7%) survived without any sequelae, while the remaining 26 patients (62%) had persistence of sequelae in one form or another. Of this group, 12 (46%) had pseudotumor cerebri and 14 (53%) had cognitive and/or behavioral disabilities. In patients with cognitive and/or behavioral disabilities associated epilepsy was found in 3 (21.4%) patients, visual disturbances in 2 (14.3%) patients and hemiparesis in 2 (14.3%) patients.[21] Studies have shown that only a small proportion (14.3%) of patients who have seizures during the acute presentation have seizures later in life.[19]

The most common causes of death are hemorrhagic infarction with raised intracranial pressure, cerebral edema, status epilepticus, sepsis, pulmonary emboli, and severity of underlying etiological systemic disease. The highest mortality is found among those who presented comatose, had a very rapid onset of symptoms or had involvement of the cortical, deep, and cerebellar veins. The patients presenting in the extreme age groups, namely infants and the elderly, also have a higher mortality rate.[20]

Children presenting with CVST and a Glasgow coma score of <12 are significantly associated with death, while older age, lack of parenchymal abnormality, anticoagulation, and lateral or sigmoid sinus involvement are independent predictors of good cognitive outcome. Involvement of the lateral or sigmoid sinus does, however, predict the development of pseudotumor cerebri.[21] Further studies on the long-term outcome need to be done.

The recurrence risk of cerebral sinus thrombosis is estimated at 12%, and data would suggest that children with chronic conditions such as anemia or congenital nephrotic syndrome have an increased risk of recurrence of CVST over a long period of time.[10,20,21]

Summary
CVST is a rare condition with a varied presentation, which can easily be missed. It is therefore important to maintain a high index of suspicion, particularly in those with predisposing illnesses.

Learning points
- Inotropes should be considered after 40 ml kg^{-1} of fluid boluses have been given and ongoing resuscitation is required.
- Heparin should be started as soon as the diagnosis is suspected.
- A high index of suspicion of CVST should be maintained in patients with predisposing conditions such as nephrotic syndrome.
- Fluid management should be reviewed frequently with the aid of biochemistry to adjust fluid regime.
- In patients with abnormal neurology neuroimaging should always be performed before a lumbar puncture is performed.
- Neuroimaging in children can be notoriously difficult to interpret and, where at all possible, the opinion of a neuroradiologist should be sought.
- When transporting a patient from a remote area, air transport should be considered.

References
1. Ameri A, Bousser MG. Cerebral venous thrombosis. *Neurol Clin* 1992; **10**(1): 87–111.
2. Barnes C, Newall F, Furmedge J, Mackay M, Monagle P. Cerebral sinus venous thrombosis in children. *J Paediatr Child Health* 2004; **40**(1–2): 53–5.
3. Belman AL, Roque CT, Ancona R, Anand AK, Davis RP. Cerebral venous thrombosis in a child with iron deficiency anemia and thrombocytosis. *Stroke* 1990; **21**(3): 488–93.
4. Bogousslavsky J, Pierre P. Ischemic stroke in patients under age 45. *Neurol Clin* 1992; **10**(1): 113–24.
5. Bonduel M, Sciuccati G, Hepner M *et al.* Factor V Leiden and prothrombin gene G20210A mutation in children with cerebral thromboembolism. *Am J Hematol* 2003; **73**(2): 81–6.
6. Bousser MG, Chiras J, Bories J, Castaigne P. Cerebral venous thrombosis – a review of 38 cases. *Stroke* 1985; **16**(2): 199–213.

7. Crassard I, Bousser MG. Cerebral venous thrombosis. *J Neuroophthalmol* 2004; **24**(2): 156–63.

8. de Bruijn SF, Budde M, Teunisse S, de Haan RJ, Stam J. Long-term outcome of cognition and functional health after cerebral venous sinus thrombosis. *Neurology* 2000; **54**(8): 1687–9.

9. de Bruijn SF, Stam J. Randomized, placebo-controlled trial of anticoagulant treatment with low-molecular-weight heparin for cerebral sinus thrombosis. *Stroke* 1999; **30**(3): 484–8.

10. deVeber G, Andrew M, Adams C *et al.* (Canadian Pediatric Ischemic Stroke Study Group) Cerebral sinovenous thrombosis in children. *N Engl J Med* 2001; **345**(6): 417–23.

11. deVeber G, Chan A, Monagle P *et al.* Anticoagulation therapy in pediatric patients with sinovenous thrombosis: a cohort study. *Arch Neurol* 1998; **55**(12): 1533–7.

12. Einhaupl KM, Villringer A, Meister W *et al.* Heparin treatment in sinus venous thrombosis. *Lancet* 1991; **338**(8767): 597–600.

13. Ferro JM, Canhao P, Stam J, Bousser MG, Barinagarrementeria F. (ISCVT Investigators) Prognosis of cerebral vein and dural sinus thrombosis: results of the International Study on Cerebral Vein and Dural Sinus Thrombosis (ISCVT). *Stroke* 2004; **35**(3): 664–70.

14. Finelli PF, Carley MD. Cerebral venous thrombosis associated with epoetin alfa therapy. *Arch Neurol* 2000; **57**(2): 260–2.

15. Hartfield DS, Lowry NJ, Keene DL, Yager JY. Iron deficiency: a cause of stroke in infants and children. *Pediatr Neurol* 1997; **16**(1): 50–3.

16. Johnson MC, Parkerson N, Ward S, de Alarcon PA. Pediatric sinovenous thrombosis. *J Pediatr Hematol Oncol* 2003; **25**(4): 312–5.

17. Keane S, Gallagher A, Ackroyd S, McShane MA, Edge JA. Cerebral venous thrombosis during diabetic ketoacidosis. *Arch Dis Child* 2002; **86**(3): 204–5.

18. Meena AK, Naidu KS, Murthy JM. Cortical sinovenous thrombosis in a child with nephrotic syndrome and iron deficiency anaemia. *Neurol India* 2000; **48**(3): 292–4.

19. Preter M, Tzourio C, Ameri A, Bousser MG. Long-term prognosis in cerebral venous thrombosis. Follow-up of 77 patients. *Stroke* 1996; **27**(2): 243–6.

20. Renowden S. Cerebral venous sinus thrombosis. *Eur Radiol* 2004; **14**(2): 215–26.

21. Sebire G, Tabarki B, Saunders DE *et al.* Cerebral venous sinus thrombosis in children: risk factors, presentation, diagnosis and outcome. *Brain* 2005; **128**(Pt 3): 477–89.

22. Stam J. Thrombosis of the cerebral veins and sinuses. *N Engl J Med* 2005; **352**(17): 1791–8.

23. Stam J, de Bruijn SFTM, De Veber G. Anticoagulation for cerebal sinus thrombosis. *The Cochrane database of Systematic Reviews* 2001; (4): CD002005.

24. van Den Belt AG, Prins MH, Lensing AW *et al.* Fixed dose subcutaneous low molecular weight heparins versus adjusted dose unfractionated heparin for venous thromboembolism. *Cochrane Database Syst Rev* 2000; (2): CD001100.

25. van Gijn J. Cerebral venous thrombosis: pathogenesis, presentation and prognosis. *J Roy Soc Med* 2000; **93**(5): 230–3.

Index